Protocols
for
Nurse Practitioners
in
Gynecologic Settings

Joellen W. Hawkins

RNC, Ph.D., F.A.A.N., Professor, Boston College
Nurse Practitioner, Crittenton Hastings House

Diane M. Roberto-Nichols

B.S., APRN-C, Nurse Practitioner/Administrator
Ellington Obstetrics and Gynecology Associates

J. Lynn Stanley-Haney

M.A., APRN-C, Nurse Practitioner
Planned Parenthood of Connecticut
Ellington Obstetrics and Gynecology Associates

Seventh Edition

THE TIRESIAS PRESS, INC.

DEDICATION

To our families and friends, our students, and our clients.

Table of Contents

PART II: APPENDIXES

BIBLIOGRAPHIES

Preface to the Seventh Edition

THIS EXTENSIVELY revised and updated edition of *Protocols for Nurse Practitioners in Gynecologic Settings* is designed to be used as a guide for nursing management of the common gynecological conditions women present within community-based settings. These include such concerns as sexually transmitted diseases, fear of HIV exposure, vaginitis and vaginosis, contraceptive needs across the reproductive lifespan, life transitions including menarche and menopause, preconception care and desire for pregnancy, and sexual assault and domestic violence. The protocols and teaching materials were originally prepared for the Women's Clinic at the Student Health Services of the University of Connecticut. Those protocols and teaching materials still form the core of this constantly evolving book.

The three principal authors are nurse practitioners practicing in women's health settings. All were actively involved in the original book's development and are responsible for its continual updating. Two protocols (Cervical Cap and Natural Family Planning) were developed by advanced practice nurses in other settings who were chosen for their expertise with those methods.

This seventh edition has a number of special features to assist you in your practice. In addition to an up-to-date bibliography for each protocol, it contains new information on contraceptive methods, STDs, smoking cessation, assessing risk of heart disease, osteoporosis assessment and prevention, management of abnormal Papanicolaou smears, pediculosis, scabies, hepatitis, hormone therapy, breast conditions and breast cancer risk, and emergency contraception. The new patient materials include information on scabies, Norplant®, syphilis, pediculosis, smoking cessation, assessing risk of heart disease, and emergency contraception. New protocols include osteoporosis and smoking cessation.

As we go to press, several promising new contraceptives are on the horizon. These include injectable monthly combination estradiol cypionate and medroxyprogesterone acetate contraceptives, with FDA approval anticipated in late 1999, progestin-only injectable with microspheres or microcapsules in 1, 3 and 6-

month formulations, contraceptive vaginal ring with progestin or progestin and estrogen, transdermal cream, new oral contraceptives, progesterone antagonist, vaccines, new two-rod, one-rod and biodegradable implants, and intrauterine devices, including one designed to release progestin for up to 5 years, one with a frameless design, and a threadless IUD./ New barrier and spermicidal methods include the Femcap and Lea's shield, as well as a sponge now on the market in Canada. Male methods under study include incapacitators targeting sperm producing cells, hormones to decrease sperm counts, implants to release hormones, antifertility vaccines, and a nonlatex condom PolyMAXX. RU486 may be ready for the U.S. market by the end of 1999.

The book's design, with wide margins and plenty of white space, allows you add to or change each protocol to suit your individual practice. A sample evaluation form is included so that you can evaluate and update your protocols as needed and in response to any legal requirements for practice in your state or country under the legislation, rules and regulations affecting the practice of nurse practitioners, nurse-midwives and clinical specialists, and the policies of your clinical setting.

— JWH, DMR-N, JLS-H

Acknowledgments

The authors wish to express their gratitude to colleagues who, over the years, have worked with them to develop, evaluate, and rewrite the protocols as they are being tested in clinical practice. Gratitude is also due to the many graduate students who have worked with the protocols and teaching materials and offered important suggestions. Our clients, too, have been very helpful in suggesting changes for the educational materials and in expressing a need for information that led to the development of some of the materials.

Special thanks go to the late Eleanor Tabeek and to Nancy Keaveney for materials on natural family planning, R. Mimi Clarke Secor for information on the cervical cap, Kathleen K. Furniss and Jacqueline Campbell for consultation on the domestic violence protocol, Richard Ferri for the HIV/AIDS Risk Self-Assessment, Martha Sternberg who co-authored the urinary tract protocol, and Cheryl Stene Frenkel for use of the protocols evaluation tool she developed.

And, finally, we wish to thank the late Helen Behnke for her intelligent and skillful editing of the original manuscript of this book.

Introduction

NURSE PRACTITIONERS in any area of practice need to consider the issues surrounding the use of protocols. Many states mandate that nurse practitioners practice under written protocols. There is growing support for such legislation; some agencies and institutions already require the use of protocols by nurse practitioners, and may even specify by whom the protocols are to be developed. Furthermore, protocols or practice guidelines are being required in some states where nurse practitioners have prescription writing privileges in order for nurse practitioners to be approved to do so. Managed care systems, too, often mandate use of clinical protocols by their practitioners.

Of course, controversy exists as to whether protocols should be used at all. Opponents argue that protocols are too rigid, that they stifle creativity and the development of problem-solving ability, and that they run counter to individualization of care. Some types of protocols do not require the skills of an advanced practitioner of nursing, to be sure, and there are some who would protest that protocols prolong the dependency syndrome of nurse practitioners, particularly when the protocols are prepared by physicians and there is little or no nursing input. Protocols can be unrealistic for some practitioners in some settings with some clients. If used as a measure of care from a legal perspective, such protocols could open up the practice to malpractice charges.

Proponents argue that protocols offer a wealth of research data for use in validating nursing management strategies. By providing a guide for standardization of data collection, a record audit can be done to determine whether client outcomes are beneficial. Protocols can be written so as to build in problem solving, and can serve as guidelines rather than a rigid set of rules. They can be used with a record-keeping system such as Weed's problem-oriented medical record system. Protocols can facilitate continuity and coordination of care, as well as enhance documentation of the clinical decision-making process. As such, they can prove extremely valuable in quality improvement programs and in measuring clinical outcomes. They can be developed to reflect the confidence level and needs of the nurse practitioners using them and delineate areas of competence and responsibility for the various health care professionals in a multidisciplinary setting.

The protocols in this book were designed originally for a particular setting and thus take into account the common presenting problems in a woman's clinic, who was going to use the protocols (nurse practitioners), the setting in which they would be used (a woman's clinic in a student health service), the availability of physician colleagues and other health care professionals for consultation, the referral system already in place, the laboratory facilities available, the basis for nurse practitioner practice in the state, and the nurse practice act. The authors now practice in other settings, so the protocols reflect those settings and the women's needs. As each protocol is now developed and tested in their clinical practices, the authors record ideas for the annual revision and updating of the material. A search of the literature is done for each protocol and is updated yearly as well.

The protocols that appear in this book are the result of an ongoing effort at writing and rewriting and of testing in clinical practice by the authors, their colleagues, and graduate students. We hope they will be useful to you in your practice as you adapt, revise, and update them to meet the needs of your clients.

REFERENCES

Courtney, R. (1997). Working with protocols. *American Journal of Nursing, 97(2):16E-16F, 16H*

Hawkins, J.W. & Roberto, D. (1984). Developing family planning nurse practitioner protocols. *Journal of Obstetric, Gynecologic, and Neonatal Nursing,* 13(3):167-170.

Mahoney, D.F. (1992). Nurse practitioners as prescribers: Past research trends and future study needs. *The Nurse Practitioner,* 17(1):44,47-48,50-51.

Moniz, D.M. (1992). The legal danger of written protocols and standards of practice. *The Nurse Practitioner,* 17(9):58-60.

Pearson, L.J. (1997). Update: How each state stands on legislative issues affecting advanced nursing practice. *The Nurse Practitioner, 22(1):18-86.*

Stock, C.M. (1995). Ten tips for writing and using practice protocols. *Contemporary Nurse Practitioner, 2(1):51-52.*

Weed, L.L. (1969). Medical Records, Medical Education, and Patient Care. Chicago: Year Book Medical Publishers.

PART I. PROTOCOLS

Methods of Family Planning

Oral Contraceptives*

I. Definition and Types

A. Oral contraceptives (OC) (also known as birth control pills) are pills that when taken by mouth produce systemic changes that prevent conception

B. Types of pills
1. A combination of synthetic estrogen and progestin
2. Progestin only (also known as mini-pills)
3. See Table 1 (pages 23-26) for oral contraceptives marketed in the U.S.

C. Directions for use (combination)
1. The pill is taken for 21 days, and an inert pill (or no pill) for 7 days, during which time withdrawal bleed should occur; some packets have 21 oral contraceptive pills only, so the woman then takes no pills for 7 days
2. A tri-cycle regimen is widely used in Europe and is becoming more widely used in the United States. This regimen, 3 packs of a monophasic pill used consecutively, may be considered in certain situations, including
    a. headaches regularly occurring during withdrawal cycles
    b. heavy withdrawal bleeds
    c. endometriosis after work-up
3. A regimen of 21 combination pills, 2 inert pills (days 22 and 23) and 5 days of ethinyl estradiol (days 24-28)

---

* Sections I through IV of this protocol were synthesized from a variety of sources including R.H. Hatcher, J. Trussell, F. Stewart, W. Cates, G.K. Stewart, F. Guest, and D. Kowal (1998), *Contraceptive Technology*, 17th ed., New York: Ardent Media; M.S. Policar, Oral contraceptive update, unpublished paper, 1993; R.P. Dickey (1998), *Managing Contraceptive Pill Patients*, 9th ed.; Durant, O.K., Essential Medical Information Systems.

D. Directions for use (progestin only)
Progestin only pills are taken continuously

II. Physical Changes Occurring with Use of the Pill
A. Ovulation is suppressed
B. The endometrium becomes deciduous making it unreceptive to implantation
C. The cervical mucus is altered, so it is hostile to sperm
D. Transport of the ovum may be altered
E. Possible luteolysis
F. Possible inhibition of capacitation of sperm

III. Effectiveness
A. 99.6% effectiveness rate for combination pill
B. 97% effectiveness rate for progestin only pill

IV. Contraindications
A. Absolute contraindications to combination pills
   1. Thromboembolic disorder (or history thereof) including postpartum deep vein thrombosis, pulmonary embolism or thromboembolism
   2. Thrombotic cerebrovascular accident (or history thereof)
   3. Coronary artery disease (or history thereof); current angina pectoris; structural heart disease complicated by pulmonary hypertension, atrial fibrillation, or bacterial endocarditis
   4. Known or suspected carcinoma of the breast
   5. Major surgery with prolonged immobility or any surgery on the legs
   6. Known impaired liver function at present time, liver problems, benign hepatic adenoma, liver cancer or history of active viral hepatitis, severe cirrhosis
   7. Known or suspected estrogen dependent neoplasm (or history thereof)
   8. Diabetes with clinical vascular disease (nephropathy, neuropathy, retinopathy, peripheral); diabetes of > 20 years duration

9. Over 35 and currently a heavy smoker (more than 15 cigarettes/day)
10. Headaches including classic migraines with neurological symptoms
11. Triglyceride level greater than 350 mg/dl
12. Known or suspected pregnancy
13. Chronic hypertension and smoking or uncontrolled hypertension

B. Relative contraindications
1. Severe headaches or common migraines, which start or worsen with initiation of pill use
2. Hypertension with resting diastolic BP of 90 or more, or resting systolic BP of 140 or more on 3 or more separate visits, or an accurate measurement of 110 diastolic BP or more on a single visit
3. Impaired liver function (i.e., mononucleosis, acute phase, medication induced changes)
4. Undiagnosed abnormal vaginal/uterine bleeding
5. 35 years or older and a light smoker (less than 8-10 cigarettes per day)
6. Hypertriglyceridemia; worrisome LDL:HDL ratio
7. Gallbladder disease: medically treated, current biliary tract disease, history of OC-related cholestasis

C. Other considerations (advantages of OC generally outweigh disadvantages)
1. Diabetes: without vascular disease
2. Congenital hyperbilirubinemia (Gilbert's disease)
3. Failure to have established regular menstrual cycle (without prior work-up) [See amenorrhea protocol]
4. Conditions likely to make it difficult for woman to take OCs correctly and consistently (learning disability, major psychiatric problems, alcoholism or other drug abuse, history of repeatedly taking oral contraceptives or other medications incorrectly
5. Major surgery with no prolonged immobilization
6. Undiagnosed breast mass
7. Cervical cancer awaiting treatment; CIN

V. Explanation of Method
A. Ways in which oral contraceptives are taken*
1. Start oral contraceptive on day 1 (first day of menses) or on Sunday of week menses start
2. Oral contraceptive must always be taken at the same time of day (within an hour either way)
3. Back-up contraception is necessary for 7 days (first cycle only)
4. Missed pills
   a. One pill missed: woman to take pill when she remembers, and then take scheduled pill at regular time
   b. Two pills missed in first 2 weeks: take 2 pills at regular time for 2 days. Use back-up contraception x 7 days
   c. Two or more pills missed in third week, or 3 or more pills missed any time (and women starts on Sundays), she should keep taking a pill each day until Sunday, then start a new packet that Sunday. Instruct woman to use a back-up method for 7 days. If woman does not start on Sundays, she should throw out pill pack and start a new pack that day. **A back-up method of birth control should be used for the first 7 days of this new pill pack**
   d. If 1 or more pills are missed and no back-up contraception is used and no withdrawal bleed, woman should be instructed to call to discuss possible pregnancy test
B. Laboratory
1. Lipid screen
   a. Lipid screen prior to starting OC
   Significant immediate family history
      1) Under age 50—stroke, coronary, or sudden death. Do lipid screen. If levels abnormal, consult with M.D. before starting OC. If normal levels, start OC and repeat test in 2 years

----

*FDA recommendation for standardizing pill use instructions; Potter, L. (1994), Will the new OC instructions increase compliance? *Advance for Nurse Practitioners*, 2(11):11-13.

    b. Lipid screen strongly advised if parents or siblings have hypertension, vascular disease, myocardial infarction, arteriosclerotic heart disease, and/or hyperlipidemia before age 50 or are on medication for hypertension
2. Consider fasting blood sugar and/or 2 hour postprandial blood sugar if parents or siblings are diabetic
3. Liver profile if woman has had mononucleosis or mono-like illness within past year or if patient has history of hepatitis or other liver disease or drug or alcohol history

VI. Complications of Method
A. Considerations for discontinuing pill use (identify problem as clearly pill related)
1. Visual problems
    a. Loss of vision, even for short periods
    b. Blurring of vision, double vision
    c. "Spots" before eyes or flashing lights
2. Numbness or paralysis in any part of the face or body, even if temporary
3. Unexplained chest pain
4. Phlebitis or painful inflamed areas along veins
5. Severe recurrent headaches or new headaches associated with pill use. (Use form on pages 21-22 for headache evaluation. If yes is answered to any question, consider consultation or referral to a gynecologist or neurologist)
6. Marked increase in blood pressure and/or with diastolic pressure more than 90
7. Marked fluid retention or weight gain
8. Severe mood changes or depression
9. Patient dissatisfaction with method
10. Development of any condition for which oral contraception is contraindicated
11. If surgery is scheduled, woman should consult the surgeon regarding pill use; discontinue for leg surgery
12. Migraine headaches which have increased in frequency or severity. (Use headache evaluation form). If yes is checked for any question, consider consult with or referral to gynecologist or neurologist)

13. Long leg cast for lower extremity
14. Exacerbation of varicosities
B. Procedure for pill-related bleeding problem, i.e., amenorrhea, scant menses, break-through bleeding
   1. Rule out the following
      a. Faulty OC taking (review packet)
      b. Pregnancy
      c. Uterine or cervical pathology-leiomyomata, polyp, cancer
      d. Pelvic or vaginal infection
      e. Drug interference
      f. Gastrointestinal problems
      g. Endometriosis
   2. Based on information gained, treatment as follows
      a. Amenorrhea or scant menses
         1) Reassure woman
         2) Consider pill change or
         3) Consider adding 20 mcg. of ethinyl estradiol, 1-2 mg. estradiol, or 0.625 mg conjugated estrogen
      b. Breakthrough bleeding
         1) During the first 3 months of OC use, reassure only
         2) Consider pill change
         3) Consider adding exogenous estrogen (20 mcg ethinyl estradiol, 1-2 mg estradiol, or 0.625 conjugated estrogen) beginning the first day of breakthrough bleed x 7 days regardless of where the woman is in her cycle; woman should continue to take OC as scheduled
         4) If treatment for a or b is unsuccessful and symptoms persist, consult with gynecologist
C. For post-pill amenorrhea
   1. Pregnancy test
   2. If amenorrhea continues after six months, refer to amenorrhea protocol for work-up
D. Adverse oral contraceptive-drug interaction (see Table 2)
   1. Management
      a. All women prior to starting oral contraception and on a yearly follow-up basis should review and re-sign informed consent for oral contraceptive use—emphasizing drug interaction and knowledge of danger signs
      b. If a woman is on any medications that decrease contra-

ceptive effect, she should be offered the option of back-up contraception such as condoms and/or spermicidal protection. Decisions about oral contraceptive use with medications (see Table 2) should be individualized. If there is any question regarding drug interaction and interference of OCs with other drugs, refer woman to gynecologist or pharmacist

VII. Indications for Using Progestin-only Pill
A. Indications
1. Is a good choice in situations where estrogen is contra-indicated
   a. Smokers
   b. Lactation
   c. History/current deep vein thrombosis/pulmon-ary embolism
   d. Surgery with immobilization
   e. Valvular heart disease
   f. Severe headaches including migraine without focal neurological symptoms
   g. Gallbladder disease
   h. Seizure disorders
   i. Elevated blood pressure ≥ 140/90
B. Contraindications
1. Undiagnosed abnormal vaginal bleeding when a serious condition is suspected
2. Breast cancer
3. Pregnancy or possibly pregnant
C. Other considerations (advantages may outweigh risks)
1. Undiagnosed breast cancer
2. CIN or cervical cancer
3. Gallbladder disease while on combined OCs
4. Diabetes without vascular involvement (Type 1 or 2)
5. Diabetes with nephropathy, retinopathy, neuropathy
6. History of current ischemic heart disease
7. History of cerebrovascular accident
8. Severe headaches, including migraines, with focal neurological symptoms
9. Mild cirrhosis (uncompensated)
10. Undiagnosed hypertension (not hypertension in preg-

nancy)
11. Irregular, heavy, or prolonged vaginal bleeding
D. Women who fit the above criteria after appropriate screening and physical exam may be candidates for this oral contraceptive, bearing in mind that irregular bleeding may present a major clinical problem. Since number of pills varies with manufacturer, careful instruction on use and review of pill packet

VIII. Procedure for Pill Check for Either Combination or Progestin-only Pills
A. All women will have routine screening of
  1. Blood pressure, weight
  2. Urine, for protein and glucose
  3. Last withdrawal bleed
B. Review side effects and danger signals
C. In some settings at 6-month check: bimanual examination, breast examination; repeat Papanicolaou as indicated by history, previous findings
D. Allow time for client to ask questions
E. If problems are elicited or suspected, consultation with other nurse practitioners and/or physician as necessary

See Appendix E for consent form and informational handout on oral contraceptives for clients.

See Bibliography 3.

NOTE

Tables 1 and 2 (pages 23-30) provide guidelines on possible drug interactions/interferences with oral contraceptives and information on contraceptives currently marketed in the United States.

Evaluation of Headaches Occurring
While on Oral Contraceptives*

Current pill Used _____ Length of Time on Pill _____

Name _____ ID _____ Date _____

Subjective Findings (to be filled out by client, interviewer, or clinician)

	Yes	No	Don't Know
1. Have your headaches been worse in the past 48 hours?	—	—	—
2. Have you started having headaches or have your headaches become worse since you started taking birth control pills?	—	—	—
3. Do you have light headedness, dizziness, or nausea at the same time as you have headaches?	—	—	—
4. Do you ever vomit at the time of your headaches?	—	—	—
5. Have you ever been told you have high blood pressure (hypertension)?	—	—	—
6. Do you have spots in front of your eyes, double or blurred vision when you have your headaches?	—	—	—
7. Do you ever lose your vision, that is, become blind or partially blind?	—	—	—
8. Do your headaches usually occur on just one side of your head?	—	—	—
9. Do you note watering of one or both eyes at the time of your headaches?	—	—	—
10. Have you ever been told you had migraine headaches?	—	—	—

	Yes	No	Don't Know
11. Does anyone in your family have a history of migraine headaches?	—	—	—
12. Are your headaches throbbing headaches?	—	—	—
13. If you use aspirin or an aspirin substitute, do your headaches continue even after you take the aspirin or aspirin substitute?	—	—	—
14. Do any foods seems to bring on headaches?	—	—	—
15. Do alcohol (such as red wine), caffeine, and/or any drugs worsen or cause headaches?	—	—	—
16. Do you have a history of or have sinusitis?	—	—	—
17. Do you have a history of or do you now have postnasal drip?	—	—	—
18. Have you ever seen a physician for your headaches? If so, what were the results?	—	—	—
19. Allergies	—	—	—
20. Have you ever had numbness or tingling of face or extremities (arms, legs, feet, hands) associated with headaches?	—	—	—

21. What bothers you most about your headaches? _____

_____

Objective Findings: B/P ____ / ____ Fundi: _____
Other Findings:_____
Localized Tenderness: _____
Assessment: _____
Plan:_____
Nurse Practitioner: _____

*Adapted from Emory University Family Planning Program. Used with permission.

Table 1. Oral Contraceptives Marketed in the United States: Formula and Dosage

* Progostin Content
Estrogen Content

Product	Norethindrone (Estrogenic Effect 1.0 / Androgenic Effect 1.0)	Ethynodiol Diacetate (Estrogenic Effect 3.4 / Androgenic Effect 0.6)	Norethindrone Acetate (Estrogenic Effect 1.5 / Androgenic Effect 1.6)	Norgestrel (Estrogenic Effect 0 / Androgenic Effect 4.2)	Norgestimate (Estrogenic Effect 0 / Androgenic Effect 1.9)	Levonorgestrel (Estrogenic Effect 0 / Androgenic Effect 8.3)	Desogestrel (Estrogenic Effect 0 / Androgenic Effect 3.4)	Mestranol µg	Ethinyl Estradiol µg	Number of Hormonal Pills	Number of Other Pills
Alesse 28 (Levlite same)						0.10			20	21	7 inert
Brevicon-21 & 28	0.5								35	21	7 inert
Demulen 1/35-21 & 28		1.0							35	21	7 inert
Zovia 1/35		1.0							35	21	7 inert
Demulen-21 & 28		1.0							50	21	7 inert
Desogen							0.15		30	21	7 inert
Genora 0.5/35	0.5								35	21	7 inert
Genora 1/35-21 & 28	1.0								35	21	7 inert
Genora 1/50-21 & 28	1.0								50	21	7 inert
Levlen						0.15			30	21	7 inert
Levora						0.15			35	21	7 inert
Jenest 28	0.5 mg(7), 1.0 mg(14)								35	21	7 inert
Loestrin FE 1/20**			1.0						20	21	7 iron
Loestrin FE 1.5/30			1.5						30	21	7 iron

*Gestodene is on the market in Europe but has not yet been approved in the U.S.

**Also available as Loestrin 1/20 and 1.5/30 with 7 inert.

Table 2 is adapted from Hatcher, Robert A., et al. (1998), *Contraceptive Technology*, 17th ed., Ardent Media, New York; R. Dickey (1998), *Managing Contraceptive Patients*, 9th ed. Durant, OK; Essential Medical Information Systems (EMIS); *Nurse Practitioners' Prescribing Reference*, Winter, 1998-09.

Table 1. (continued)

	Progestin Content							Estrogen Content			
	Norethindrone (Estrogenic Effect 1.0 / Androgenic Effect 1.0)	Ethynodiol Diacetate (Estrogenic Effect 3.4 / Androgenic Effect 0.6)	Norethindrone Acetate (Estrogenic Effect 1.5 / Androgenic Effect 1.6)	Norgestrel (Estrogenic Effect 0 / Androgenic Effect 4.2)	Norgestimate (Estrogenic Effect 0 / Androgenic Effect 1.9)	Levonorgestrel (Estrogenic Effect 0 / Androgenic Effect 0.3)	Dosogostrel (Estrogenic Effect 0 / Androgenic Effect 3.4)	Mestranol µg	Ethinyl Estradiol µg	Number of Hormonal Pills	Number of Other Pills
Lo/Ovral-21 & 28				0.3					30	21	7 inert
Modicon-21 & 28	0.5								35	21	7 inert
(Necon .05/35 same)									35	21	7 inert
Nelova 1/35E	1.0								35	21	7 inert
Necon 1/35 same									35	21	7 inert
Nelova 0.5/35E	0.5								35	21	7 inert
Nelova 1/50M	1.0							50		21	7 inert
Nelova 10/11 (NEE,	1.0(10 days)								35	10	7 inert
10/11 same)	0.5(11 days)								35	11	
Norcept E 1/35	1.0								35	21	7 inert
Nordette 21 & 28						1.5			30	21	7 inert
Levora, same									35	21	7 inert
Norethin 1/35E	1.0								35	21	7 inert
Norethin 1/50M	1.0							50		21	7 inert
Necon 1/50M same								50		21	7 inert
NEE 0.5/35			0.5						35	21	7 inert
NEE 1/35			1.0						35	21	7 inert
Norinyl 1/35	1.0								35	21	7 inert
Norinyl 1+50/21 & 28	1.0							50		21	7 inert
Norlestrin 2.5/50-21			2.5						50	21	
Norlestrin 2.5/50-FE			2.5						50	21	7 inert

Table 1. (continued)

	Progestin Content														Estrogen Content			
	Norethindrone Estrogenic Effect 1.0	Norethindrone Androgenic Effect 1.0	Ethynodiol Diacetate Estrogenic Effect 3.4	Ethynodiol Diacetate Androgenic Effect 0.6	Norethindrone Acetate Estrogenic Effect 1.5	Norethindrone Acetate Androgenic Effect 1.6	Norgestrel Estrogenic Effect 0	Norgestrel Androgenic Effect 4.2	Norgestimate Estrogenic Effect 0	Norgestimate Androgenic Effect 1.9	Levonorgestrel Estrogenic Effect 0	Levonorgestrel Androgenic Effect 8.3	Desogestrel Estrogenic Effect 0	Desogestrel Androgenic Effect 3.4	Mestranol µg	Ethinyl Estradiol µg	Number of Hormonal Pills	Number of Other Pills
Norlestrin 1/50-21 & 28						1.0										50	21	7 inert
Norlestrin 1/50-FE						1.0										50	21	7 iron
Ortho-Cept														0.15		30	21	7 inert
Ortho-Cyclen										0.250						35	21	7 inert
Ortho-Novum 1/35 21 & 28	1.0															35	21	7 inert
Ortho-Novum 10/11/21 & 28																		
Necon 10/11 same																		
White tablets	0.5(10)															35	21	7 inert
Peach tablets	1.0(11)																	
Ortho-Novum 1/50-21 & 28	1.0														50		21	7 inert
Ovcon-35	0.4															35	21	7 inert
Ovcon-50	1.0														50		21	7 inert
Ovral 21 & 28								0.5							50		21	7 inert
Zovia 1/50			1.0												50		21	7 inert
Mircette													—	0.15		20(21) / 10(5)	26	2 inert
MINI (Progestin only)																		
Micronor	0.35																28	
Nor-Q-D	0.35																42	
Ovrette								0.075									28	

Table 1. (continued)

	Progestin Content							Estrogen Content			
	Norethindrone Estrogenic Effect 1.0 / Androgenic Effect 1.0	Ethynodiol Diacetate Estrogenic Effect 3.4 / Androgenic Effect 0.6	Norethindrone Acetate Estrogenic Effect 1.5 / Androgenic Effect 1.6	Norgestrel Estrogenic Effect 0 / Androgenic Effect 4.2	Norgestimate Estrogenic Effect 0 / Androgenic Effect 1.9	Levonorgestrel Estrogenic Effect 0 / Androgenic Effect 8.3	Desogestrel Estrogenic Effect 0 / Androgenic Effect 3.4	Mestranol µg	Ethinyl Estradiol µg	Number of Hormonal Pills	Number of Other Pills
TRIPHASICS											
Estrostep 21			1mg						20(5), 30(7), 20(9)	21	—
Estrostep®FE			1mg						20(5), 30(7), 35(9)	21	7 inert
Triphasil 21 & 28 (Tri-levelen, Trivora, same)						0.050(6), 0.075(5), 0.125(10)			30(6), 40(5), 30(10)	21	7 inert
Ortho-Novum 7/7/7/21 & 28	0.5(7), 0.75(7), 1.0(7)								35	21	7 inert
Tri-Norinyl 21 & 28	0.5(7), 1.0(9), 0.5(5)								35	21	7 inert
*Tri-Cyclen					0.180(7), 0.215(7), 0.250(7)				35, 35, 35	21	7 inert

*Tri-Cyclen is the only OC currently indicated to treat acne vulgaris in women 15 and older who have no contraindications to OC use, want contraception, have achieved menarche, and have not responded to topical antiacne medications.

Table 2. Possible Interactions Between Oral Contraceptives and Other Drugs*

Interacting Drugs	Adverse Effects	Comments and Recommendations
When in doubt, consult with a pharmcist		
Antipyretics and analgesics Acetaminophen, aspirin, meperidine, antipyrine	Possible decrease in pain relief (increased metabolism)	Monitor pain-relief response; may have to adjust analgesic dosage
Alcohol	Possible increased effect of alcohol (↓ metabolism)	Caution patient
Antibiotics Troleandomycin Cyclosporine	↑ serum levels, risk to liver	choose alterna- tive method
Anticoagulants (oral)	Decreased anticoagulant effect (↑ factor VII & X)	Use alternate contraceptive
Antidepressants Tricyclics amitriptyline, desipra- mine, imipramine, nortriptyline	Possible increased antidepressant effect (↓ metabolism)	Monitor antidepressant effect
Anti-infectives: sulfonamides	Possible decreased contraceptive effect; possible breakthrough bleeding	Use back-up method during treatment
Barbiturates/Anticonvul- sants (phenobarbital, primidone, carbamazepine, phenytoin, topirimate, succimide)	Decreased contraceptive effect (↑ metabolism)	Avoid simultan- eous use; alternative con- traceptives for long course of treatment; consider 50 mcg ethinyl estradiol OC

*Adapted from: R.A. Hatcher, J. Trussell, F. Stewart, W. Cates G.K. Stewart, F. Guest and D. Kowal (1998), *Contraceptive Technology* (17th ed.), New York: Ardent Media; R.P Dickey (1998), *Managing Contraceptive Patients* (9th ed.), Durant, OK: Essential Medical Information Systems (EMIS); *Nurse Practitioner's Drug Handbook* (1996), Springhouse, PA: Springhouse; L.A. Eisenhauer & M.A. Murphy (1998). *Pharmacotherapeutics and Advanced Nursing Practice.* New York: McGraw-Hill.

Table 2 (con't). Possible Interactions Between Oral Contraceptives and Other Drugs

Interacting Drugs	Adverse Effects	Comments and Recommendations
Benzodiazepine Tranquilizers such as: diazepam (Valium), nitrazepine, chlordiazepoxide (Librax, Librium), alprazolam (Xanax)	Possible increased or tranqilizer effects including psychomotor impairment and possibly impairs elimination due to ↓ clearance	Use with caution. Greatest impair ment during menstrual pause in contraceptive dosage
Beta-blockers such as: propranolol (Inderal) atenolol (Tenormin) metoprolol (Lopressor) pindolol (Visken) Nadolol (Corgard)	Possible increased blocker effect (↓ metabolism)	Monitor cardiovascular status; ↓ drug dosage if necessary
Betamimetics: isoproterenol (Isuprel, Aerolone, Vaso-Iso)	↓ response due to ee	Adjust drug dose, monitor closely
Cholesterol Lowering Agents: clofiborate, gemtibrozil	↑ clearance rate	May need to ↑ dose, monitor lipid profile
Corticosteroids (cortisone, prednisone)	Possible increased corticosteroid toxicity (may impair elimination of drug)	Possibly need to ↓ dosage
Griseofulvin (Fulvicin, Grisactin Grifulvin, others)	Decreased contraceptive effect (↑ metabolism)	Use alternative contraceptive
Guanethidine (Ismelin)	Decreased guanethidine effect (mechanism not established)	Avoid simultaneous use
Methyldopa (Adoril, Aldomet, Amodopa, Dopamet, Apomethyldopa, Novomedopa)	Decreased hypertensive effect	Avoid simultaneous use

Table 2 (con't). Possible Interactions Between Oral Contraceptives and Other Drugs

Interacting Drugs	Adverse Effects	Comments and Recommendations
Oral Antidiabetics such as: chlonopropamide (Diabinese), glipizide (Glucotrol), tolazamide (Tolinase), tolbutamide (Tolinase)	Possible decreased hypoglycemic effect	Monitor blood glucose using low dose estrogen & progestin; consider other birth control
Penicillins	Decreased contraceptive effect possible; breakthrough bleeding	Low but unpredictable incidence; use alternative contraceptive during treatment
Phenytoin (Mesantoin); mephenytoin. (Dilantin) phenytoin sodium (Di-Phen, Diphenylan)	Decreased contraceptive effect; possible decreased phenytoin effect	Use alternative contraceptive; 50 meq. ethinyl estradiol; monitor phenytoin concentration
Rifampin (Rifadin, Rimactane)	Decreased contraceptive effect ($\uparrow$ metabolism of progestins)	Use alternative contraceptive
Tetracycline/ ampicillin short-term<10 days	Decreased contraceptive effect	Use back-up contraceptive during and then x 7 days after treatment.
Theophyllines (Aerodate, Bronkodyl, Slo-bid, Slo-Phyllin, Theobid, Theolair, Theophyl, Theo-Dur, others)	Increased theophylline effect ($\downarrow$ clearance by 30-40%)	Monitor theophylline concentration; use with caution
Troleandomycin (TAO)	$\uparrow$ risk of hepatotoxicity $\uparrow$ effects of TAO	Avoid simultaneous use

Table 2 (con't). Possible Interactions Between Oral Contraceptives and Other Drugs*

Interacting Drugs	Adverse Effects	Comments and Recommendations
Vitamins C, B1, B$_2$, B$_6$, B$_{12}$, folic acid, calcium, magnesium, zinc	Decreased serum concentration; ↑ serum concentration of estrogen with ≥ 1 gram vitamin C/day	Adjust dietary sources ↑
Vitamin A, copper, iron	Decreased serum concentration	Adjust dietary sources; use supplements with caution

Individual practitioner evaluation is important to assure that women can choose the best contraceptive method and avoid adverse effects.

Contraceptive Injectable (Depo-Provera ®)

I. Definition
Synthetic hormonal substance (depot-medroxyprogesterone acetate or DMPA) that acts by blocking gonadotropin, thus preventing ovulation from occurring. Also decreases sperm penetration through cervical mucus, decreases tubal motility, and causes endometrial atrophy preventing implantation. Injected intramuscularly every 12 weeks into the muscle of the upper arm or buttocks.

II. Etiology
Effects include suppression of ovulation for at least 91 days by inhibiting gonadotropin production.

III. Effectiveness
A. Failure rate of less than one pregnancy per 100 women per year

IV. Background to Electing the Method

A. Consideration of, or use of, other methods; side effects or other undesirable characteristics precluding their use
B. Desire for long-term contraceptive
C. Desire for reversible method
D. Desire for method disconnected from intercourse
E. Contraindication to estrogen containing hormonal contraceptives
F. Administration can be highly confidential

V. Contraindications for Use of Method

A. Known or suspected pregnancy or as a diagnostic test for pregnancy
B. Unexplained abnormal vaginal bleeding suspicious of serious pathology
C. Known breast malignancy
D. Known sensitivity to Depo-Provera or any of its ingredients (check any allergic reaction to local anesthetics for dental or other procedures = same ingredient in the carrier substance of local anesthetics and Depo-Provera)

VI. Use with Caution; Careful Monitoring May Be Necessary

A. Depression
B. Kidney disease
C. Abnormal mammogram
D. Planned pregnancy in near future
E. Mentally handicapped woman with menstrual hygiene problems
F. Hypertension
G. Gallbladder disease
H. Mild cirrhosis

VII. Advantages of Depo-Provera® for Women Who Have the Following Situational Conditions

A. Can reduce or control endometriosis
B. Sickle cell (can reduce pain or crisis)
C. Smokers any age regardless of numbers of cigarettes/day
D. Breastfeeding
E. Immediate postpartum use
F. Cholestasis of pregnancy

G. Benign ovarian cysts
H. Irregular heavy or prolonged vaginal bleeding
I. Epilepsy (may decrease seizures)
J. Iron deficiency anemia
K. Use of rifampicin, griseofulvin, phenytoin, carbamezapine, barbiturates, primidone
L. Current long-term antibiotic use (acne)

VIII. Complications and Side Effects

A. 1. Menstrual irregularity, irregular cycles and spotting, amenorrhea in 50% of women after one year, >75% by end of second year; first 3 months most women are irregular and many women have amenorrhea by the second dose
   2. If menstrual irregularity is heavy or prolonged, consider use of 10-21 days of oral estrogen, i.e., conjugated estrogen (Premarin) 1.25 to 2.5 mg)
B. Weight gain in two-thirds of women due to increased appetite; average 5 pounds; weight loss in 10%
C. Long-term use possibly contributes to lower bone mineral density
D. Breast tenderness
E. Headaches
F. Abdominal bloating
G. Tiredness, fatigue, weakness
H. Dizziness, nervousness
I. Depression: rare but important in women without previous endogenous depression; mood changes
J. Post use infertility for a mean of 10 months (range=4-31 months)
K. Thromboembolic disorders
L. Visual disturbances—loss of vision (total or complete), protosis, diplopia, migraine with accompanying visual symptoms
M. Nausea
N. Increased hair growth on face or body, or alopecia
O. Increased or decreased libido
P. Skin rash or increased acne

IX. Explanation of Method and Assessment

A. Depo-Provera is injected intramuscularly (in gluteal or deltoid muscle) in the first 5 days of the menstrual cycle (after onset of menses), within 5 days postpartum, or, if breastfeeding, at 4-6 weeks postpartum. The injection consists of one 150-milligram dose every 12 weeks for as long as contraceptive effect is desired. If time between injections is greater than 13 weeks, do pregnancy test before administration. Inject with 1.5" up to 3" needle (depends upon size of woman since it needs to be deep intramuscular) and do not rub the site as rubbing breaks up the micro crystals and increases absorption. Depo-Provera is now available in 150 mg/ml pre-filled syringes as well as single and multiple-dose vials

B. Review of personal and family history for contraindications and precautions with use; review with physician as appropriate for precautions

C. Physical examination
   1. Complete examination including pelvic exam, Pap smear and breast exam

D. Discussion of effects and side effects of drug
   1. Drug interactions with bromocriptine. Check with pharmacist for other possible interactions before taking any other prescription drug (see VIII)
   2. Warning signs:
      Sharp chest pain, coughing of blood, sudden SOB
      Sudden severe headaches, vomiting, dizziness, or fainting
      Visual disturbance or speech disturbance
      Weakness or numbness in arm or leg
      Unusually heavy vaginal bleeding
      Severe pain or swelling in calf
      Severe pain or tenderness in lower abdomen, pelvic area
      Persistent pain, pus or bleeding at injection site
   3. Use back-up contractive method for 7 days after first injection
   4. Vasovagal response occurs rarely with injection, so be sure clinician giving drug can manage this response (some sites have emergency meds ready as part of injec-

tion protocol)
E. Laboratory
1.   Papanicolaou smear annually
2.   Liver function studies if jaundice appears subsequent to use
3.   Other as indicated by history and physical findings
4.   Consider checking estradiol levels after 2 years of continuous use over age 40

X. Follow-up
A. Visit every 12 weeks for injection
B. Review of side effects, danger signs to report
C. Review of menstrual cycles
D. Papanicolaou smear annually along with complete physical examination including pelvic and breast examinations
E. If greater than 13 weeks, do very sensitive pregnancy test before injection
F. Teach about calcium in diet and supplements for recomended daily amount; exercise to build or maintain bone mass
G. Consider exogenous estrogen for long-term use.

See Appendix F for a combined client information and consent form for using Depo-Provera. See Bibliography 11.

Diaphragm

I. Definition/Mechanism of Action
A diaphragm is a shallow rubber or silicone cap with a flexible rim which is placed in the vagina so as to cover the cervix. It serves as both a mechanical barrier and a receptacle for (contraceptive) spermicidal cream or jelly which must be used to insure effectiveness.

II. Effectiveness and Benefits
A. Method: 97% effectiveness rate
B. User: 80-85% effectiveness rate

C. May be inserted up to four hours prior to intercourse
D. May have some protective effect against transmission of certain sexually transmitted diseases
E. Effective form of contraception for women who have infrequent intercourse or in whom there are contraindications for other methods

III. Side Effects and Complications
A. Allergic reaction of client or her partner to rubber or to the spermicidal agent (a silicone diaphragm is available)
B. Inability to achieve satisfactory fitting
C. Inability of client to learn correct insertion and/or removal technique
D. Use may be associated with an increased incidence of urinary tract infection due to upward pressure of the rim of the diaphragm against the urethra
E. Pelvic discomfort, cramps, pressure on the bladder or rectum can occur if
   1. Diaphragm is too large
   2. Patient has chronic constipation
F. Toxic shock syndrome: severe cases occurring immediately after use have been reported in diaphragm users during menses (although these appear to be related to damage to vaginal walls during scanty flow by tampon use rather than diaphragm use per se)
G. Foul-smelling vaginal discharge may occur if the diaphragm is left in too long

IV. Types (Representative of Several Manufacturers)
A. Arcing spring
   1. Sturdy rim with firm spring strength (spiral, coiled spring)
   2. Firm construction allows diaphragm to be kept in place despite rectocele, cystocele, mild pelvic relaxation, uterine retroversion
   3. Folds in an arc-shape
B. Coil spring
   1. Spring in rim is spiral, coiled, and sturdy

    2. Best suited for women with good vaginal tone and no uterine displacement

    3. Folds flat for insertion

C. Wide-seal

    1. Cuff inside rim

    2. Available in arcing and coil spring; also in silicone

V. Fitting

A. Most diaphragms are available in sizes ranging from 50 or 55 millimeters to 95 or 100 millimeters (available sizes in 5 millimeter gradations)

B. Fit should be snug between the posterior fornix, pubic symphysis and lateral vaginal walls, but should cause no pressure or discomfort

C. The client may review and sign informed consent form (see Appendix G)

D. After a diaphragm has been fitted, instructions have been given, and the client has demonstrated her ability to insert and remove it, she may be given an appointment for a follow-up visit in one week. During this week the client is instructed to practice wearing the diaphragm for at least 8-hour intervals. (In many settings, one-week follow-up may be unrealistic, so diaphragm fitting and use will be taught at one visit and the client given the prescription or kit.) It is helpful for the client to be given a phone number and times to call about any concerns or problems.

E. At follow-up appointment

    1. Diaphragm is checked for fit and proper insertion

    2. Instructions are again reviewed and client is given an opportunity to ask questions

F. If above criteria are met, client is then given prescription for diaphragm

G. Yearly diaphragm check is recommended, but the client should return for recheck sooner if she

    1. Gains or loses 10-15 pounds (although some sources query the necessity of this and suggest return if diaphragm does not seem to fit well or can be displaced)

    2. Has any pelvic surgery

3. Has miscarriage, abortion, or wishes to resume using diaphragm after giving birth
4. Is having problems with use

Appendix G may be photocopied and used as an informational handout on the diaphragm, as well as a consent form, for your clients. See Bibliography 5 on the diaphragm and Bibliograpy 23 on toxic shock syndrome.

Intrauterine Devices (IUDs)

I. Definition/Mechanism of Action
A. A sterile foreign body placed in the uterus to prevent pregnancy. This is accomplished through several mechanisms:
   1. A local sterile inflammatory response to the foreign body (IUD) causes a change in the cellular makeup of the endometrium; with the copper devices there is an effect on the endometrium of interfering with the enzyme systems, and with the progesterone device, an effect over time of a less well-developed endometrium
   2. A possible increase in the local production of prostaglandins that may increase endometrial activity
   3. Alteration in uterine and tubal transport
   4. IUDs probably exert an antifertility effect beyond the uterus and interfere with fertility before an ovum reaches the uterus
   5. Alteration of cervical mucus causing a barrier to sperm penetration (progesterone IUD)
B. The exact mechanisms of action are not completely understood. One thing that has become clear is that the IUD does not act as an abortifacient.
C. Different types of IUDs use varying mechanisms of action to prevent pregnancy

II. Effectiveness
A. Theoretically: 97-99% effectiveness rate
B. User: 90-96% effectiveness rate

The range is close since the client's participation is low and therefore there is little possibility of patient error

III. Contraindications

A. Absolute contraindications
1. Active pelvic infection (acute or subacute), including known or suspected gonorrhea or chlamydia
2. Known or suspected pregnancy
3. Recent or recurrent pelvic infection
4. Purulent cervicitis; untreated acute cervicitis or vaginitis
5. Undiagnosed genital bleeding
6. Distorted uterine cavity (bicornuate; severely flexed)
7. History of ectopic pregnancy (Progesterone IUD)
8. Diabetes mellitus (Progesterone IUD only)
9. Allergy to copper (known or suspected) or diagnosed Wilson's Disease (Paragard only)
10. Abnormal pap smear; cervical or uterine malignancy or premalignancy (endometrial hyperplasia, cervical intraepithelial neoplasia or cancer)
11. Impaired responses to infection (diabetes, steroid treatment, immunocompromised patients)
12. Presence of previously inserted IUD
13. Genital actinomycosis

B. Relative contraindications (benefits usually outweigh risks)
1. Multiple sexual partners or partner has multiple partners
2. Emergency treatment difficult to obtain should complications occur; this would primarily be a problem in very rural areas or developing countries
3. Cervical stenosis
4. Impaired coagulation response (ITP anticoagulant therapy, etc.)
5. Uterus sounding less than 6 cm or more than 10 cm
6. Endometriosis
7. Leiomyomata
8. Endometrial polyps
9. Severe dysmenorrhea (Progestasert IUD may be therapeutic).

10. Heavy or prolonged menstrual bleeding without clinical anemia; consider oral iron or nutritional alterations to prevent with IUD
11. Impaired ability to check for danger signals
12. Inability to check for IUD string
13. Concerns for future fertility
14. Postpartum endometriosis or infected abortion within the past three months
15. History of PID
16. Valvular heart disease (potentially making woman susceptible to subacute bacterial endocarditis); for insertion and removal woman needs to receive:
    a. Oral: Amoxicillin 2 grams 1 hour before procedure
    b. Parenteral: Ampicillin 2 grams IM or IV within 30 minutes before the procedure; Gentamicin (Garamycin, and others) 1.5 mg/kg (120 mg max) IM or IV 30 minutes before the procedure
    c. Penicillin allergy: Vancomycin (Vancocin, and others) 1 gram IV infused slowly over 1 hour beginning 1 hour before the procedure; Gentamicin 1.5 mg/kg (120 mg. max) IM or IV 30 minutes before procedure

IV. Insertion Technique
A. Procedure
   1. Woman is scheduled for appointment for insertion only during menses and after
      a. Negative Papanicolaou smear (within 6 months)
      b. Negative gonorrhea/Chlamydia testing
      c. Appropriate medical and menstrual history is obtained
   2. Client should be instructed to eat before coming to an appointment
   3. Take oral analgesic or nonsteroidal anti-inflammatory 30-60 minutes before procedure
   4. IUD consent form (see Appendix H) and minor surgical consent form must be reviewed and signed at the time of an IUD consultation and evaluation, after discussion of
      a. Procedure
      b. Mechanism of the device

    c. Side effects and complications

    d. Relationship to woman's needs

5. Atropine 0.5 mg should be available at the time of insertion for severe vasovagal response

6. Anxious woman, or woman for whom it is deemed necessary to perform a paracervical block and/or use IV atropine (to decrease likelihood of vasovagal reaction), should be referred to a gynecologist for insertion

7. Insertion under sterile technique

    a. Bimanual examination to determine uterine position and size; insert warmed speculum

    b. Cleanse the vagina, cervix, and endocervical canal with iodine solution (unless allergic to iodine)

    c. Xylocaine gel or hurricane spray could be used to decrease discomfort of tenaculum

    d. Use tenaculum to straighten the uterine body and cervical canal

    e. Sound the uterus (depth less than 6 cm. or more than 10 cm. is contraindication)

    f. Insert specific IUD as instructed by manufacturer

    g. Spasm of the internal cervical os may occur; it is usually relieved by simply waiting. *Never* force entry of the sound or applicator

    h. After insertion, observe the client for weakness, pallor, diaphoresis, either bradycardia or tachycardia, hypotension and syncope which may occur (check blood pressure several times following insertion)

    i. If client has mild cramping, the following may be used:

        1) Aspirin 325 mg x q 4 hours (in some settings aspirin is not used due to its effect on clotting), or

        2) Non-aspirin analgesic 650 mg every 4 hours, or

        3) A prostaglandin inhibitor (NSAID) such as Motrin® 400 mg p.o., qid

    j. Explain to client that the IUD is effective immediately. In some settings it is recommended that the client abstain x 1 day due to disruption of cervical mucus barrier

    k. Instruct client to check for presence of IUD string post menstruation or after unusual cramping prior to relying on device for continued contraception effect

    l. Follow-up with appointment in 6 weeks; at that time be sure the woman can feel the IUD strings

V. Complications Following Insertion and What to Do about Them

A. Immediate, severe vasovagal response
1. Notify physician
2. Place patient in shock position
3. Monitor pulse and blood pressure until stable
4. Administer oxygen as needed
5. Atropine 0.4 mg subcutaneously or intramuscularly may be administered if appropriate

B. Severe immediate cramping: remove IUD

C. Excessive pain or bleeding is often a sign of perforation (fundal); physician consult for management

D. Side effects or later complications
1. Two or more missed periods: recommend a serum pregnancy test. Pregnancy is rare but when this happens, there is a 50% chance of miscarriage. If IUD is removed, this drops to 25%
2. Pregnancy occurring while IUD is in place: it is now recommended that, due to risk of infection, the IUD should be removed at the time of diagnosis whether the pregnancy is continued or terminated. There should be consultation with a gynecologist prior to removal of the IUD by the gynecologist or nurse practitioner
3. Break-through bleeding related to IUD: use the following guidelines for removal:
   a. Bleeding is associated with endometritis
   b. Hematocrit falls 5 points
   c. There is a hematocrit of 30-32% or lower
   d. The IUD is partially expelled
   e. The client wants the IUD removed
4. Cramping and pelvic pain
   a. Rule out ectopic pregnancy

       1) Obtain a serum pregnancy test
       2) Consider ultrasound and surgical consult (physician consult)
  b. Pain or cramping caused by or associated with
       1) Partial expulsion of IUD
         a) Remove IUD
       2) Pelvic inflammatory disease (a long-standing foul-smelling discharge in an IUD wearer is presumed to be PID until proven otherwise)
         a) Remove IUD
         b) Treat infection; culture and sensitivity at time of removal and adjust treatment as indicated
         c) Consult a physician prior to inserting another IUD (some sources advise waiting a year)
       3) Spontaneous abortion
5. Expulsion
  a. Objective findings when the cervix is visualized
       1) The IUD is seen at the cervical os or in the vagina
       2) The IUD string is lengthened (partial expulsion)
       3) The IUD string is absent (complete expulsion)
       4) The IUD cannot be located using various methods of probing (physician consult)
       5) The IUD is absent on ultrasound of abdomen
  b. Removal and reinsertion of IUD
       1) If partial expulsion occurs, IUD should be removed. IUD may be reinserted immediately if there is no infection or possibility of pregnancy, or with the next menses
       2) If completely expelled, a new IUD may be reinserted as outlined above
6. Lost IUD strings
  a. Referrals for locating IUD include
       1) Exploration of canal with gentle probing; if not found, then
       2) Ultrasound
       3) Flat plate of abdomen
       4) Hysterosalpingogram
7. Difficulty in removing IUD

The following techniques may help in the removal of IUDs
   a. Remove only during menses
   b. Employ gentle, steady traction, remove IUD slowly. If IUD does not come out easily, physician consult is in order
   c. If IUD strings are not visible, nurse practitioner may probe for them in the cervical canal with narrow forceps
8. Uterine perforation (fundal or cervical), embedding of the IUD
   a. Objective findings include
      1) Absence of IUD string
      2) Inability to withdraw IUD if string is still present
      3) Demonstration of displaced IUD by ultrasound, hysteroscopy, or x-ray
   b. If perforation or embedding is suspected, referral to physician is in order
   c. Reinforcement of education that multiple partners increase the risk of infection, including HIV infection

VI. Follow-up
A. Yearly Papanicolaou test and pelvic examination with removal and reinsertion as the particular IUD requires (Progestasert® yearly; ParaGard T 380A® 10 years)
B. As needed for any of above-mentioned complications with physician consultation as necessary.

Appendix H may be photocopied for your clients as an informational handout as well as a consent form for using an IUD.
See Bibliography 6.

Contraceptive Spermicides and Condoms

Spermicides

I. Definition
Spermicides are substances used alone or with a vaginal barrier to prevent sperm from reaching the uterus. All contain an inert base or carrier substance and an active ingredient, most commonly the surfactant nonoxynol-9, which disrupts the integrity of the sperm cell membrane.

II. Effectiveness and Benefits
A. Method: 96% effectiveness rate
B. User: 60% effectiveness rate
C. Inexpensive and readily available
D. Some protective effect against the transmission of sexually transmitted disease, including possibly the AIDS virus (HIV)

III. Side Effects and Disadvantages
A. Local irritation from spermicide or allergy to spermicide or carrier substance
B. Can necessitate interruption of love-making for application
C. Emotional reaction to touching one's own body

IV. Types*
A. Creams, jellies, gels
B. Foams
C. Foaming tablets
D. Suppositories
E. Vaginal contraceptive film
F. Bioadhesive gel
G. Water soluble lubricant with spermicide

---

*Koromex® cream and Ortho Gynol® have Octoxynol as the spermicide. Concentration of spermicide varies from 1-12.5% depending on the product. Some spermicides are flavored and some are colored. Protectaid sponge has nonoxynol-9, sodium cholate, and benzalkonium chloride—available OTC in Canada.

V. How to Use
A. Instructions should be read prior to using any spermicide. Method of insertion, time of effectiveness, time needed prior to intercourse, etc., varies with each type
B. A new insertion of spermicide is needed before each act of intercourse
C. Wash the applicator with soap and water after each use
D. When the woman uses a spermicide alone, the partner should always use a condom

VI. Follow-up
Yearly physical examination including Papanicolaou smear is recommended.

See Appendix I for patient handout on spermicides and condoms and Bibliography 7 for references.

Condoms

I. Definition
Condoms are thin sheaths, most commonly made of latex but is also made of sheep intestine or polyurethane*, which prevent the transmission of sperm from the penis to the vagina. The female condom (vaginal pouch) is made of polyurethane.

II. Effectiveness
A. Method: 97-98% effectiveness rate
B. User: 70-94% effectiveness rate; 85% for female condom (range 74.0-91.1%)
C. Inexpensive and readily available
D. Offer protection against the sexually transmitted diseases, including the AIDS virus (HIV)
E. Encourage male participation with birth control (conventional male condom)
F. Female condom is polyurethane (fewer allergic reactions as compared with latex

---

*Avanti® polyurethane condoms (male) are now being marketed in the U.S.

III. Side Effects and Disadvantages
A. Allergic reactions to latex (rare) or lubricant or spermicide on products with either of these in place
B. Use necessitates interruption of love-making for application
C. May decrease tactile sensation
D. Psychological impotency may occur
E. Only latex condoms can be considered effective protection against the AIDS virus (HIV); the polyurethane vaginal pouch (female condom) is twice as thick as latex and viral permeability may be less than latex
F. Polyurethane male condoms are more likely than latex to break or slip off, but they are useful for persons who don't like latex condoms or are latex sensitive

Use of both vaginal spermicides and condoms has an effectiveness rate in the high nineties when both methods are used correctly

IV. Types
Condoms (male) vary in color, texture (smooth, studded, or ribbed), shape, size, and price. They come lubricated or non-lubricated, impregnated with spermicide or plain. Some are extra strength, some are sheerer and thinner, and some are uniquely shaped or scented

V.a. How to Use the Male Condom
A. The male condom should always be put on an erect penis before there is any sexual contact, and used in every act of intercourse
B. The male condom should not be pulled tightly over the end of the penis; about one inch should be left for ejaculation fluid and to avoid breakage; some condoms have a reservoir tip
C. The penis should be withdrawn before it becomes limp, and the open end of the male condom should be held tightly while withdrawing to prevent spilling the contents
D. The partner should always use a contraceptive spermicide when a male condom is used
E. Condoms should be used only once

V.B. How to Use the Female Condom (comes prelubricated)

A. Pinch ring at closed end of pouch and insert like a diaphragm, covering the cervix; adding 1 or 2 drops of additional lubricant makes insertion easier and decreases or eliminates squeaking noise and dislocation during intercourse

B. Adjust other ring over labia

C. Can be inserted several minutes to 8 hours prior to intercourse

D. Remove after intercourse before standing up by squeezing and twisting the outer ring and pulling out gently

VI. Follow-up

A. Annual examination, Papanicolaou smear, mammogram as appropriate to age.

NOTE: Clinicians should remind clients that if a condom breaks or slips off, emergency contraception is available.

Appendix I has information on contraceptive spermicides and condoms that you may wish to photocopy for distribution to your clients. See Bibliography 7.

Cervical Cap*

I. Definition

The cervical cap is a thimble-shaped, deep-domed barrier device that fits over the cervix, and is used in combination with a spermicidal preparation. The cervical cap is FDA approved for general use as a birth control method in the United States.

II. Effectiveness and Benefits

A. Current use effectiveness rates range from 92-96%

---

*This protocol was developed by R. Mimi Clarke Secor, R.N., C.S., F.N.P., M.Ed., M.S., Certified Family Nurse Practitioner, and is used with her permission.

B.   May be inserted up to 12 hours before intercourse and kept in place for several days, and additional spermicide is not necessary with repeated lovemaking (intercourse with ejaculations)
C.   Possible option for women unable/not desiring to use other methods of contraception
D.   Increased comfort and reduced risk of cystitis as compared to the diaphragm
E.   Less disruption of sexual response compared to diaphragm

III. Side Effects and Complications of Use
A.   Inability to achieve satisfactory fitting due to anatomic abnormalities, normal variations of cervix or vagina, and limited sizes and designs of caps (only 50-70% of women can be fit)
B.   Inability of client to learn correct insertion and/or removal techniques (rare)
C.   Partner's or woman's complaints of discomfort (rare)
D.   Allergic reaction to rubber or spermicidal agent (very uncommon)
E.   Lack of trained practitioner to fit cap

IV. Types
A.   Prentif Cavity Rim Cervical Cap, imported from England; four sizes: 22, 25, 28, and 31 mm (inner diameter)
B.   Additional styles have been developed and are being researched currently including a silicone cap

V.   Fitting
A.   Review of medical history
  1. Allergies (including spermicidal agents)
  2. Current medications
  3. Past or present illness/medical condition
  4. Past surgery
  5. Review of systems, noting especially history of constipation, which may lead to cap dislodgement
B. Review of gynecologic history
  1. Menstrual history (cap should be fitted when woman is not

menstruating)

2. Contraceptive history, past and present (reasons for choosing or changing methods)
3. Papanicolaou smear history (most recent Pap should be normal for cap fitting to occur)
4. Past/current genitourinary infections (resolve before cap fitting or use)
5. History of toxic shock or other serious infections, especially any associated with hospitalization
6. Sexual history (especially vaginal/digital foreplay, as this may cause cap dislodgement)
7. Pregnancy history, including if currently breast feeding. (After vaginal delivery, woman should wait 6-8 weeks for initial cap fitting or refitting; should be refit after breast feeding is discontinued as size may have changed)
8. Vaginal health: self-care habits such as douching, use of tampons or pads

C. Informed consent

Since FDA approval of the cap, an informed consent statement is optional but recommended. This consent statement should include: explanation of the current status of the cap and its effectiveness, potential side effects, contraindications, and recommended guidelines for use and follow-up care. A statement regarding willingness to use a back-up method of birth control the first 1-3 months is also recommended. Some sources suggest back-up birth control only the first six times the cap is used. There are no clear guidelines on this issue; it is suggested that each clinician examine the data and reach a consensus among clinicians with whom they work

D. Pelvic examination

1. Speculum examination
   a. Observe for vaginal or cervical abnormalities/infections
   b. Observe cervical characteristics, including size, shape, position, length and color, and characteristics of the cervical os
   c. Think about suitability for cap and consider which size cap might be appropriate

2. Bimanual examination
   a. Note any uterine or adnexal pathology
   b. Note position of cervix relative to the vaginal axis (parallel, oblique, perpendicular*)
   c. Note any vaginal abnormality such as a partial septum
   d. Evaluate vaginal tone and muscle supports, presence of cystocele or rectocele, uterine prolapse, or extreme vaginal laxity
   e. Estimate the length and diameter of the cervix and the vagina (note if cervix is proximal or distal to the vaginal introitus)
   f. Again consider suitability for cap and which size might be appropriate
   g. Note any rectal condition such as hemorrhoids, fissures, constipation
E. Cap assessment: criteria for suitable cap fitting
   1. Cervical characteristics
      a. Cervical length of at least 1.5 cm (there are certain exceptions to this, but such cases should be reserved for the experienced cap fitter)
      b. Cervical width of at least 1.0 cm and no more than 3.0 cm
      c. Cervical angle should be as nearly parallel to the axis of the vagina as possible (parallel, best angle; oblique, usually acceptable; perpendicular, relative contraindication)**
      d. Other cervical characteristics (or abnormalities)
   2. Vaginal characteristics
      a. The general tone of the vaginal tissues determines, in part, the quality of the cap fit, affecting the degree of suction present
      b. In addition, a vagina tapering toward the cervix pro-

---

* *Parallel:* cervix and os angled toward the vaginal opening
  Oblique: cervix angled down toward the floor of the vagina
  Perpendicular: cervix and os angled toward the tailbone/rectum at 90-degree right angle to vaginal axis
** However, fitters disagree regarding this recommendation.

provides better cap suction and therefore is a desirable characteristic (this anatomical feature requires experience to evaluate properly)

 c. The vaginal walls should be free of lesions or structural abnormalities such as septal wall defects. (Vaginal infections are a temporary contraindication and should be resolved before a cap fitting is attempted)

 d. Vaginal length should be adequate to ensure that the cervix is distal enough from the introitus to prevent dislodgement or partner complaints (this requires experience to evaluate properly)

3. General considerations

 a. The candidate should be in good health at the time of the fitting and be free of genitourinary infection or abnormal conditions (such as abnormal Papanicolaou smear)

 b. The candidate should be comfortable touching her body, especially her cervix and vagina. As needed, preteaching and counseling is recommended prior to the cap fitting appointment

 c. The more a candidate is involved in the cap fitting process and gains experience in using the cap, the greater the effectiveness is likely to be

 d. There is no correlation between the size diaphragm a woman wears and the size cap she will wear

F. Fitter characteristics

It takes time to develop expertise in fitting cervical caps. Until you have fit several dozen women with cervical caps it is best to have a more experienced person check your fittings. The following are suggestions which may help in the evaluation process:

1. Evaluate the position of the cap immediately after you initially insert it for the woman. Attempt to dislodge or loosen the cap from the cervix. Note the resistance or tension present

2. Allow the cap to remain in position for 3 to 5 minutes and then reevaluate the cap's suction in the manner described

above

3. During the waiting period, the woman may be instructed to locate various landmarks on the cap such as the soft dome, the thick rim, and the sometimes elusive notch on the side of the cap. You may want to insert the cap incorrectly so the patient can practice distinguishing correct from incorrect positioning. The client may also practice turning the cap. This is done by pushing a finger against the rim of the cap and rotating it sideways, 1/4 to 1/2 turn. Some fitters believe this step enhances the suction. Compare the suction before and after turning the cap. Pushing against the notch on the side of the cap makes turning the cap easier

4. Each time the patient practices inserting the cap the fitter should check for proper position and the quality of suction

5. Generally, the cap's suction improves with increasing time worn. In some women the cap seems to create suction immediately whereas in others the suction may increase markedly after 5 minutes. Occasionally, it may take up to 30 minutes to establish suction. If you doubt the quality of suction, suggest the woman wear her cap when coming to your office, having inserted it at home at least 30 minutes in advance of her appointment

6. Rating the cap's suction: The following is a rating scale (known as the Secor Scale) suggested and developed by the author of this section to assess and rank the quality of a cap's suction, using a scale of 0 to 3+, 3+ being the best cap fitting possible. A description of each category follows:

   a. O fit: cap has no suction or ability to remain over the cervix; falls off immediately upon attempted placement over the cervix

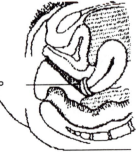

CERVICAL CAP

   b. 1+ fit: the cap stays

on the cervix but it requires very little effort to dislodge the cap from the cervix. This is considered less than a minimally acceptable fit and unpredictable

c. 1-2+ fit: may be minimally acceptable (unpredictable) fit. Little resistance present when the cap is loosened from the cervix. Slightly more resistance than with the 1+ fit. Do not give cap to woman. Require refitting in 2 weeks to reassess quality of fit

d. 2+ fit: minimally acceptable. Requires moderate amount of finger strength to loosen the cap from the cervix

e. 2-3+ fit: above average cap fit. Requires more than moderate amount of force to loosen the cap, but is still relatively easy to remove. (Do not rely on woman's perception of difficulty because she may think the suction is good and it is simply her lack of experience which is causing the difficulty removing the cap)

f. 3+ fit: extremely snug fit. Requires unusual amount of strength to remove the cap; you may have to use all the finger strength you can muster to loosen it (this tension is not harmful and it may be helpful to tell the woman this). This quality of fit may be deceptive. Sometimes the cap will fit too snugly over the cervix and, in some women, may cause cramping. It may also increase the possibility of cap dislodgement if the cap is so snug that it covers only the tip of the cervix and not the base. In this case, it is better to increase the cap size to lessen the snugness of the cap against the cervix)

NOTE:

As the quality of cap suction improves, so will the tendency of the cap, once loosened from the cervix, to reposition itself back onto the cervix. This is what the author calls the cap's "homing" instinct. This characteristic, when present, may indicate an enhanced fit

7. Assessing snugness of the cap to the cervix. Also known as gap. This is an area of controversy. Some fitters have suggested the cap should fit as snugly as possible. Others have

theorized that there should be a small amount of room around the base of the cervix to accommodate the cervical size variability that occurs throughout a woman's menstrual cycle. How much the cervix varies is not known. Some clinicians suggest women be fit with the cap when they are at midcycle; however, this is not always feasible and, therefore, for most offices and clinics it becomes an impractical requirement. There should probably be a few mm of space between the inside rim of the cap and the cervical base. If the cervix is parallel to the vaginal axis, a gap of 2-3 mm may be acceptable. If the cervix is perpendicular, a gap of no more than 1 mm is ideal (this is because a cap fit to this cervix is more vulnerable to dislodgement). Experience is required to assess this measurement with confidence.*

8. Assessing the coverage of the cap over the cervix. Initially, the fitter should search completely (360°) around the rim of the cap, reaching as high as possible to feel if the base of the cervix is covered completely by the cap. This is usually impossible for the woman to perform but should be assessed scrupulously by the fitter at the time of the fitting. If the base of the cervix is uncovered, especially anteriorly, the patient may experience dislodgement and possible pregnancy, even without complete dislodgement. The cap is much like a condom and must be positioned completely over the cervix and seal itself against the posterior fornices of the vagina.

NOTE:

A nearly adequate fit with the cap is never satisfactory because the cap can act as a sperm cup if it becomes dislodged or if not properly located over the cervix initially.

G. Sequence of events for fitting the cervical cap

1. To be accomplished by the woman before the actual fitting:

   a. Read literature on the cervical cap including brief history, effectiveness data, skill sheet, and the consent form

---

* Fitters vary in their recommendations regarding this guideline.

      b. Achieve familiarity with one's anatomy, particularly the vagina and location of the cervix. The fitter provides assistance and encouragement as needed

      c. Complete a written health history questionnaire. This affords more time for discussion of cap-related concerns at the time of the fitting

  2. Actual cervical cap fitting

      a. Schedule at least 45 minutes for the visit

      b. Perform a complete physical exam and review woman's health history

      c. Obtain a Papanicolaou smear, gonorrhea and/or Chlamydia culture, and other diagnostic tests as indicated

      d. Determine proper cervical cap size

      e. Encourage woman to practice inserting and removing cap until she can insert and remove it properly twice without coaching. Woman must also be able to identify if the cap is improperly positioned (fitter inserts cap improperly and asks woman to identify its position)

H. Follow-up visit for the cervical cap

  1. If the fitter is uncertain about the quality of the cap fit, request the woman to return in 2 weeks or consider having a more experienced fitter recheck the cap with you

  2. Encourage the woman to return within 3 months to reassess the cap fit and her skill level

  3. Reevaluate the cervical cap fit yearly or according to protocol or clinician's recommendations

  4. Some fitters recommend reevaluating the cap fit with weight change greater than 15 pounds

  5. Evaluate fit after any pregnancy, D&C, gyn surgery of the cervix or uterus

I. Suggestions for the clinician fitting the cap

  1. Encourage the woman to view her cervix during the examination

  2. Use of plastic speculum offers an unobstructed view of the vagina and cervix, which can be very helpful to the woman using a cervical cap

  3. Initially insert the cap for the woman and then instruct her to locate the cap and its major features: the soft dome, the

firm rim, the notch on the side of the cap

4. Remove the cap for the woman and then walk her through the insertion procedure. (Remind her to locate her cervix each time before inserting the cap. Also remind her to keep the outside rim of cap dry for best control during insertion)

5. Review the removal procedure, then encourage the woman to attempt removal. (Fingernails must be short to prevent injury and to enable client to reach the cap rim with ease.) Suggest she not be delicate in removing the cap; in fact, she may be most successful if she thinks of arm wrestling with the cap. Squatting and bearing down as if having a bowel movement may also ease removal by shortening the vagina and lowering the cervix.

J. Inability of patient to develop the necessary skills

1. Difficulty inserting the cap

   a. Suggest the woman, in the comfort of her home, reread the instructions and practice feeling her cervix and visualizing the skills needed to insert and remove the cap. Then ask her to return for another 30-minute practice session. More than an hour of practice at the time of the initial visit may be exhausting and frustrating for the woman

   b. Suggest the woman maintain contact with the cap continuously during the insertion process. This will lessen the chance of the cap attaching itself to the vaginal wall improperly and will help the woman guide the cap to its proper location over the cervix

2. Difficulty removing the cap

   a. Assist the woman with removal and encourage her to try inserting the cap again. Sometimes more practice and greater familiarity with the cap are all that's needed

   b. Suggest the woman

      1) Bear down and at the same time squat

      2) Try using different fingers and either hand; sometimes the thumb is effective

      3) Try pulling on the soft dome of the cap; this will not tear the material of the cap

   c. Rarely, a loop may be needed to help the patient

remove the cap. Reassure her this is a temporary solution and she will probably soon develop skills to remove the cap without the loop. An effective loop may be made by threading 10 lb. nylon fish line through the side of the notch of the cap, being careful not to puncture the dome portion of the cap. Tie a secure knot (one square knot works well with one extra tie added). Trim the ends no shorter than 1 cm (shorter may irritate the partner and longer is unnecessary). The loop should be approximately 2 cm long; too long, it may become wrapped around the dome of the cap making it difficult to locate. If the loop comes off, another loop may be added. Dental floss should not be used as it may harbor bacteria and is also difficult to identify when moist

    d. Occasionally, a woman may not be able to master the necessary skills to use the cap successfully. If this is the case despite repeated practice sessions, accept the situation and reassure her that she may use one of many other effective methods of birth control

K. Controversies in the literature

    1. Turning the cap may improve its suction. A 1/4 to 1/2 turn is probably sufficient, although some clinicians recommend more extensive turning. Some experts claim a cap that won't turn is a better fit than a cap that will turn. This is an area of controversy. All criteria should be applied when judging the fit. It is the author's opinion that the ability to turn the cap is not necessarily a sign of an unacceptable fit.

    2. Checking proper placement of the cap. The only reliable way to evaluate the position of the cap is by sweeping the entire rim (360°) feeling for the uncovered cervix. The cervix cannot be reliably palpated through the cap dome.

Appendix J contains information on the cervical cap which you may wish to photocopy for distribution to your clients.

See Bibliography 8.

Vaginal Contraceptive Sponge*

I. Definition
A. Description: The vaginal contraceptive sponge looks like a small doughnut with a hollow in the center. The hollow area fits over the cervix (opening to uterus). It measures about one- and three-quarters of an inch in diameter. Across the bottom is a string loop which provides for easy removal. The sponge is polyurethane and contains a spermicide called Nonoxynol 9®
B. Method of action
1. Provides a barrier between sperm and the cervix
2. Traps sperm within the sponge
3. Releases spermicide contained within the sponge to inactivate sperm over a 24-hour period

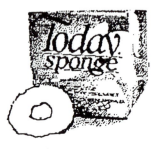

II. Effectiveness and benefits
A. 89-90.8% method; 84.5-86.7 use effectiveness
B. Readily available, over the counter, no prescription needed
C. Sexual intercourse may be repeated within a 24-hour period without adding extra cream, jelly, or foam
D. Spermicides are thought to have a protective effect against the transmission of sexually transmitted diseases

III. Side Effects and Disadvantages
A. Irritation or allergic reactions to the spermicide (Nonoxynol 9®
B. Inability to learn correct insertion technique
C. Difficulty removing sponge

---

*As this book went to press, Allendale Pharmaceuticals announced it will bring back the Today® sponge by fall of 1999. Protectaid® sponge with F-5Gel® is available over the counter in Canada.

D. May have a relationship to development of toxic shock syndrome if not used as directed

IV. Procedure to use

A. Insertion
   1. The sponge may be inserted any time up to 24 hours before sexual intercourse. There is no need to add additional cream or jelly once the sponge has been moistened under water and inserted into the vagina
B. Removal
   1. Read the sponge instructions carefully
   2. Remember to remove sponge slowly to avoid tearing it
   3. Do not flush sponge down the toilet
   4. Special removal instructions:
      a. If sponge appears to be stuck, simply relaxing the vaginal muscles and bearing down should make it possible for the client to remove the sponge without difficulty
      b. The sponge may turn upside down in the vagina thus making the string loop more difficult to find. The woman can find the string by running a finger around the edge on the back side of the sponge until she feels the string. If she cannot find the loop, the woman should grasp the sponge between her thumb and forefinger and remove it slowly
      c. If the sponge tears during removal, the woman may remove any small pieces of sponge that may remain inside the vagina by running a finger around the upper vault of the vagina
      REMEMBER: The sponge cannot get lost in the vagina.

V. Additional Information

A. It is recommended that the client wash her hands with soap and water before inserting the sponge to avoid introducing infective organisms into the vagina
B. It is okay to wear the sponge while swimming or bathing
C. The sponge may only be used once and then should be

discarded

D. Annual check-ups are recommended.

CAUTION: Some concern has been expressed about the relationship between use of the sponge and the development of toxic shock syndrome if not used as directed. Therefore, an alternate method of contraception should be used during menses. Danger signals of toxic shock that occur with the menstrual period are fever (101° and above), diarrhea, vomiting, muscle ache, rash (sunburn-like). (See Bibliography 23.)

Appendix K contains information on the vaginal sponge that you may wish to photocopy for your clients. See Bibliography 9.

Natural Family Planning*

I. Definition

Natural family planning is a method of controlling family size through the use of normally occurring signs and symptoms of ovulation and the entire menstrual cycle, for both the prevention and achievement of pregnancy.

II. Etiology

Effects of hormones on basal body temperature, cervical mucus, the position of the cervix, the cyclical nature of the ovulatory and endometrial cycles, and the physical process of the release of an egg make possible knowledge of occurrence of ovulation.

III. Background for Electing the Method

A. What the client presents with
1. Motivation to learn natural signs and symptoms of ovulation for purposes of fertility regulation
2. Often a history of previous use of other methods of family planning
3. Failure, dissatisfaction, or lack of harmony in values

---

*This protocol was developed by the late Eleanor Tabeek, R.N., Ph.D., C.N.M., and is used with her permission and that of her family. Updates by Nancy Keaveney, R.N., B.S.

with other methods
4. Cultural, ethnic, religious values and personal beliefs harmonious with natural family planning
5. Medical contraindications to the use of one or more other methods
B. Additional background information to be obtained from the client
1. Medical/surgical history
2. Obstetrical history
3. Gynecological history including menstrual history
4. Family planning method currently being used
5. The client's knowledge about the female human body, especially the ovulation cycle
6. Family history

IV. Physical Examination
A. Vital signs
1. Temperature   2. Pulse   3. Blood pressure
B. Complete physical examination
C. External examination of genitalia
D. Vaginal examination utilizing a speculum
Position of cervix; observation of mucus
E. Bimanual examination, noting
1. Adnexal pain   2. Masses   3. Tenderness

V. Laboratory Test
A. Papanicolaou smear if none within past year; cultures, wet mount as appropriate or per protocol
B. Mammography as recommended

VI. Differential Diagnosis
Preference for other method

VII. Teaching about Natural Family Planning
See Appendix M, Teaching Natural Family Planning
A. Fertility awareness
B. General introduction to natural family planning
C. Basic information about natural family planning and methods

1. Ovulation method
2. Temperature method (BBT)
3. Fertile and infertile periods
4. Cervical palpation
5. Symptothermal methods
6. · Keeping and interpreting a chart

D. Aspects of method having to do with interpersonal and intimate relationships

VIII. Complications
A. Inability of client to interpret signs and symptoms
B. Lack of acceptability of method to partner
C. Unplanned pregnancy

IX. Consultation/Referral
To specialist or program for teaching of natural family planning

X. Follow-up
A. Annual examination and Papanicolaou smear
B. Evaluation of effectiveness of the method
C. Evaluation of client satisfaction

See Appendixes L and M.
See Bibliography 10.

Contraceptive Norplant® Implants

I. Definition
Flexible, nonbiodegradable tubes filled with a synthetic hormone of the progestin family (levonorgestrel), placed under the skin on the inside of the upper arm, and designed to release progestin at a constant rate for five years

II. Etiology
Effects of progestin include suppression of ovulation, thickening of cervical mucus and making it more scanty, and suppression of endometrial proliferation

III. Effectiveness
A. 99+% method effectiveness first 5 years; decreases significantly after 5 years and should be replaced

IV. Background to Electing the Method
A. What the client presents with
  1. Motivation for use of method
  2. Often history of previous use of one or more methods
  3. Failure of previous methods, dissatisfaction with methods and/or lack of harmony with lifestyle
  4. Medical contraindications for one or more methods
  5. Not completed childbearing but desires long-term spacing
B. Additional background information to be obtained from client
  1. Medical history
  2. Pregnancy history
  3. Family planning method(s) currently in use; use history
  4. LMP—it is recommended that insertion be performed within 7 days from the onset of menstruation
  5. Gynecological history including menstrual history
  6. Client's knowledge about her body

V. Physical Examination
A. Vital signs
  1. Temperature   2. Pulse   3. Blood pressure
B. Complete physical exam including mammography if over 35
C. External examination of genitalia
D. Vaginal examination utilizing speculum
E. Bimanual examination noting
  1. Adnexal masses   2. Adnexal pain, tenderness

VI. Laboratory Tests
Papanicolaou smear if none within one year; cultures, wet mount as appropriate

VII. Differential Diagnosis
Preference for other method

Consider a trial of Ovrette® (norgestrel) or combination oral contraceptive with levonorgestrel for three months to evaluate tolerance of progestin in Norplant (if no contraindication to estrogen)

VIII. Contraindications to Method
A. Known or suspected pregnancy
B. History of known or presently suspected breast cancer
C. Undiagnosed abnormal vaginal bleeding — suspicious for serious pathology

IX. Other Considerations (Use with Caution)
A. Abnormal mammogram   C. Hypertension
B. Allergy or intolerance   D. Diabetes
   to local anesthetic

X. Advantages for Women With These Conditions/Situations
A. Smokers of any age regardless of number of cigarettes/day
B. Breastfeeding
C. Immediate postpartum
D. Immediate post abortion
E. Endometriosis
F. Benign ovarian cysts
G. Cholestasis in pregnancy
H. Iron deficiency anemia
I. Long-term antibiotic use
J. Hyperlipidemia

XI. Teaching about Method
A. Insertion
B. Removal
C. How the method works
D. Stress with client that
   she will have menstrual cycle changes
E. Side effects
F. Dangers
G. Have client review and sign informed consent

XII. Insertion Technique
A. Have client lie on her back on the examination table with her less dominant arm flexed at the elbow and externally rotated

so that her hand is lying by her head

B. The optimum insertion area is the inside of the upper arm about 8-10 cm above the elbow crease

C. Make insertion graph prior to cleansing the area with an antiseptic solution

D. Open sterile Norplant® system package. Place sterile drapes above and below the insertion area

E. After determining the absence of allergies to the anesthetic agent, fill a 5 ml syringe with local anesthetic. Anesthetize the insertion area by first inserting the needle under the skin and releasing a small amount of anesthetic, then anesthetize the six areas on the graph

F. Use the scalpel to make a small shallow incision through the skin (approximately 2 mm)

G. Insert the tip of the trocar through the incision beneath the skin at a shallow angle. Once the trocar is inserted, it should have the bevel up toward the skin to keep the capsules in a superficial plane. It is important to keep the trocar subdermal by tenting the skin with the trocar

H. When the trocar has been inserted the appropriate distance, remove the obturator and load the first capsule into the trocar using the thumb and forefinger. Gently advance the capsule with obturator toward the tip of the trocar until you feel resistance

I. Never force the obturator

J. Release of the capsule can be checked by palpation

K. Do not remove the trocar from the incision until all capsules have been inserted

L. After the insertion of the sixth capsule, palpate the capsules to make sure all six have been inserted, then remove trocar

M. Press the edges of the skin together and close the incision with a skin closure (steri-strips); some advise firm pressure over the site right after insertion to decrease bruising

N. Cover the insertion area with a dry compress and wrap gauze around the arm to ensure hemostasis

0. Advise the client to keep the insertion area dry for 2-3 days. Remove gauze after 1 day and the steri-strips after 3 days.

P. Advise the woman to avoid lifting heavy objects for 48 hours

XII. Removal of Implant (Norplant®)

A. Recommendations of manufacturer (Wyeth)
1. Position, drape and cleanse client's arm as in insertion technique
2. Locate the implanted capsules by palpation, possibly marking their position with a sterile skin marker; cleanse skin with iodine solution
3. Apply a small amount of local anesthetic under the capsule ends nearest the original incision site. This will serve to raise the ends of the capsules. Anesthetic injected over the capsules will obscure them and make removal more difficult.
4. Make a 4 mm incision with the scalpel close to the ends of the capsules. Do not make a large incision.
5. Push each capsule gently toward incision with fingers.
6. When the tip is visible or near the incision, grasp it with a mosquito forceps
7. Use the scalpel very gently to open the tissue sheath that has formed around the capsule
8. Remove capsule from incision with a second mosquito forceps
9. After the procedure is completed, the incision is closed with steri-strips and a pressure dressing is applied

B. Emory method*
1. Advantage of method: less removal time (approximately 10 to >30 minutes); less pain; less post-removal bruising
2. Use 6-7 cc of Xylocaine (more than manufacturer recommends) (can also use lidocaine with 1:100,000 epinephrine buffered with 1 mEq sodium bicarbonate: 10 ml lidocaine to decrease pain of injection)
3. Make incision 8 mm to 1 cm (larger incision)
4. Attempt vigorous disruption of adhesions using a small curved hemostat (more disruption of adhesions prior to attempting removal)

XIII. Complications and Side Effects

A. Inability to site implants properly: select another method

---

* As taught by S. Surma, M.D., Emory University; tips from Klaisle & Darney (see Bibliography 11)

B. Inability to tolerate presence of implants: select another method
C. Hypermenorrhea: oral estrogen (with gynecologist consult); usually diminishes within a year
D. Headaches: non-narcotic analgesics, evaluate with headache history and for neurological signs
E. Weight change: diet history, counseling, exercise (average = 5 pounds)
F. Mastalgia: supportive bra, vitamin E 200-400 mg/day
G. Galactorrhea: decrease nipple stimulation; evaluate if persistent for breast pathology unrelated to contraceptive implants
H. Acne: diet, skin cleaners, topical antibiotics
I. Irregular menses: reassurance; assessment if bleeding is heavy, menses prolonged or more frequent than q 21 days consider ethinyl estradiol 30 micrograms qd until bleeding stops and advise women that bleeding may resume after estrogen therapy is ended. Reevaluate method for woman and consider supplemental oral contraceptives x 3 months (see Abnormal Vaginal Bleeding protocol)
J. Papilledema
K. Difficult removal: trauma to site; broken implant; bruising; pain; inability to locate all 6 implants

XIV. Consultation/Referral
To nurse practitioner, nurse midwife, or physician trained in implant technique, for insertion, removal, problems

XV. Follow-up
A. Return for check of insertion in 2 weeks
B. Consider return to check for side effects and problems in 3 months
C. Annual examination. Papanicolaou smear. Mammogram as age-appropriate
D. Evaluate effectiveness of method, side effects
E. For removal if pregnancy desired, for replacement at expiration if method continuation desired

See Appendix NN and Bibliography 11.

Emergency Contraception

I. Definition
Emergency contraception (EC), often known as the "morning after pill,"* is pharmacologic or mechanical intervention after exposure to the possibility of conception with no or uncertain contraceptive protection. Such intervention is based on inhibiting fertilization or implantation. The means for intervention are either mechanical (an intrauterine device) or hormonal (high-dose, short-term oral contraceptives or progestational agents).

II. Etiology
Disruption of fertilization or of implantation beginning within 72 hours after unprotected intercourse is based on several theoretical premises:
A. Progestational agents will change or interfere with sperm migration or the capacity of a sperm to penetrate the egg
B. Progestational agents are thought to inhibit motility of the fallopian tubes
C. Estrogen, specifically ethinyl estradiol, is thought to reduce plasma level of progesterone and may, therefore, interfere with the function of the corpus luteum or possibly the function of luteinizing hormone, thereby disrupting ovulation
D. Progestational agents and estrogen (estradiol) are known to shorten the luteal phase of the cycle
E. IUDs, specifically copper bearing devices, are thought to interfere with the enzyme systems of the endometrium and perhaps alter the permeability of the endometrial microvasculature, perhaps interfering with implantation

III. Effectiveness
Used within 72 hours, hormonal emergency contraception reduces risk of pregnancy by 75% for those women who would have become pregnant (8 of 100), so 2 of 100 will become pregnant

---

* The FDA has approved labeling of some oral contraceptives for emergency contraception use.

IV. History
A. What the client presents with
   1. Last act of unprotected intercourse within the past 72 hours
   2. Desire to inhibit fertilization or implantation
B. Additional information to be obtained
   1. Cycle history and any previous use of contraceptives
   2. Estimated day(s) of exposure to sperm without any protection or with known method failure (i.e., condom broke, slipped off; IUD expelled; cervical cap or diaphragm displaced; missed 7 or more combination birth control pills in past 2 weeks, or missed 2 or more progestin only pills)
   3. Contraindications to hormone or IUD use
   4. Circumstance of unprotected exposure—rape, possible STD exposure; teratogen exposure
   5. Other acts of unprotected intercourse during this cycle

V. Physical Examination
A. Pelvic exam—speculum and bimanual—if appropriate
B. Collect specimens following rape/sexual assault protocol (pages 232-244) as necessary/desired by woman; complete the assessment for evidence

VI. Laboratory Diagnosis
A. Pregnancy test
B. STD testing as warranted by history

VII. Differential Diagnosis
A. Consider alternatives should woman desire to keep a pregnancy if one should occur
B. Sexual assault—consider rape counseling
C. Pregnancy already established prior to current exposure with unprotected intercourse

VIII. Treatment
A. Combined oral contraceptives must be initiated within 72 hours of exposure (Yuzpe method)

1. Ovral 2 white pills p.o. stat, followed by 2 white pills in 12 hours
2. Lo-Ovral 4 white pills p.o. stat, followed by 4 white pills in 12 hours
3. Nordette 4 light orange pills p.o. stat, followed by 4 light orange pills in 12 hours
4. Levlen 4 light orange pills p.o. stat, followed by 4 light orange pills in 12 hours
5. Triphasil 4 yellow pills p.o. stat, followed by 4 yellow pills in 12 hours.
6. Tri-levlen 4 yellow pills stat, followed by 4 yellow pills in 12 hours
7. Alesse 5 pink pills stat and 5 pink pills in 12 hours
8. Levlite 5 pink pills stat and 5 pink pills in 12 hours
9. Levora 4 white pills stat and 4 white pills in 12 hours
10. Trivora 4 pink pills stat and 4 pink pills in 12 hours

B. Preven* — 2 light blue pills stat then 2 light blue pills in 12 hours (0.05 mg ethinyl estradiol and 0.25 mg levo-norgestrel)
C. Progestational agents; treatment must be initiated within 72 hours** and causes less nausea and vomiting
D. Mechanical agents
   1. Copper IUD insertion within 5-7 days of exposure with precautions for IUD use, STD exposure, risk factors for IUD use; some protocols specify prophylactic antibiotics with insertion

IX. Explanation of Method

A. Education: for each woman specific for postcoital intervention method including side effects of intervention and danger signs; if IUD is inserted, instructions about IUD use, danger signs, and complications and potential for 10 years of protection against pregnancy
B. Education about resumption of menses: based on woman's cycle history, if hormones are taken during follicular phase,

---

* Preven available in an emergency contraception kit.
**A 2-pill kit (Postinor-2) is available in Europe; each pill is equivalent to 20 Ovrette pills; FDA approval being sought.

menses will follow about day 21; if during ovulation, around day 26, and if in luteal phase, about day 29

X. Complications and Side Effects
A. Pelvic infection with IUD use (see protocol for PID)
B. Ectopic pregnancy: possible increased risk with hormone use (up to 10% of pregnancies); copper IUD use won't inhibit tubal implantation (see information on ectopic pregnancy in the protocol "Acute Pelvic Pain")
C. Pregnancy
   1. Decision-making regarding continuation or termination of pregnancy
D. Nausea and vomiting
   1. Drink glass of milk or eat a snack with each oral dose to reduce risk of nausea and vomiting
   2. Compazine 25 mg rectal suppository q 12 hours or 10 mg p.o. qid
   3. Tigan, 200 mg suppository q 12 hours
   4. Meclizine hydrochloride (Antivert, Dramamine II) 25 mg 1 hour before EC pills
   5. Give extra tablets of oral contraceptives in event of vomiting dose; instruct woman to take repeat dose if vomiting within one hour after taking the dose and pills are visible in vomitus

XI. Consultation and Referral
A. For pregnancy exposure as the result of sexual assault/rape, refer to rape crisis center, rape counseling
B. For complications of postcoital intervention as necessary

XII. Follow-up
A. No menses within 3 weeks after intervention, return for evaluation for continued pregnancy (failure of emergency contraception or preexisting pregnancy); to rule out ectopic pregnancy
B. For a contraceptive method chosen by woman for use following the emergency contraception

The Emergency Contraceptive Hotline, 1-800 NOT-2-LATE, is a 24-hour toll-free service offered in English and Spanish. Callers can get names, phone numbers, and location of 3 local providers. Internet access: http://opr.princeton.edu.ec

See Appendix CC and Bibliography 4.

Sterilization

I. Definition

Sterilization in women is the purposeful occlusion of the fallopian tubes by surgical disruption. Several methods are practiced through closed laparoscopy, open laparoscopy, or suprapubic mini-laparotomy. The method of tubal occlusion depends on the surgical route. These occlusion methods include excision of a portion of each tube and suturing of the ends; excision of the fimbriated end; excision of a portion and then suturing of the proximal end into the muscle of the uterus and the distal end in the broad ligament; banding with silastic or titanium rings or clips; ligation of a loop of the tubes with non-absorbable suture material; occlusion by unipolar or bipolar electrocoagulation.

II. Background for Electing Sterilization

Decision by the woman to seek permanent sterilization through tubal ligation as a means of fertility regulation

III. History

A. What the woman presents with:
1. History of use of one or more methods of contraception
2. Dissatisfaction with available methods and/or method failure
3. Experiencing problems with one or more methods and decision not to have any more children
4. Medical contraindications for use of one or more methods
5. Psychosocial contraindications for use of one or more methods
6. Desire to have no more children or no children; need/desire for permanent method

    7.   Premenopause, less than one year without a period
B. Additional information to be obtained
    1.   Knowledge about all family planning methods used
    2.   Psychosocial and cultural aspects: size of family desired, beliefs about sterilization, family attitudes
    3.   Knowledge about the sterilization procedures available and beliefs about reversibility
    4.   History of any previous pelvic surgery, partial or total hysterectomy, oophorectomy, salpingectomy, laparoscopy, plastic surgery such as tubal reconstruction
    5.   Medical/surgical history, present use of medications
    6.   Type of anesthesia for previous surgeries; any untoward effects
    7.   Gynecologic and obstetric history: pregnancies, live births, abortions, ectopic pregnancies, endometriosis, uterine anomalies, presence of adhesions, uterine leiomyomas (fibroids)
    8.   Menstrual history to the present; last period; PMS; character of menses and menstrual cycle
    9.   Contraceptive use to present and reasons discontinued

IV. Physical Examination

A. Vital signs
    1.   Blood pressure   2. Pulse
B. General physical exam: lungs, heart, neck, abdomen, breasts, extremities, thyroid

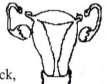

TUBAL LIGATION

C. Pelvic examination
    1.   External: Skene's glands, Bartholin's glands, urethra
    2.   Vaginal examination: walls, discharge, cervix; inspect for cystocele, rectocele, urethrocele
    3.   Uterus: masses, tenderness, enlargement, possible pregnancy
    4.   Adnexa: masses, tenderness, palpable ovaries or tubes, enlargement

V. Laboratory (for preoperative work-up only or for symptoms of problem)

A. Urinalysis, culture if signs of urinary tract infection

B. Complete blood count
C. Pregnancy test
D. Gonorrhea culture

E. Chlamydia test
F. Papanicolaou smear

VI. Differential
None

VII. Treatment
Teaching
A. Methods of sterilization and possible failure
B. Chance of future reversal; choice of method of sterilization related to this
C. Information on informed consent
D. Risks and benefits
E. Discussion of regret
F. Information on waiting period
G. Postoperative implications, i.e., restrictions
H. Sexual adjustments following procedure
I. Information on possible post-tubal ligation syndrome

VIII. Complications
Conditions contraindicating procedure or choice of procedure such as previous surgery or extensive adhesions; allergy or untoward response to anesthesia

IX. Consultation/Referral
To provider who does tubal ligations if the procedure is not offered in the practice setting

X. Follow-up
A. Postoperative care

See Bibliography 12.

Sterilization: Postoperative Care

I. Definition
Follow-up care after the performance of sterilization by tubal ligation or occlusion; time of follow-up will vary depending upon the procedure performed

II. Etiology
A. Transabdominal surgical procedure: ligation and resection; electrocoagulation
B. Laparoscopy and electrocoagulation, clips or rings

III. History
A. Type of procedure done, when, anesthesia
B. Any sutures to be removed
C. Menstruation: last menstrual period, character
D. Resumption of sexual activity, response; change in sexual habits
E. What client may present with
   1. Pain, fever, bleeding or discharge from operative site
   2. Abdominal pain; pelvic pain
   3. Vaginal discharge
   4. Urinary symptoms: frequency, dysuria, hematuria
   5. Any new symptoms/concerns with menstrual cycle not experienced prior to tubal ligation such as endocrine manifestations

IV. Physical Examination
A. Vital signs
   1. Blood pressure 2. Pulse 3. Temperature
B. Abdominal examination
   1. Inspection: incision site(s) if any
   2. Auscultation: bowel sounds, hyper- or hypoactive
   3. Palpation: tenderness, guarding, masses
C. Pelvic examination
   1. Uterus: tender, enlarged, masses, fixed or mobile, pain on cervical manipulation
   2. Adnexa: masses, tenderness

V. Laboratory
A. Cervical culture if fever, uterine, adnexal tenderness present (gonorrhea, Chlamydia)
B. Urinalysis and culture if signs of urinary tract infection
C. CBC, differential, sedimentation rate and/or C-reactive protein if fever, tenderness
D. Pregnancy test if uterus enlarged or adnexal mass, signs of ectopic

VI. Differential Diagnosis
A. Urinary tract infection
B. Perforation of bowel
C. Pelvic infection
D. Salpingitis
E. Peritonitis
F. Tubal hemorrhage
G. Problems with sexual expression; lack of libido, responsiveness

VII. Treatment
As indicated by symptoms and diagnosis

VIII. Complications
A. Hemorrhage
B. Pregnancy
C. Perforation of bowel, bowel burns with electrocoagulation
D. Pelvic inflammatory disease
E. Urinary tract infection
F. Salpingitis
G. Infection of incision site(s)
H. Pelvic abscess
I. Peritonitis
J. Bladder damage
K. Uterineperforation
L. Post-tubal ligation syndrome
M. Regrets

IX. Consultation/Referral
A. Consultation/referral to surgeon for differential diagnosis and treatment of any problem
B. Referral for mental health counseling if experiencing sexual maladjustment, regrets

X. Follow-up
A. Return for recheck after resolution of any complications
B. Annual Pap smear, pelvic examination, health examination; mammography per recommendations

See bibliography 12.

Infertility

I. Definition
Inability to conceive after one full year or more of unprotected intercourse.

II. Etiology
A. Factors in male infertility: faulty sperm production; reproductive tract anomaly; physical and chemical agents (coal tar, radioactive substance, etc.); endocrine disorders; general state of health; blocked vas deferens; testicular infection; injury to reproductive organs/tract; nerve damage; impotence; lifestyle factors (smoking, alcohol, street drugs, etc.); incompatible immunologic factors for sperm—antispermatozoa antibodies
B. Factors in female infertility: blocked fallopian tubes; anovulatory cycles; anatomical anomalies; hormonal imbalance; obstruction of vaginal, cervical, and/or uterine cavity; hostile cervical mucus; ovarian cyst or tumor; pituitary tumor; endometriosis; previous STDs, vaginitis, vaginosis, PID, septic abortion, history of and drug treatment for thyroid disease, depression, asthma; lifestyle factors (alcohol, smoking, street drugs, etc.)
C. Factors in couple infertility: improper technique for intercourse; infrequent intercourse; emotional state; male and female factors contributing to infertility

III. History
A. What the client presents with
    1. History of failure to conceive for period of time with no use of contraception

    2. Desire for pregnancy

B. Additional information to be obtained
1. Complete medical and surgical history; family history
2. Complete menstrual history including menarche, character of menses, frequency, duration, last menstrual period, post-menarche amenorrhea
3. Gynecologic history: anomalies, problems, infections, surgery, DES exposure, endometriosis, fibroids, abnormal Paps
4. Contraceptive history to the present including post-method amenorrhea
5. Obstetrical history: any previous conceptions; number of children, abortions, stillbirths; complications
6. Partner's reproductive history; medical, surgical history
7. Employment history: exposure to radiation, viruses, other substances known to cause sterility; teratogens
8. Sexual history: techniques, frequency and timing of intercourse in relation to the menstrual cycle; use of lubricants, douches, sex stimulants or toys; trauma
9. Report of any previous infertility testing, work-ups; diagnoses; interventions; genetic evaluation
10. Lifestyle history: use of recreational (street) drugs, prescription drugs, alcohol, tobacco, caffeine, eating habits, saunas or hot tubs, exercise (including biking and running); stress
11. Age of patient/partner may determine timing of intervention

IV. Physical Examination

A. Vital signs
1. Temperature
2. Pulse
3. Blood pressure

B. Complete physical examination; observation of secondary sex characteristics

C. External examination (careful observation for signs of

infection, lesions, or anomalies)

1.	Clitoris	2.	Labia
3.	Skene's glands	4.	Bartholin's glands
5.	Vulva	6.	Perineum

D. Pelvic examination
1. Length of vagina
2. Position and character of cervix
3. Any anomalies
4. Sounding of uterus
E. Bimanual examination (examine for palpable masses, tenderness, anomalies, signs of trauma)

1.	Uterus	2. Ovaries	3.	Adnexa

V. Laboratory
A. Papanicolaou smear, maturation index; mammogram as appropriate
B. N. gonorrhea culture; RPR status (syphilis), TB status, HIV, hepatitis status; Rubella titre
C. Chlamydia smear
D. Pregnancy test in amenorrhea
E. Complete blood count; erythrocyte sedimentation rate
F. Mycoplasma and ureaplasma culture
G. Endometrial biopsy during luteal phase
H. Serum progesterone level days 21-23 of cycle
I. Wet mounts, vaginal cultures
J. Prolactin level, FSH, LH, TSH, Rh factor, blood type

VI. Differential Diagnosis
A. Partner infertility, sterility
B. Sterility
C. Anomaly, absence of reproductive organs
D. Cause(s) of intertility

VII. Treatment
A. Infertility work-up for the woman
1. Basal body temperature charts, may use test for LH surge instead

2. Commercially available ovulation tests or devices and fertility monitoring devices*
3. Postcoital test—serial if antispermatozoa antibodies
4. Cervical mucus test, sperm antibody level; sperm agglutination test; sperm immobilization test; endometrial biopsy 2-3 days before menstruation
5. Hysterosalpingogram after menses, before ovulation
6. Hormonal assay (serum) such as FSH, LH, prolactin, estrogen DHEA-S, testosterone, urinary LH 4-5 days at midcycle
7. Tuboscopy
8. Ultrasound
9. Laparoscopy with chromotubation, hydrotubation; hysteroscopy; salpingoscopy

B. Work-up of partner involving tests done by specialist
C. For complete work-up, referral may be in order

VIII. Complications
A. Risks associated with certain tests; costs of testing
B. Persistent infertility, discovery of sterility
C. Effects on couple's relationship

IX. Consultation/Referral
To gynecologist or infertility specialist; reproductive technology centers; genetic counseling

X. Follow-up
Long-term process for work-up that is staged, so client would be asked to return for next phase of testing if conception not achieved

See bibliography 13.

---

* Examples are OvuGen®; Clear Plan Easy®, First Response®, OVu Quick® Self Test for detecting luteinizing hormone (LH) in urine; Clear Plan Easy Fertility Monitor®

Vaginal Discharge, Vaginitis, and Sexually Transmitted Diseases

Checklist for Vaginal Discharge Work-up

Subjective Data

A. Social history
  1. Age
  2. Occupation
  3. Partner status
     a. Frequency of sexual contact
     b. Last sexual act and type
     c. Age of first intercourse
  4. Pregnancy history
  5. Sexual preference
  6. Number of sexual partners; known partner history; history of new partner within past month
  7. Documented STD history including HIV status
  8. Recent weight change
B. Previous gynecologic surgery including abortion, tubal ligation, D&C
C. Past or current medical illness; chronic diseases
D. Family history of diabetes, personal history of Type 1, 2
E. Diet, alcohol, cigarettes, recent change in habits; use of street drugs; use of sex toys, stimulants
F. Medications (past and present); recent antibiotics; use of vaginal medications (OTC and prescription)
G. Past history of similar problems
  1. Dates   2. Treatment   3. Follow-up

H. Vaginal discharge
   1. Onset
   2. Color
   3. Odor
   4. Consistency
   5. Amount
   6. Constant vs. intermittent
   7. Related to sexual contact
   8. Relationship to menses
   9. Relation to other life events
I. "Sores": anywhere on the body; rashes
J. Genital itching, swelling, or burning; genital sores or tears
K. Abdominal or pelvic pain
L. Fever, chills
M. Achy joints
N. Nausea and vomiting; diarrhea
O. Dyspareunia
P. Known contact with sexually transmitted disease; AIDS risk*
Q. Birth control (including recent changes in method or products used)
   1. Oral contraceptive: type and length of use
   2. Intrauterine device: type, how long in place
   3. Diaphragm; cervical cap
   4. Norplant®, Depo Provera®
   5. Condom (male or female); foam, jelly, cream, vaginal film, tablets, suppositories, gels
R. History of douching; use of soaps, chemicals
S. Personal hygiene
   1. Use of feminine hygiene sprays or deodorant tampons, panty liners, or pads
   2. Poor personal hygiene
T. Clothing: consistent wearing of tight-crotched pants; type of underwear; pantyhose
U. Last menstrual period
V. Urinary problems
   1. Frequency
   2. Dysuria
   3. Urgency
   4. Hematuria: other debris in urine
   5. Odor
   6. Dark or cloudy urine; color
W. Allergies to drugs: reactions
X. Partner problems

---

*See Appendix DD.

Objective Data

A. Vital signs: blood pressure, pulse, respiration, temperature
B. Inguinal lymph nodes
C. Abdominal examination: rebound, bowel sounds, suprapubic tenderness, masses, organomegaly, enlarged bladder, costo-vertebral angle (CVA) tenderness
D. External genitalia: Bartholin's glands, Skene's glands, "sores," rash, genital warts, swollen reddened urethra, urethral discharge
E. Vaginal examination (speculum)
   1. Inspection of vaginal walls, vaginal lesions, tears, discharge
   2. Inspection of cervix: friability, ectropion, cervical erosion, discharge from os, cervical tenderness; color
   3. Discharge: if present, characteristically is thick, mucus at cervical os, difficult to remove
F. Bimanual examination: pain on cervical motion, fullness or pain in adnexa, tenderness of uterus, size of uterus

Assessment and Plan

A. Normal discharge: usually clear or white, non-irritating or non-pruritic, pH 3.8-4.2, doesn't pool, has body, can write initials in it
B. Diagnosis
   1. Wet prep will be negative
   2. Gram stain will be negative
   3. pH within normal range
C. Treatment: none required
D. Patient education
   1. Reassurance
   2. If clinical and/or laboratory findings are not within normal limits, refer to protocol for suspected organism(s) for further work-up

Hints on Preparation of a Wet Smear*

A. Collect a copious amount of vaginal discharge from the

---

*Adapted from material developed by R. Mini Clarke Secor (1997) Vaginal microscopy, *Clinical Excellence for Nurse Practitioners 1(1)29-34,* and from Fischbach, F., *A Manual of Laboratory and Diagnostic Tests,* 5th ed., Philadelphia: Lippincott, 1996.

lateral walls with a wooden Pap spatula (some say a cotton swab moistened with saline); repeat so you have two samples to work with

B. Place a drop of the specimen mixture at each end of a clean glass slide, or on 2 separate slides, when you are ready to read the slides; or place a drop of saline on one slide and a drop of KOH on a second before collecting specimens; place in cardboard slide holders if available

C. Add a drop of KOH* (10%) to one specimen or stir one specimen into the KOH on the slide and sniff immediately for the characteristic "fishy" odor of bacterial vaginosis (+ whiff test)

D. Cover both specimens with cover slips once you reach the microscope. Plan to view the plain saline specimen first to allow time for the KOH to lyse cells prior to looking for Candida.** If you suspect trichomonas, you may want to examine slide without a cover slip, as the slip can sometimes immobilize the trich. Warming the slide will also increase the possibility of seeing trichomonads

E. With the 10X objective in place on the microscope, the light on low power and the condenser in the lowest position, place the slide on the stage and lower the objective until it is as close to the slide as possible

F. Adjust the eyepieces until a single round field is seen. Turn the coarse focus knob until the specimen is focused. Use the fine focus knob to bring the specimen into sharp focus

G. Be sure to use subdued light and a lowered condenser for a wet specimen. Try increasing the light and raising the condenser while viewing the specimen to see how the cells and bacteria disappear from view

H. Move the slide until you have a general impression of the number of squamous cells. Switch to high power (40X); it may be necessary to increase the amount of light slightly

I. Evaluate the slide for bacteria, WBCs, clue cells, trichomon-

----

* Note that KOH should be used with care, since it is very damaging to the microscope.

**Candida torulopsis glabrata does not have the same characteristics as Candida albicans so KOH will be negative.

ads, and Candida. Even if one organism is identified, continue to scan the slide systematically to fully evaluate the specimen. Vaginitis/vaginosis may have multiple causes

J. Move the KOH slide into position; switch back to low power to scan the slide for Candida. If hyphae are noted, switch to high power to confirm the impression

K. Be sure to wipe spilled fluid from the stage. If the objective becomes contaminated, clean it only with special lens paper

L. To perform gram staining:

1. Spread a *thin* smear of the specimen on a glass slide. Air dry the slide completely, or dry it carefully high above a flame

2. After the specimen is dry, fix it by passing it through a flame several times (with the specimen side away from the flame). Allow it to cool completely; otherwise the reagents used in the staining process may precipitate on the slide

3. Flood the slide with Gram crystal violet. Wait 10 seconds, then rinse with tap water

4. Flood the slide with Gram iodine. Wait 10 seconds, then rinse with tap water

5. Wash the slide with decolorizer just until the fluid dripping from the slide changes from blue to colorless, then immediately rinse the slide with tap water. This step is crucial to ensure correct decolorizing

6. Flood the slide with Gram sufranin. Wait 10 seconds, then rinse the slide with tap water

7. Allow the slide to air dry, or blot dry. Place the slide on the microscope stage and put a small drop of oil on the stained specimen. With the oil power objective in place, the condenser up and the diaphragm open (for bright field illumination), focus and examine several fields on the slide

8. When finished, remove the oil from the lens with lens paper

Appendix O contains information on vaginal discharge to copy or adapt for your clients. See bibliography 14.

Work-up for Vaginal Discharge and Odor

I. Definition

Vaginal discharge that may or may not have a distinctive odor may be a vaginitis or vaginosis.

Vaginitis: Inflammation of the vagina, characterized by an increased vaginal discharge containing many white blood cells (WBCs).

Vaginosis: Characterized by increased discharge without inflammatory cells (WBCs).

II. Etiology

A. Foreign body (i.e., forgotten tampon, retained cap, condom, or diaphragm)
B. Allergy to soap or feminine hygiene spray
C. Deodorants
D. Scented toilet tissue
E. Vaginal contamination through oral or rectal intercourse
F. Poor personal hygiene
G. Sensitivity to contraceptive spermicides or lubricants
H. Condom allergy. (Hint: If woman is allergic to latex, then use latex condom with animal skin or polyurethane condom over; if man is allergic to latex, use animal skin condom or polyurethane with a latex condom over)
I. Presence of a pathogen

III. History

A. What client may present with
    1. Vaginal discharge, may be chronic
    2. Vaginal odor
    3. Vulvar/vaginal irritation, pruritus, and/or burning made worse by urniation, intercourse
    4. Post-coital bleeding
    5. Difficulty urinating or pain with urination
B. Additional information to be considered
    1. Relationship of discharge to birth control method: any

ended

3. Relationship of discharge to sexual contact: recency; partner affected; recent change in partners
4. Relationship of discharge to personal hygiene: any recent change in hygiene products or toiletries; douching
5. Any history of vaginal infection associated with sexually transmitted disease or pelvic inflammatory disease
6. History of
   a. Previous infection or STD
   b. Chronic cervicitis
   c. Cervical surgery
   d. Abnormal Papanicolaou
   e. Diethylstilbestrol (DES) exposure
7. Description of discharge
   a. Color
   b. Onset
   c. Odor
   d. Consistency
   e. Constant vs. intermittent
   f. Color of discharge on underwear; changes

IV. Physical Examination

A. External examination: external genitalia
   1. Erythema
   2. Excoriations
   3. Lesions
   4. Edema
B. Vaginal examination (speculum)
   1. Presence of foreign body
   2. Erythema and edema of the vaginal vault
   3. Inspection of cervix
      a. Erythema
      b. Erosion
      c. Severe physiological ectropion
      d. Friability
      e. Serous sanguineous discharge
      f. Lesions
C. Bimanual examination if indicated

V. Laboratory Examination

A. As indicated by findings
   1. Wet saline prep; KOH slide
   2. Gram stain
   3. Gonorrhea culture if indicated
   4. Chlamydia test if indicated
   5. Urinalysis if indicated
   6. Herpes culture if indicated
   7. Cervical culture
   8. pH with nitrazine paper
   9. HIV testing

VI. Differential Diagnosis

A. Normal physiological discharge
B. Diethylstilbestrol (DES) exposure
C. Chlamydia
D. N. gonorrhea
E. Candida albicans or other Candida infection; bacterial vaginosis
F. Urinary tract infection
G. Condylomata
H. Herpes simplex
I. Contact dermatitis
J. Tinea or other fungus

VII. Treatment

A. General measures
   1. Removal of causative factor
   2. Education as to
      a. Personal hygiene
      b. Avoidance through use of alternatives to causative factors
B. Medications
   1. No treatment, depending on evaluation of clinical data
   2. If a pathogen is identified, treat via appropriate protocol
   3. If after one week of no treatment, try Aci-jel®, one application intravaginally at h.s. for 7-14 days or until tube is used up

VIII. Complications

Abnormal Papanicolaou smear resulting from continuing irritation; reparative process

IX. Consultation/Referral

Unresolved symptomatology

X. Follow-up

A. One week if indicated, then prn
B. If no improvement at one week after treatment of Aci-jel®, referral to physician

See Appendix O and Bibliography 14.

Candidiasis

I. Definition
Candidiasis, or monilia, is a microscopic yeast-like fungal infection of the vagina usually caused by Candida albicans (90%). Candida tropicalis, Torulopsis glabrata, Candida Krusei, Candida parapsilosis and other lesser known Candida species are also clinically implicated.

II. Etiology
A. A fungus of the genus Candida, species albicans, tropicalis, or Torulopsis glabrata, part of the normal flora of the mouth, gastrointestinal tract, and vagina; may become pathogenic under variable conditions, such as change in the vaginal pH, which encourage an overgrowth of the organism
B. Incubation period: about 96 hours

III. History
A. What client may present with
   1. Pruritus
   2. Vulvar and vaginal swelling
   3. Vulvar excoriation
   4. Vulvar burning with urination
   5. Dyspareunia or burning during and/or after intercourse
B. Additional information to be considered
   1. Previous vaginal infections or vaginosis; diagnosis, treatment and compliance with treatment
   2. Chronic illness (diabetes); immunocompromised
   3. Sexual activity
   4. History of sexually transmitted disease or pelvic inflammatory disease
   5. Last intercourse; changes in frequency
   6. Last menstrual period
   7. Method(s) of birth control
   8. Other medications
      a. Antibiotics   b. Steroids   c. Estrogens
   9. Description of discharge

     a. Color
     b. Onset
     c. Odor
     d. Consistency
     e. Constant vs. intermittent
     f. Relationship to sexual contact
     g. Relationship to menses
     h. Use of vaginal deodorant sprays, deodorant or scented tampons, panty liners, or pads, douches, perfumed toilet tissue
     i. Change in laundry soaps, fabric softener, body soap (amount of soap used and application inside labia)
     j. Clothing: consistent wearing of tight-crotched pants; wearing nylon underwear, panty hose under slacks; wearing underwear to bed
10. "Jock" itch (partner), athlete's foot (self or partner), itchy rash on thighs, buttocks, under breasts; oral candidiasis (thrush)
11. Diet high in refined sugar

IV. Physical Examination
A. External examination
   Observe perineum for excoriation, erythema, edema, ulcerations, lesions
B. Vaginal examination (speculum)
   1. Inspection of vaginal mucosa: may be erythematous, irritated, with white patches along side walls
   2. Cervix
   3. Discharge: characteristically thick, odorless, white, curd-like, resembling cottage cheese, with pH remaining in the normal range of 3.8-4.2 (nitrazine paper)
C. Bimanual examination

V. Laboratory Examination*
A. Wet prep microscopic examination to visualize hyphae, pseudohyphae, spores or buds

*Biomed Diagnostic has introduced In Tray Colorex Yeast Test to differentiate the 4 species. 1-800-964-6466.

B. Consider vaginal or cervical culture.
C. Consider fasting blood sugar and 2° post-prandial on women with chronic yeast infections
D. Further laboratory work as indicated by history including HIV testing

VI. Differential Diagnosis
A. Herpes genitalis
B. Chemical vaginitis
C. Contact dermatitis
D. Normal physiologic discharge
E. Candidiasis 2° to diabetes, pregnancy, + HIV status
F. Candida Torulopsis glabrata or Candida tropicalis or lesser known species (C. Krusei, C. parapsilosis, other C. species)
G. Trichomonas, bacterial vaginosis,Chlamydia, or gonococcal infection

VII. Treatment
A. Medications (some of these are now over the counter)* ‡
   1. Butoconazole 2% cream 5 grams intravaginally x 3 days OR
   2. Clotrimazole (Gyne-Lotrimin®, Lotrimin®, Mycelex®, Mycelex-G®) 1% cream 5 grams (1 applicator full) intravaginally qhs x 7-14 days OR
   3. Clotrimazole 100 mg vaginal table qhs x 7 days OR
   4. Clotrimazole 100 mg vaginal tablet, 2 tablets for 3 days OR
   5. Clotrimazole 500 mg vaginal tablet 1 single dose OR
   6. Miconazole (Monistat®) 2% cream 5 grams (1 applicator full) intravaginally x 7 days OR
   7. Miconazole 200 mg vaginal suppository 1 each for 3 days OR

---

*Imidazole drugs (Miconazole, Clotrimazole, Econazole, Butaconazone) are not as effective for non-Candida albicans infections as are triazole compounds including terconazole and tioconazole.

‡ Note serious adverse effects can occur; use with caution when patient is taking other drugs, so check carefully for drug interactions before recommending or prescribing.

8. Miconazole 100 mg vaginal suppository 1 each for 7 days OR
9. Nystatin® 100,000 unit vaginal tablet, 1 table qd for 14 days OR
10. Tioconazole (Vagistat-1®) 6.5% ointment 5 grams intravaginally single dose hs (pregnancy category C) OR
11. Terconazole (Terazol®) 0.4% cream 5 grams (1 applicator full) intravaginally x 7 days OR
12. Terconazole 0.8% cream 5 grams (1 applicator full) intravaginally x 3 days OR
13. Terconazole 80 mg suppository 1 each x 3 days
14. Oral therapy: Fluconazole (Diflucan®) 150 mg oral tablet, one tablet in a single dose (pregnancy category C)
15. In pregnancy: use only topical azole therapies; most effective in pregnancy are butoconazole, clotrimazole, miconazole, and terconazole; most experts recommend 7-day therapy
16. Miconazole cream (Monistat-Derm®) or chlotrimazole cream (Mycelex®) can be used for external irritation
17. If treatment is unsuccessful, may refill script x 1; if still unsuccessful, consider treating partner and/or fasting blood sugar and 2° postprandial. Review history carefully with woman
18. If fasting blood sugar and 2° postprandial are within normal limits several options may be considered
    a. Clotrimazole® 1 applicator full intravaginally every other week x 2 months. If patient remains symptom free, reduce treatment to q month, the week prior to menses
    b. If 9 is not successful, Candida torulopsis glabrata or Candida Tropicalis should be considered. If lab confirms diagnosis, treat with gentian violet one tampon q hs x 12 days; triazole compounds have also been found to be effective (Terazol®—terconazole)
    c. Boric acid capsules. 600 mg 1 capsule 2 x/week intravaginally for recurrent candida vaginitis (4 or > epiisodes year) as organism may be Torulepsis glabrata (less sensitive to fluconazole or imidazoles)

    d. Clove of garlic in gauze placed in vagina for 10-12 hours; other complementary therapies (see Biography 32)

B. General measures
  1. No intercourse until symptoms subside; then use condoms until end of treatment
  2. No douching
  3. Stress importance of continuing medication even if menses begin
  4. **Do not** use tampons during treatment
  5. Stress hygiene, cotton underwear, loose clothing, no underpants while sleeping, wipe front first and then back
  6. Do not use feminine hygiene sprays, deodorants, etc.
  7. Treat athlete's foot, "jock"" itch, or rash with OTC antifungals (such as Lotrimin®, Tinactin®) or prescription Dual-action Lotrisone®
  8. Consider the use of: vitamin C 500 mg BID→QID to ↑ acidity of vaginal secretions or oral acidophilous tablets 40 million to 1 billion units QD (1 tablet)

VIII. Complications
Drug interactions; adverse reactions to treatment

IX. Consultation/Referral
A. No response to treatment as outlined above
B. Elevated fasting blood sugar or 2° postprandial
C. Presence of concurrent systemic disease

X. Follow-up
None necessary unless
A. Symptoms persist after treatment
B. Symptoms recur or exacerbate

Appendix P has information on candidiasis which you may wish to photocopy or adapt for your clients.

See Bibliography 14.

Trichomoniasis

I. Definition
Infection with the organism Trichomonas, usually sexually transmitted; found in the vagina and urethra of women and the urethra of males.

II. Etiology
The parasitic protozoan flagellate, Trichomonas vaginalis

III. History
A. What the client may present with
   1. Foul-smelling vaginal discharge, often fishy
   2. Burning and soreness of vulva, perineum, thighs
   3. Vaginal and perineal itching
   4. Dyspareunia, dysuria
   5. Postcoital bleeding
   6. Possibly no objective symptoms
B. Additional information to be considered
   1. Previous vaginal infection, vaginosis; diagnosis, treatment; compliance with treatment
   2. Sexual activity; partner preference (do not disregard possibility of women having sex with women)
   3. History of sexually transmitted disease or pelvic inflammatory disease
   4. Last menstrual period
   5. Last intercourse, sexual contact
   6. Method of birth control; other medications
   7. History of chronic illness (especially seizure disorders)
   8. Description of discharge
      a. Color   f. Constant vs intermittnet
      b. Onset   g. Relationship to menses
      c. Odor   h. Relationship to sexual contact
      d. Consistency
      e. Amount
   9. Partner has symptoms

IV. Physical Examination
A. External examination
   Observe perineum for excoriation, erythema, edema, ulceration, lesions
B. Vaginal examination (speculum)
   1. Inspection of vaginal walls; red papules may appear
   2. Inspection of cervix: strawberry appearance of cervix and upper vagina due to petechiae
   3. Discharge: greenish, yellow, malodorous, frothy with >4.5 pH (5.0-7.0)
C. Bimanual examination

V. Laboratory Examination
A. Wet prep microscopic examination; should see highly motile cells, slightly larger than leukocytes, smaller than epithelial cells; > 10 WBCs/high power field
B. Gonococcus culture, Chlamydia test, serology testing for syphilis if history indicates; culture for T. vaginalis; DNA probe for T. vaginalis
C. CBC should be done if more than two courses of Metronidazole® taken within 2-month period
D. KOH "whiff" test: sometimes fishy but not always

VI. Differential Diagnosis
A. Candidiasis
B. Bacterial vaginosis
C. Urinary tract infection
D. Gonorrhea
E. Chlamydia infection

VII. Treatment*
A. Medications
   1. Metronidazole (Flagyl®, Metryl®, Protostat®, Satric®) 2 grams orally in single dose (review history for seizure disorder)
   2. Metronidazole 500 mg BID x 7 days (recommended for treatment failures)

---

*Vaginal gel Metronidazole® is not recommended for trichomoniasis as the protozoa are multifocal including the urethra, Skene's glands, and so on.

    3. Metronidazole capsules 375 mg BID x 7 days*
    4. In pregnancy, Metronidazole 2 grams orally in single dose

B. General Measures
    1. Stress importance of not drinking alcohol during treatment or for 48 hours after treatment
    2. Metronidazole® can cause gastrointestinal upset; also causes urine to darken
    3. Stress avoidance of intercourse during treatment; if intercourse does occur, condoms should be used
    4. Stress importance of completing medication
    5. Stress personal hygiene; cotton underpants, no underpants while sleeping, wipe front first, and then back
    6. Client should be given informational handout to deliver to sexual partner advising need for partner's treatment
    7. Comfort measures for severe symptoms: sitz baths
    8. Stress that if partner is not treated before next act of unprotected intercourse, reinfection can occur

VIII. Complications

A. Of the disease
    Spread of the infection to urethra, or prostate in the male
B. Untreated Trichomonas vaginalis may result in atypia on Papanicolaou smear; may also be associated with adverse pregnancy outcomes (premature rupture of membranes and preterm delivery); ↑ susceptibility to HIV acquisition
C. Of the treatment
    1. Nausea
    2. Neurological symptoms: seizures
    3. Vomiting (may be severe) if alcohol is consumed while on treatment or within 48 hours after treatment
    4. Possibility of blood dyscrasia post treatment

---

*Not yet approved by CDC—not in guidelines but approved by the FDA with pharmacological equivalency of metronidazole 250 mg tid for 7 days; no clinical data available to demonstrate clinical equivalency.

IX. Consultation/Referral
A. Refer to physician if woman has seizure disorder prior to initiating therapy
B. Consult if treatment (VII. A. 1. and 2.) fails

X. Follow-up
None necessary unless symptoms persist or recur after treatment

See Appendix Q and Bibliography 14.

Bacterial Vaginosis

I. Definition
A clinical syndrome characterized by an overgrowth of anaerobic bacteria, genital mycoplasmas, and gardnerella vaginalis (including bacteroides, peptostreptococcus, mobiluncus curtesii and decease in lactobacilli).

II. Etiology
A. Bacterial vaginosis (BV) is a vaginosis rather than vaginitis. As such, there is usually little or no inflammation of epithelium associated with the syndrome (relative absence of polymorphonuclear leukocytes). It is not caused by a single pathogen, but is probably a disturbance of the vaginal microbial ecology, with a displacement of normal lactobacillary flora by anerobic microorganisms
B. It is a sexually associated rather than a sexually transmitted syndrome. (Bacterial vaginosis is found more often in sexually active women.) A male version of BV has not been identified

III. History
A. What the client may present with
   1. Vaginal odor (fishy)
   2. Increased vaginal discharge—white, thin adherent discharge

    3. Vaginal burning after intercourse

    4. No symptoms in many clients

B. Additional information to be considered

    1. Previous vaginal infections; diagnosis, treatment; compliance with treatment

    2. Chronic illness; careful history of seizure disorders

    3. Sexual activity; partner preference

    4. History of sexually transmitted disease or pelvic inflammatory disease

    5. Last intercourse

    6. Last menstrual period

    7. Method of birth control; other medications

    8. Description of discharge

        a. Onset

        b. Color

        c. Odor stronger during intercourse

        d. Consistency

        e. Constant vs. intermittent

        f. Relationship of symptoms to sexual contact

        g. Relationship of symptoms to menses

        h. Amount

    9. Use of vaginal deodorant sprays, deodorant tampons, panty liners, or pads, douches, perfumed toilet tissue

   10. Change in laundry soaps, fabric softener, body soap

   11. Clothing: consistent wearing of tight-crotched pants; nylon underwear, underwear to bed

   12. Personal hygiene

   13. Recent change in lifestyle (stress, personal crisis)

   14. Partner symptoms

IV. Physical Examination

A. External examination

Perineum usually has a normal appearance

B. Vaginal examination (speculum)

    1. Inspection of vaginal walls

    2. Inspection of cervix

    3. Discharge: characteristically adherent homogenous, whitish in color, and of a fishy, musty odor with pH>4.5.

Take smear from lateral walls of vagina, not cervix, for accurate pH (use nitrazine paper for test)
C. Bimanual examination if indicated

V. Laboratory Examination May Include
A. Diagnosis (3 of 4 — Amsel criteria)
   1. White, thin adherent discharge
   2. ph ≥ 4.5
   3. + whiff test (fishy amine odor from vaginal fluid mixed with 10% KOH)
   4. Clue cells on wet mount: epithelial cells dotted with large numbers of bacteria that obscure cell borders, should see ≥ 20% clue cells
B. Few WBCs seen on wet mount; decreased Lactobacilli
C. Further laboratory work as indicated by history or wet prep results

VI. Differential Diagnosis
A. Trichomoniasis   B.   Presence of foreign body

VII. Treatment
A. Medications
   1. Vaginal preparation
      a. Metronidazole gel (MetroGel®) 0.75% one applicatorful (5 grams) intravaginally BID x 5 days or one applicatorful 8 HS x 5 days (if additional treatment is necessary within 2 months, a CBC will be necessary)
      b. Clindamycin phosphate cream (Cleocin® vaginal cream 2% one applicatorful, 5 grams) intravaginally HS x 7 nights. Clindamycin is contraindicated with colitis, other chronic bowel disease. *Note:* the mineral oil in Cleocin® vaginal cream may weaken latex or rubber products such as condoms or vaginal diaphragms. Use of these products within 72 hours following treatment is not recommended
   2. Oral preparation:
      a. Metronidazole (Flagyl® ER) 750 mg orally   1 qd

    x 7 days*

    b. Metronidazole (Flagyl®) 500 mg orally BID x 7 days

3. Alternative treatment:
    a. Metronidazole 2 grams orally single dose
    b. Clindamycin 300 mg orally BID x 7 days
    c. Clindamycin cream 2% 5 grams once a day HS for 7 days

4. In pregnancy:
    For women at high risk (previous preterm delivery)
    a. Metronidazole 250 mg orally TID for 7 days
    b. Metronidazole 2 grams orally single dose
    c. Clindamycin 300 mg orally BID for 7 days
    For women a low risk (no history of preterm delivery)
    a. Metronidazole 250 mg p.o. TID for 7 days
    b. Metronidazole 2 grams p.o. in single dose
    c. Clindamycin 300 mg orally BID for 7 days
    d. Metronidazole gel 0.75% one applicatorful (5 grams) intravaginally BID for 5 days
    e. Second trimester Clindamycin 2% 5 grams x 7 nights

5. Treatment for partner not recommended (no decrease in recurrences with partner treatment and no effect on cure rates)

6. **Note:** If bacterial vaginosis coexists with candidiasis:
    a. Treat a predominant organism first. If symptoms persist, recheck and treat as indicated
    b. Consider local treatment for candidiasis concurrently with oral treatment for bacteria vaginosis as above
    c. Cleocin® also kills lactobacilli, so candidiasis is common after treatment. Consider sequential treatment

B. General measures
  1. Stress avoidance of intercourse until symptoms subside, then use condoms until end of treatment; condom therapy

---

*FDA approved but data on equivalency with other clinical regimens not published.

for 4-6 weeks (without antibiotic treatment) often results in resolution of BV
2. Stress no douching during treatment or after
3. Stress necessity of completing course of medication
4. Nausea, vomiting, and cramps can occur (if patient is on Metronidazole®). Stress no alcohol intake during treatment and for 48 hours after completing medications
5. Stress appropriate choice of medications if pregnant/possibly pregnant
6. Stress hygiene: cotton underwear, loose clothing, no underpants while sleeping, wipe front first and then back, no feminine deodorants or hygiene sprays
7. Careful history of seizure disorders
8. Metronidazole® can cause GI upset even with no alcohol

XIII. Complications
Bacterial vaginosis has been associated with PID, endometritis, cervicitis, inflammation or ASCUS on Pap smears, possible link to LGSIL on Pap smears, preterm rupture of membranes, preterm labor, low birth weight, chorioamnitis; ↑ risk of HIV acquisition

IX. Consultation/Referral
If no response to treatment as discussed above

X. Follow-up
None necessary unless:
A. Symptoms persist after treatment
B. Symptoms recur

See Appendix R and Bibliography 14.

Chlamydia Trachomatis Infection

I. Definition
Chlamydia trachomatis infection is a parasitic sexually transmitted disease of the reproductive tract mucous membrane of either sex.

II. Etiology

A. The causative organism is a small, obligate, intracellular, bacterium-like parasite (Chlamydia trachomatis or C. trachomatis) that develops within inclusion bodies in the cytoplasm of the host cells.

B. The incubation period is unknown

III. History

A. What the client may present with
  1. Female
     a. Vaginal discharge
     b. Dysuria
     c. Pelvic pain
     d. Changes in menses
     e. Intermenstrual spotting
     f. Postcoital bleeding
     g. Frequently asymptomatic
     h. Mucupurulent discharge in cervical os
  2. Male
     a. Dysuria
     b. Thick, cloudy penile discharge
     c. Rarely asymptomatic
B. Additional information to be considered
  1. Previous vaginal infections; diagnosis, treatment; compliance with treatment
  2. Chronic illness
  3. Sexual activity; new partner(s)
  4. History of sexually transmitted disease or pelvic inflammatory disease
  5. Known contact
  6. Last intercourse, sexual contact
  7. Method(s) of birth control, other medications
  8. Description of discharge
     a. Onset
     b. Color
     c. Odor
     d. Consistency
     e. Amount
     f. Constant vs intermittent
     g. Relationship to sexual contact
     h. Relationship to menses
  9. Use of vaginal deodorant sprays, deodorant tampons, panty liners, pads, perfumed toilet tissue, douches
  10. Change in laundry soaps, fabric softener, body soap

11. Clothing: consistent wearing of tight-crotched pants
12. Personal hygiene
13. Any drug allergies

IV. Physical Examination
A. Vital signs
   1. Blood pressure   2. Temperature
B. Abdominal examination: check for guarded referred pain, rebound pain
C. External examination
   Observe perineum for edema, ulcerations, lesions, excoriations, erythema, enlarged, tender Bartholin's glands
D. Vaginal examination (speculum)
   1. Inspection of vaginal walls
   2. Cervix (cervicitis), friability
   3. Discharge: if present, is characteristically mucopurulent
E. Bimanual examination
   Pain on cervical motion (positive Chandelier sign), fullness in adnexa, tender uterus

V. Laboratory Examination
A. DFA: secretions fixed on slide and stained with fluorescein-labelled monoclonal antibody specific for Chlamydial antigens
B. Laboratory test for Chlamydia (sensitivities and specificities vary):
   1. Enzyme-linked immunoassays (EIA) detection of Chlamydial antigens
   2. DNA probe (Genprobe®) (PRC + LCR = amplified tests done on Genprobe®)
   3. Polymerase chain reaction (PCR)
   4. Ligase chain reaction (LCR)
C. Endocervical culture (only 100% specific test in transport media — do in medico-legal cases (rape, child sexual abuse)
D. Serology test for syphilis if history indicates
E. Consider HIV testing
F. Consider hepatitis B & C testing
G. GC culture

VI. Differential Diagnosis

A. Gonorrhea   B. Appendicitis   C. Cystitis

VII. Treatment

A. Medication
   1. Azithromycin 1 gram orally in a single dose *OR* Doxycycline 100 mg orally BID x 7 days or Doryx (coated Doxycyline) 100 mg BID x 7 days (causes less nausea)
   2. Alternative regimens
      a. Erythromycin base 500 mg orally QID x 7 days
      b. Erythromycin ethylsuccinate 800 mg orally QID x 7 days
      c. Ofloxacin 300 mg orally BID x 7 days
      d. Zithromax (category B pregnancy) 1 gram oral suspension syrup p.o. in 2-3 ounces of water. Follow with 2-3 ounces of water (not in CDC Guidelines but useful clinically especially for pre-abortion patients)
   3. In pregnancy
      a. Erythromycin base 500 mg orally QID x 7 days
      b. Amoxicillin 500 mg orally TID x 7-10 days (for erythromycin intolerance)
      c. Zithromax 1 gram oral suspension syrup p.o. in 2-3 ounces of water (category B pregnancy). Follow with 2-3 ounces of water (common practice but not in CDC Guidelines 1998)
   4. Alternative regimens in pregnancy
      a. Erythromycin base 250 mg orally QID x 7 days
      b. Erythromycin ethylsuccinate 800 mg QID x 7 days
      c. Erythromycin ethylsuccinate 400 mg orally QID x 14 days
      d. Azithromycin 1 gram orally in single dose
B. For contacts
   1. Offer Chlamydia test prior to treatment
   2. Start treatment prior to results of testing
   3. Treat same as for woman; do follow-up culture or testing per CDC Guidelines
   General measures
   1. Stress partner should be treated

2. Stress no intercourse or condom use until both partners are treated
3. Condom for back-up birth control method for remainder of cycle if on oral contraceptives
4. Stress importance of completing medication for woman and partner
5. Stress no use of feminine hygiene sprays, deodorants, douches
6. Stress possibility of increased photosensitivity with Doxycycline®
7. Inform patient taking tetracycline that medication should be taken 1 hour before or 2 hours after meals and/or consumption of dairy products, antacids, mineral-containing products
8. Return for reevaluation if symptoms persist or return after treatment

VIII. Complications
A. Women
  1. Pelvic inflammatory disease
    a. Pelvic abscess (ovarian)
    b. Infertility
  2. Abnormal Papanicolaou smear with cervicitis
  3. Postpartum infection
B. Men
  1. Epididymitis
C. Reiter's syndrome (primarily men) — arthritis symptoms
D. Perihepatitis
E. Newborn
  1. Conjunctivitis
  2. Pneumonia

IX. Consultation/Referral
A. If no response to treatment as discussed above
B. If complications develop

X. Follow-up
A. If no response to treatment or possibility of reinfection

B.   Test of cure not routinely required per CDC Guidelines, but if done, should be 3-4 weeks post-treatment. If symptoms persist or reinfection is suspected, consider retesting women after treatment. (↑ rate of reinfection)
C.   Consider retesting 3 weeks after completion of treatment with erythromycin
D.   Repeat Pap if abnormal prior to treatment
E.   Gonorrhea cultures if not done
F.   Serology test for syphilis
G.   In some states, Chlamydia is a reportable disease

Appendix S has information on Chlamydia trachomatis infection to photocopy or adapt for your clients.

See Bibliography 16.

Genital Herpes Simplex

I. Definition
Genital herpes simplex is a recurrent viral infection of the skin and mucous membranes of the genitalia, characterized by eruptions on a lightly raised erythematous base.

II. Etiology
A.   Herpes simplex virus (HSV). There are two HSV strains:
1.   HSV Type I: commonly causes herpes labialis ("cold sores") and herpes keratitis
   a.   Usually seen in childhood (as acute gingivostomatitis)
   b.   May be seen in adults who engage in oral sex, kissing
   c.   Incubation period 3-7 days, course 1-3 weeks
   d.   May be recurrent and has no cure
2.   HSV Type II
   a.   Genital counterpart of acute gingivostomatitis Primarily sexually transmitted
   b.   Incubation period 4-7 days, course may last 2-3 weeks

    c. May be recurrent and has no cure
3. Both HSV I (10%) and II (90%) have been implicated in genital infections and vice versa

III. History
A. Genital herpes
    1. Primary infection (may actually be caused by Type I or II); mean duration 12 days
        a. Multiple lesions
            1) Male: penis, buttocks, thigh
            2) Female: labia, fourchette, cervix, buttocks, thigh, nipples
        b. Myalgia
        c. Arthralgia
        d. Malaise
        e. Fever
        f. Dysuria, male and female (urinary retention may occur, especially in women with lesions close to meatus)
        g. Dyspareunia
        h. Headache (can be sign of herpes meningitis)
    2. Recurrent genital lesions
        a. Lesions less painful
        b. Less or no systemic symptoms
        c. Unilateral
        d. Prodromal symptoms (itching, burning, and/or tingling at site where lesions then appear)
B. Additional information to be considered
    1. Genital herpes: primary infection
        a. Known exposure
        b. Sexual preference
        c. Recent participation in oral sex with partner having herpes labialis
    2. Genital herpes: recurrent infection
        a. History of recent exposure to reactivating factors: physical trauma, exposure to sunlight, stress, menses
        b. Prodrome

1) Pruritus
2) Burning at site of previous lesion(s)
3) Tingling at site of previous lesion(s)
4) Symptoms as in 1, 2, and/or 3 across nerve tract serving site of previous lesion(s); i.e., sciatic pain with lesion on labia

IV. Physical Examination
A. Genital herpes
1. Primary infection
a. Temperature, blood pressure
b. Examination of genitalia: vesicular lesions containing cloudy liquid on erythematous base. Vesicles break, lesions coalesce forming ulcerative lesions with irregular borders, macerated if in moist areas
1) Female: lesions (painful), examination will be difficult; use of speculum may be impossible. Lesions present as described in III.A.
2) Male: lesions (painful) present in areas previously described in III.A. Urethral discharge may be present
c. Groin: inguinal adenopathy may be present
d. Abdomen: bladder distension, secondary to urinary retention may be present; more common in women
2. Recurrent infection genital herpes
As above (III.B.2.) but clinical picture is less severe

V. Laboratory Examination May Include
HSV Types I and II
A. Scrape lesion for samples for
1. Virology culture
2. Genital lesions: consider gonococcus culture, serology test for syphilis, Chlamydia test (may need to wait until follow-up visit if infection is severe)
3. Antigen detection (such as Herpchek^{TM}), cytology (less sensitive than culture)
4. ELISA and Western Blot are highly accurate
B. Consider HIV testing

VI. Differential Diagnosis

A. Syphilis

B. Chancroid

C. Lymphogranuloma inguinale

D. Granuloma inguinale

VII. Treatment Genital Herpes

A. General therapy

1. Consider immune status of patient with frequent outbreaks and/or long duration outbreaks, plus the degree of systemic involvement

2. Comfort measures

   a. Tepid water sitz baths, plain or with Betadine solution; dry carefully with cool air hair dryer making sure to hold it away from body

   b. If voiding over lesions is painful, instruct patient to void while sitting in water in bathtub

   c. Stress avoidance of tight, restricting clothing. The vulva should be exposed to air flow as much as possible (patient may wear a skirt or robe without underpants when at home)

   d. Peri-irrigation for comfort

3. Patient education

   a. Explain the disease process and route of transmission to the patient (i.e., oral/genital sex during outbreaks)

   b. Clients should be advised to abstain from sexual activity while lesions are present

   c. Explain the dangers associated with herpes during pregnancy

   d. Discuss possible factors involved with recurrences

   e. Discuss need for yearly Papanicolaou smear

   f. Support group: alt.support.herpes (usenet news group)

B. Medication

1. Initial genital outbreak

   a. Acyclovir 200 mg orally 5x day for 7-10 days

   b. Acyclovir 400 mg orally TID x 7-10 days

   c. Valacyclovir (Valtrex®) 1 gm orally BID x 7 days

   d. Famciclovir (Famvir®) 250 mg orally TID for 7-10

days
   e. Zylocaine 2% gel or cream; apply 3-4 times daily (do not use around urethra) for comfort measure
   f. Bacitracin ointment, apply locally, for secondary infection only 2-5 x daily
2. Episodic recurrent infection
   a. Episodic—infrequent outbreaks 6 times or fewer a year. Therapy should be initiated as early as possible after onset of symptoms for best effect
   b. Acyclovir 400 mg orally TID for 5 days
   c. Acyclovir 200 mg orally 5 times a day for 5 days
   d. Acyclovir 800 mg orally BID for 5 days
   e. Famciclovir 125 mg orally BID for 5 days
   f. Valacyclovir 500 mg orally BID for 5 days
3. Suppressive therapy* for chronic outbreaks more than 6x/year
   a. Acyclovir 400 mg orally BID
   b. Famciclovir 250 mg orally BID
   c. Valacyclovir 250 mg orally BID (per package insert)
   d. Valacyclovir 500 mg orally QD
   e. Valacyclovir 1000 mg orally QD
4. In pregnancy (report treatment—see CDC 1998 Guidelines)
   a. First clinical episode—treat with oral acyclovir
   b. In life-threatening maternal HSV infection, treat with IV acyclovir
5. Unresolved herpes—herpes outbreaks lasting several weeks or more
   a. Immunological status should be evaluated with physician consultation
6. Oral lesions—treat with Idoxuridine (Stoxil, Herplex), Peridin-C (ascorbic acid, Hesperidin methyl Chalcone, and Hesperidin Complex); penciclovir cream 1% (Denavir)

---

*Daily suppressive therapy ↓ frequency of HSV recurrences by at least 75% for persons with >6 episodes a year; this treatment does not totally eliminate symptomatic or asymptomatic viral shedding or potential for transmission of virus.

VIII. Complications
A. Secondary infection of lesion
B. Keratitis (keep fingers away from eyes)
C. Generalized herpetic skin eruptions
D. Meningitis
E. Encephalitis
F. Pneumonitis
G. Hepatitis
H. Fetal/neonatal infection
I. Spread to other persons at risk of developing disseminated herpes
  1. Immunosuppressed or deficient individuals including persons with HIV
  2. Patients with open skin lesions, e.g., burns, atopic dermatitis
  3. Infants, small children

IX. Consultation/Referral
A. Secondary infections
B. Urinary retention if unable to void in bathtub
C. Suspected ocular lesion
D. Severe primary episode
E. Poor fluid intake associated with severe primary episode
F. Persistent headache, nausea, vomiting, photophobia, convulsions, pain in upper right quadrant, chest pain, SOB
G. Unresolved outbreaks lasting several weeks or more
H. Life-threatening episode in pregnant woman

X. Follow-up
As needed

See Appendixes T and FF for information you may want to photocopy or adapt for your clients.

See Bibliography 14.

Condylomata Acuminata (Genital Warts)*

I. Definition
Condylomata acuminata is a sexually transmitted condition (but it may also be a fomite) caused by a virus, Human Papilloma Virus (HPV), and characterized by the formation of warty excrescences on the external genitalia, and on the cervix, vagina, anal area, nipples, umbilicus, pharynx. Virus does not always cause a lesion; subclinical infection occurs on cervix and externally.

II. Etiology
A. The cause of the condition is a DNA virus of the Papilloma group (HPV)—more than 80 types of HPV have been identified; for anogenital warts, types 6, 11 are most common
B. Incubation period: 1 to 6 months; may be much longer (up to 30 years); up to 70% may regress spontaneously
C. Period of communicability is unknown

III. History
A. What the client may present with
   1. "Feeling a lump" in vulvar area
   2. Increased vaginal discharge
   3. Vulvar itch
B. Additional information to be considered
   1. Previous vaginitis/vaginosis; diagnosis, treatment
   2. Sexual activity, last intercourse, sexual contact
   3. Last menstrual period: any chance of pregnancy
   4. Method of birth control
   5. Previous history of condylomata, herpes simplex
   6. Known contact; consider any contact with person with condylomata on any body part
   7. History of sexually transmitted disease or pelvic inflammatory disease
   8. Description of discharge (odor, consistency, amount, color)

---

* A reportable disease in at least one state (Massachusetts) at time of publication.

9. Any drug allergies
10. History of abnormal Papanicolaou smear
11. Reactivation of subclinical infection with sexual activity
12. Self-infection from condyloma on any body part
13. Lifestyle: smoking, sexual practices such as anal intercourse, sex toys, exposure to utraviolet light, nutrition

IV. Physical Examination

A. External Examination
   1. Small, pink, soft papillomatous or raised "warty" lesion visualized in
      a. Periclitoral area
      b. Vestibule
      c. Posterior perineal and perianal areas
      d. Extragenital areas
   2. Confluence of many individual warts may give impression of a single, fleshy, proliferative lesion
   3. Secondary infection of lesions (from scratching)
B. Vaginal examination (speculum); observe for same lesions as above
   1. Vaginal walls
   2. Cervix (more often subclinical and no visible lesions on inspection)

V. Laboratory Examination May Include

A. Visual examination (classic appearance, as above); often visible after application of 5% acetic acid (white vinegar)
B. Gonococcal culture
C. Chlamydia smear
D. Serology test for syphilis
E. Other laboratory work as indicated by history and examination
F. Colposcopy
G. Papanicolaou test
H. DNA testing—DNA probe (Hybrid Capture II®)
I. Biopsy of cervix or unresponsive lesion on vulva for histologic examination
J. HIV testing

VI. Differential Diagnosis
Condylomata lata (associated with syphilis), molluscum contagiosum, lipomas, fibroma, adenomas, squamous cell carcinoma,
nevi, seborrheic keratoses, psoriatic plaques, carcinoma in situ,
micropapillometosis labialis, giant condyloma (Buschke-Löwen-
stein tumor), Bowenoid papulosis, malignant melanoma

VII. Treatment
A. Medical treatment
   1. Patient applied
      a. Podofilox (Condylox®) 0.5% solution or gel BID for
         3 days; no therapy 4 days; repeat prn
      b. Imiquimod (Aldara®) (an immune response modifier
         inducing cytokines), 5% cream 3 times a week h.s.
         for as long as 8-16 weeks (may weaken rubber in dia-
         phragms, condoms); needs to be washed off after 6-10
         hours
   2. Provider applied
      Apply trichloracetic (TCA) or bichloracetic (BCA) acid*
      (topical) or podophyllin resin (podophyllin), 25% usually
      in benzoin (10%) and isopropyl alcohol: allow to dry; (ap-
      ply vaseline collar with podophyllin**)
      a. No need to wash trichloracetic acid off; wash podo-
         phyllin off in 3-4 hours
      b. May burn on application
      c. Only use once a week x 8-12 weeks
      d. Intralesional interferon
      e. 5FU (Ffudex, Fluroplex) to lesions (especially for
         vulvar, perianal, penile and meatal warts)
   3. Pregnancy: Podofilox, imiquimod, podophyllin and 5-FU
      should NOT be used in pregnancy.
B. Surgical treatment
   1. Cryotherapy with liquid nitrogen or cryoprobe
   2. CO_2 laser vaporization

---

* No data on BCA efficacy are available.
**Podophyllin is now considered ineffective; its use has been discontinued
in many settings. Use should be limited to >0.5 ML or <10CM^2/session to ↓
potential systemic effects

3. Surgical excision
4. LEEP (Loop electrosurgical excision procedure)
C. General measures
   1. Sexual partner(s) should be checked if lesions are present; CDC recommends that the role of reinfection is probably minimal but partner might benefit from counseling
   2. Stress importance of personal hygiene
D. Use of condoms to help prevent further infection with partners likely to be uninfected (note precaution with imiquimod)
E. Education that even after treatment and elimination of visible warts, the potential for transmission exists

VIII. Complications

A. Lesions can become numerous and large requiring more extensive treatment
B. Literature is showing evidence of a linkage between condylomata and abnormal paps, cervical and vulvar cancer with HPV6, 11, 16, 18, 31, 33, 35, 39, 42, 43, 44, 45, 51, 52, 56, and 59, but more than 20 types have been found in cervical and other anogenital cancers
C. Laryngeal papillomatosis in infant
D. Men with HPV are at increased risk for dysplastic changes and cancers in the penile and anorectal areas

IX. Consultation/Referral

Refer to or consult with physician
A. After 8-12 treatments for evaluation
B. If warts are present on vaginal walls or cervix or rectal mucosa (see VII.C.)
C. Extensive or deep anorectal warts for proctologic examination; urethroscopy as indicated
D. If any wart is over 2 cm in size or for large cluster of warts, consider referral
E. Abnormal Pap smear (per protocol)
F. For possible biopsy in older age groups; atypical appearance of lesions, poor response to treatment in younger clients
G. Pregnant women

X. Follow-up
A.   Weekly x 8-12 weeks
B.   Client advised to check self periodically and return
      if warts recur
C.   Stress importance of q 6 month Papanicolaou smear
      in woman treated for condylomata (some settings
      repeat q 3 months x 1 year, then q 6 months x 1
      year; if normal, then yearly, and some now say
      yearly if none over 1 year are abnormal)

See Appendix U on condylomata acuminata, and
Appendix V on self-treatment with Condylox and Aldara,
information you may want to photocopy or adapt for your
clients.
See Bibliography 16.

Gonorrhea

I. Definition
Gonorrhea is a sexually transmitted bacterial infection of the
urethra, anus, and/or cervix; the causative organism can also be
cultured in the nasopharynx. As many as 80% of infected women
may be asymptomatic.

II. Etiology
A. The causative organism is Neisseria gonorrhoeae, a gram
    negative, intracellular, non-motile diplococcus. Increasingly,
    plasmid-mediated penicillinase-producing N. gonorrhoeae
    (PPNG), plasmid-mediated tetracycline resistant (TRNG),
    chromosomally mediated resistant (CMRNG) and Spectino-
    mycin-resistant strains exist. Incubation: 1-13 days.

III. History
A. What client may present with

1. Females: a large percentage (perhaps 80%) of infected women are asymptomatic in the early disease stage
    a. Early symptoms
        1) Dysuria, dyspareunia
        2) Leukorrhea; change in vaginal discharge
        3) Unilateral labial pain and swelling
        4) Lower abdominal discomfort
        5) Pharyngitis
    b. Later symptoms
        1) Purulent, irritating vaginal discharge
        2) Fever (possibly high)
        3) Rectal pain and discharge
        4) Abnormal menstrual bleeding
        5) Increased dysmenorrhea
        6) Nausea, vomiting
        7) Lesions in genital area; labia pain
        8) Joint pain and swelling
        9) Upper abdominal pain (liver involvement)
        10) Pain, tenderness in pelvic organs; urethral pain
2. Males: usually symptomatic (up to 10% asymptomatic)
    a. Early symptoms
        1) Dysuria with frequency
        2) Whitish discharge from penis
        3) Pharyngitis
    b. Later symptoms
        1) Yellow or greenish discharge from penis
        2) Epididymitis
        3) Proctitis
B. Additional information to be considered
    1. Previous vaginal infections, diagnosis and treatment
    2. Chronic illness
    3. Sexual activity; number, new sexual partner(s)
    4. History of sexually transmitted disease or pelvic inflammatory disease
    5. Known contact
    6. Last intercourse, sexual contact
    7. Method of birth control, other medications

    8. Description of discharge

a.	Onset	d.	Consistency
b.	Color	e.	Amount
c.	Odor	f.	Relationship to sexual contact

    9. Any change in menses (increased flow or dysmenorrhea)
    10. Any drug allergies
    11. HIV risk or exposure

IV. Physical Examination
A. Vital signs
    1. Blood Pressure   2. Temperature   3. Pulse
B. Abdominal examination
    1. Guarding   2. Referred pain
    3. Rebound pain   4. Upper bilateral quadrant pain
    5. Bowel sounds indicating intestinal hyperactivity
C. External examination
    1. Inspection of Skene's glands
    2. Inspection of urethra
    3. Inspection of Bartholin's glands
D. Vaginal examination (speculum)
    1. Vaginal walls: discharge, redness
    2. Cervix: mucopurulent discharge
    3. Vaginal discharge
E. Bimanual examination
    1. Pain when cervix is moved by examiner
    2. Uterine tenderness
    3. Adnexal tenderness
    4. Adnexal mass
F. Throat examination
    1. Erythema including tonsils
    2. Edema of posterior pharynx
    3. Erythema

V. Laboratory Examination
A. Gonococcus culture/Chlamydia test (Thayer-Martin still the gold standard for GC); polymerase chain reaction (PCR) and ligase chain reaction (LCR) tests useful; for rectal and throat need to culture (Thayer-Martin)

B. Serology test for syphilis

VI. Differential Diagnosis
A. Chlamydia   B. Appendicitis   C. Ectopic pregnancy

VII. Treatment
A. Medication
1. Ceftriaxone 125-250* mg IM single dose, OR Ciprofloxacin 500 mg orally single dose (not in women <18) OR Ofloxacin 400 mg orally single dose PLUS (for Chlamydia coverage)
   a. Doxycycline 100 mg orally BID x 7 days OR
   b. Doryx 100 mg orally BID x 7 days OR
   c. Azithromycin 1 gram orally in a single dose OR
   d. Ofloxacin 300 mg orally for 7 days OR
   e. Erythromycin base 500 mg orally QID x 7 days OR
   f. Erythromycin ethylsuccinate 800 mg orally QID x 7 days
2. Alternative regimens
   a. Spectinomycin 2 grams IM in a single dose OR
   b. Ceftizoxime 500 mg IM single dose OR
   c. Cefotaxime 500 mg IM single dose OR
   d. Cefotetan 1 gram IM single dose OR
   e. Cefoxitin 2 grams IM single dose with probenecid 1 gram orally OR
   f. Enoxacin 400 mg orally single dose OR
   g. Lomefloxacin 400 mg orally single dose OR
   h. Norfloxacin 800 mg orally single dose
   PLUS Chlamydia regimen
3. Pregnancy: Cephalosporins such as Ceftriaxone 125 mg IM single dose; if not tolerated use Spectinomycin 2 grams IM single dose
   PLUS Chlamydia regimen for pregnancy
   Do not use quininolones (Ciprofloxacin, Ofloxacin, Enoxacin, Lomefloxacin, Norfloxacin) or tetracyclines in pregnancy

---

*In some states Ceftriaxone 250 mg IM 1 dose is the recommended treatment

    4. Pharynx
       Ceftriaxone 125 mg IM single dose OR
       Ciprofloxacin 500 mg PO single dose OR
       Ofloxacin 400 mg PO single dose
       PLUS Chlamydia regimen
    5. For contacts: verify if partner had diagnosed infection; also try to ascertain if culture was betalactinase positive or negative, then after appropriate culture treat with same regimen as client depending on history of sensitivities

B. General measures
    1. All sexual partners should be treated if last sexual contact was within 60 days of onset of symptoms in client or diagnosis of infection. If > 60 days, treat last sexual partner
    2. No intercourse until both partners are treated, or use condoms, but abstinence is preferred
    3. Stress importance of completing medication
    4. Stress personal hygiene
    5. Stress need for follow-up culture if symptoms persist, recur, or exacerbate

VIII. Complications

A. Females
    1. Pelvic inflammatory disease
      a. Pelvic abscess or Bartholin's abscess
      b. Infertility
    2. Disseminated gonococcal infections
    3. In pregnancy: spontaneous abortion, premature rupture of membranes, premature delivery, chorioamnionitis

B. Males
    1. Proctitis
    2. Infertility due to epididymitis, prostatitis and/or seminal vesiculitis
    3. Urethral stricture
    4. Disseminated gonococcal infections

C. Newborns: ophthalmia neonatorum, sepsis, arthritis, meningitis, rhinitis, urethritis, inflammation at sites of fetal monitoring

D. Males and females
   1. Meningitis
   2. Endocarditis
   3. Gonococcal conjunctivitis

IX. Consultation/Referral
A. If no response to treatment as discussed above
B. If complications develop

X. Follow-up
A. Test of cure not recommended by CDC unless symptoms recur, exacerbate, or do not resolve
B. Serology test for syphilis in 30 days
C. Chlamydia test if not done at initial visit prior to treatment
D. Consider HIV and hepatitis B and C screening

Appendix W has information about gonorrhea that you can photocopy or adapt for your clients.
See Bibliography 14.

Syphilis

I. Definition
Syphilis is a sexually transmitted systemic disease characterized by periods of active florid manifestations and periods of symptomless latency. It can affect any tissue or vascular organ of the body and can be passed on from mother to fetus.

II. Etiology
A. The causative organism is a motile spirochete, Treponema pallidum (T. pallidum)
B. Incubation period, 10-90 days; average 21 days

III. History
A. What the client may present with
   1. Primary symptoms
      a. Painless lesion (chancre) at site of entry of T. palli-

dum including vulva, labia, fourchette, clitoris, cervix, nipple, lip, roof of mouth, tonsils, bite area, finger, urethra, rectum, and smooth, firm borders of ulcer
   b. Enlarged inguinal or regional nodes; trochlear
2. Secondary symptoms that may or may not occur 2-8 weeks or as long as 6 months after initial infection (can also overlap)
   a. Generalized symmetrical papillo-squamous eruption of palms, soles or mucous membrane (condylomata lata)
   b. Alopecia; may have "moth eaten look"
   c. Loss of lateral 1/3 of eyebrow
   d. Generalized non-tender lymphadenopathy
   e. Symptoms of upper respiratory tract infection
   f. Low grade fever
   g. Malaise, anorexia, and arthralgia
   h. Mild hepatitis, splenomegaly or nephrotic syndrome in about 10% of cases
   i. Mucus patches on tongue, under foreskin
3. Latent stage
   No clinical symptoms although 25% may have recurrence of cutaneous lesion
   a. Early latency (infectious): infection within the preceding year
   b. Late latency (non-infectious): over a year from date of initial infection. Patient may remain in latent stage for remainder of his/her life; however, 1/3 will develop the tertiary form of disease
   c. Tertiary stage
      Osseous or cutaneous structures, cardiovascular system or nervous system become involved; most common developments are cardiovascular syphilis and neurosyphilis
   d. Neurosyphilis can occur at any stage from 1-30 or more years after original infection
B. Additional information to be considered
   1. Sexual preference
   2. Current sexual activity

3. Last sexual contact
4. Birth control method
5. History of known contacts
6. History of previous sexually transmitted disease
7. History of recurrent infectious illness
8. History of recurrent fever, malaise, arthralgia, or rash of unknown etiology
9. History of recurrent infectious illness (e.g., mononucleosis)
10. Current medical therapy
11. Risk for HIV exposure

IV. Physical Examination
A. Vital signs
1. Temperature   2. Blood pressure   3. Pulse
B. General examination of skin
1. Alopecia
2. Rash including soles of feet, palms, condyloma lata
C. Pharyngeal examination
D. Examine for enlarged inguinal nodes
E. External examination of genitalia
Vulvar lesions; chancre at point of inoculation
F. Internal examination (speculum)
1. Inspection of vaginal walls for lesions
2. Inspection of cervix for lesions
3. Inspection of discharge
G. Bimanual examination

V. Laboratory Examination
A. Nontreponemal: venereal disease research laboratory (VDRL) and rapid plasma reagin (RPR) (these are nonspecific serum tests) reported as titres
1. Biological false positives occur with cardiolipin antigens sometimes present in drug abuse and in such diseases and conditions as
a. Lupus erythematosus
b. Mononucleosis
c. Malaria

      d. Leprosy
      e. Viral pneumonia
      f. After smallpox vaccinations or other recent vaccinations
      g. Persons with HIV
      h. Narcotic addiction
      i. Arthritis
      j. Sclerederma
      k. Tuberculosis
      l. Chronic fatigue syndrome
      m. Pregnancy

B. Specific serum treponemal antibody tests (correlate poorly with disease activity; persons who have a reactive test will have it for life unless diagnosis and treatment are very early)
    1. Fluorescent Treponemal Antibody-Absorption Test (FTA-ABS)
    2. Microhemagglutination Assay for T. Pallidum (MHA-TP)
    3. TPHA (Treponema pallidum hemagglutination)

C. Gonococcus culture
D. Chlamydia test
E. Biopsy of the lesion
F. Darkfield microscopy exam (rarely available in free-standing clinics or offices)—most useful for males
G. Consider HIV testing; testing for Hepatitis B, C

VI. Differential Diagnosis

A. Herpes simplex   C. Chancroid
B. Condylomata acuminata   E. Lymphogranuloma venereum
C. Granuloma inguinale

VII. Treatment (with physician consult in some settings)

A. Medication (for primary and secondary syphilis
    1. Benzathine-penicillin G (BiCillin®) 2.4 million units IM stat.* CAUTION RE: Jarisch-Herxheimer Reaction: in

---

*In some states the protocol is two doses of benzathin-penicillin 2.4 million units 1 week apart.

50% of cases, 6-12 hours after injection, patient develops high fever, malaise, and exacerbation of symptoms lasting 24 hours. (This is a sign that the spirochete is breaking down)
2. For penicillin allergy: Doxycycline 100 mg orally BID x 28 days *OR* Tetracycline 500 mg orally QID x 14 days
B. For early latent syphilis (<1 year)
1. Benzathine penicillin G, 2.4 million units IM single dose
C. For late latent syphilis or unknown duration
1. Benzathine penicillin G, 7.2 million units total, in 3 doses of 2.4 million units IM each at 7-day intervals
D. For later syphilis or unknown duration
1. Benzathine penicillin G, 7.2 million units total, in 3 doses of 2.4 million units IM each at 7-day intervals
E. In pregnancy
1. Treat with penicillin regimen appropriate for stage of syphilis
2. Desensitize and treat with penicillin for allergy
F. General measures
1. Support, especially in regard to possible Jarisch-Herxheimer Reaction
2. Stress importance of completing all medication
3. Partner should be treated concurrently; all contacts within past 6 months should be interviewed

VIII. Complications
A. Progression of disease to tertiary stage
B. 100% transmission to fetus with primary and secondary in pregnancy; 50% fetal mortality. Early latent: 80% fetal infection (20% premature, 20% fetal death, 40% carriers). Late latent: 40% fetal transmission, 10% fetal death.

IX. Consultation/Referral
Positive diagnosis of disease

X. Follow-up
Serology tests for primary and secondary syphilis (nontreponemal serologic) should be obtained at 3 and 6 months (falling titer

should be demonstrated if treatment is adequate (4-fold drop by 6 months using same test). For latent syphilis, repeat testing at 6, 12, and 24 months.

See Appendix MM and Bibliography 16.

Chancroid

I. Definition
Chancroid is a bacterial infection of the genitourinary tract in which a rapidly growing ulcerated lesion forms on external genitalia. Definitive diagnosis requires the identification of H. ducreyi using special culture media. Even with the use of these media, sensitivity is ≤ 80%. Diagnosis is usually based on clinical findings.

II. Etiology
A. Causative agent is Haemophilus ducreyi, a short gram negative bacillus with rounded ends, usually found in chains and groups
B. Incubation period, 4-7 days after exposure (rare <3 or >10 days)

III. History
A. What client may present with
   1. History of a painful macule on the external genitalia which rapidly changed to a pustule and then to an ulcerated lesion; may have "kissing ulcers" from autoinoculation; can also be painless
   2. Enlarged inguinal nodes
   3. Abscess in inguinal region
   4. A sinus formed over the healed lesion
   5. New lesions forming when exposed to lesions already present
   6. Pain on voiding or defecating
   7. Rectal bleeding
   8. Dyspareunia

B. Additional information to be obtained
1. History of sexually transmitted disease or pelvic inflammatory disease
2. Previous vaginal infections; diagnosis, treatment
3. Previous urinary tract infections
4. Sexually active
5. Last sexual contact; new partner
6. Did partner complain of "sores"
7. Last menstrual period
8. Method of birth control; other medications (antibiotics may mask symptoms)
9. Any associated vaginal discharge
10. Any associated pain
11. Travel to Asia (Thailand especially), Africa, South America, Philippines in past month

IV. Physical Examination
A. Vital signs
  1. Temperature   2. Blood pressure   3. Pulse
B. Inguinal nodes
1. Size
2. Tenderness
3. Nodes matted together forming a fluctuant abscess (buboes) in groin; usually unilateral inguinal lymphadenopathy
C. External examination
1. Observe labia, fourchette, clitoris, vagina, anal area for macules, papules
2. Observe for shallow, non-indurated, painful ulcers with ragged, undetermined edges, varying in size and often coalesced; base of ulcers may be gray/bluish gray
3. Observe for sinuses which may have formed when skin over abscesses has broken down
4. Look for new lesions which may be forming as a result of autoinoculation
D. Vaginal examination (speculum); observe for lesions in vagina, on cervix
E. Bimanual examination

V. Laboratory Examination
A. Usually based on clinical findings and history
B. Cultures to laboratory; use media containing fresh defibrinated rabbit's blood or patient's own serum
C. Darkfield exam for T. pallidum or serologic test for syphilis performed at least 7 days after onset of lesions and repeated in 3 months
D. Gonococcus culture, Chlamydia test
E. Herpes culture
F. HIV testing should be done at the time of this diagnosis and again in 3 months if initial results are negative
G. Further laboratory work as indicated
H. PCR testing for H. ducreyi when it becomes available

VI. Differential Diagnosis
A. Herpes simplex
B. Syphilis
C. Lymphogranuloma venereum
D. Granuloma inguinale

VII. Treatment
A. Medications
   1. Azithromycin 1 gram orally single dose *OR*
   2. Ceftriaxone 250 mg IM single dose *OR*
   3. Ciprofloxacin 500 mg orally twice a day for 3 days (safety in children <15 years of age or in pregnancy has not been established) *OR*
   4. Erythromycin base 500 mg orally QID x 7 days
B. Medications in Pregnancy
   1. Ceftriaxone 250 mg IM single dose *OR*
   2. Erythromycin base 500 mg orally QID for 7 days
C. General measures
   1. Buboes should be aspirated through adjacent intact skin, not incised
   2. No sexual contact until course of medication is finished
   3. Stress importance of completing course of medication
   4. All sexual contacts should be examined and observed for 3 months with regular checks for sexually transmitted disease
   5. Comfort measures

    a. Tepid water sitz baths; dry carefully with cool air hair dryer making sure to hold it away from body
    b. Avoid tight, restricting clothing
    c. Expose perineum to air flow as much as possible (wear a skirt without underpants when at home)
    d. Recommend peri-irrigation set for comfort
  6. Patient education
    a. Explain disease process and route of transmission
    b. Stress that sexual partner(s) need to be checked regularly (see X.C.)

VIII. Complications
A. Phimosis in the male   D. Severe tissue destruction
B. Urethral stricture   E. Ulcers may take years to heal
C. Urethral fistula   F. Perineal fistulas

IX. Consultation/Referral
A. Physician if infection is suspected
B. If no response after 7 days of treatment, treatment as outlined above
C. Secondary infections
D. All HIV positive persons diagnosed with chancroid

X. Follow-up
A. Patient should be re-examined 3-7 days after initiation of therapy. If treatment is successful, there should be symptomatic improvement within 3 days of starting therapy. Clinical improvement should be evident within 7 days. If no improvement, consultation as above
B. It should be noted that it may take $\geq$ 2 weeks for complete healing of ulcers. The amount of time is related to the size of the ulcer
C. All sexual partners who have had sexual contact within 10 days preceding symptoms with a person diagnosed with chancroid should be evaluated and treated even in the absence of symptoms

See Bibliography 14.

Lymphogranuloma Venereum

I. Definition
Lymphogranuloma venereum is a sexually transmitted disease characterized by a transitory primary lesion followed by suppurative lymphangitis and serious local complications.

II. Etiology
A. Causative agent: Chlamydia trachomatis, serotypes, L1, L2, L3
B. Incubation period 3 days-3 weeks
C. Found mainly in tropical or subtropical climates (Asia, Africa, South America); rare in USA

III. History
A. What the client may present with
   1. "Sore" in genital area, mouth, anus, penis (of short duration, may go unnoticed); usually painless vesicle or nonindurated
   2. Fever
   3. Malaise
   4. Headaches
   5. Joint pain
   6. Anorexia
   7. Vomiting
   8. Unilateral tender enlargement of inguinal lymph node; stiffness, aching of groin
   9. Abscess in groin after 2-3 weeks
   10. Sinuses, scars in lower vagina or around introitus or (in males) on penis
   11. Rectal discharge; perirectal/perianal fistulas and strictures
   12. Vaginal discharge
B. Additional information to be considered
   1. Sexual preference; sexual practices
   2. Last sexual contact; new partner
   3. Known contact
   4. History of sexually transmitted disease or pelvic inflam-

matory disease
5. Last menstrual period
6. Method of birth control; other medications (antibiotics may mask symptoms)
7. History of chronic infections
8. Recent trip out of country or new immigrant from a country where LGV is common

IV. Physical Examination
A. Vital signs
   1. Blood pressure   2. Pulse
   3. Respiration   4. Temperature
B. Inguinal nodes
   1. First symptoms unilateral tender enlargement of nodes
   2. Disease progresses for 2-3 weeks to form a large, tender, fluctuant mass that adheres to deep tissues and has overlying reddened skin (bubo)
   3. Multiple sinuses develop with purulent or serosanguineous discharge
   4. Healing occurs with scar formation, but sinuses persist or recur
   5. Chronic inflammation causes blockage of the lymphatic vessels leading to edema, ulceration and fistula formation
C. Vaginal examination (speculum)
   1. Vaginal walls: initial lesion may be on upper vaginal wall, resulting in enlargement and suppuration of perirectal and pelvic lymphatic vessels
   2. Cervix: initial lesion could be on the cervix
D. Bimanual examination
   Tenderness in groin, vulva
E. Rectovaginal examination
   Rectal wall may be involved, resulting in ulcerative proctitis with serosanguineous rectal discharge

V. Laboratory Examination and Diagnosis
A. LGV complement fixation test: fourfold rise or single titer of≥1:64; (80% of patients have titer 1:16 or higher)
B. Serology test for syphilis, gonorrhea culture, Chlamydia test

C. Biopsy of chronic anorectal lesions to rule out carcinoma
D. Microimmunofluorescence test (microl F) measures specific antibody and distinguishes various serotypes of antibody (use if titer ≥1:512
E. In absence of microimmunofluorescence test, diagnosis may be made by careful history, clinical examination, and presence of high or rising titers of LGV complement fixation antibodies

VI. Differential Diagnosis
A. Syphilis
B. Herpes simplex
C. Carcinoma
D. Chancroid
E. Granuloma inguinale
F. Chlamydia

VII. Treatment
A. Medications
    1.   Doxycycline 100 mg orally BID x 21 days **OR**
    2.   Erythromycin base 500 mg orally QID for 21 days
B. Medications in pregnancy
    1.   Erythromycin base 500 mg orally QID for 21 days
C. General measures
    1.   Sitz bath
    2.   Stress importance of completing the course of medication
    3.   All sexual partners should be treated if contact within 30 days before onset of symptoms; examine and test for Chlamydia/gonorrhea in urethra, cervix
    4.   Comfort measures
        a. Tepid water sitz baths; dry carefully with cool air hair dryer making sure to hold it sufficiently away from body
        b. Avoid tight, restricting clothing
        c. Expose perineum to air flow as much as possible (wear a skirt or robe without underpants at home)
        d. Recommend peri-irrigation set
    5.   Patient education
        a. Explain disease process and route of transmission

    b. Stress importance of sexual partner(s) being checked regularly (see X.D.)

VIII. Complications
A. Scar formation
B. Sinuses causing blockage of the lymphatic vessels which lead to edema
C. Fistula formation: rectovaginal, vulvar, other
D. Suppuration of perirectal and lymphatic vessels
E. Rectal stricture
F. Systemic: phlebitis, hepatomegaly, nephropathy

IX. Consultation/Referral
A. With physician prior to treatment if infection is suspected
B. If no response to treatment as outlined above
C. If any of the above complications occur

X. Follow-up
A. Reevaluate 3-5 days after treatment
B. Then evaluate every 1-2 weeks until healing is complete
C. All patients should be followed for 6 months after successful treatment

    See Bibliography 14.

Granuloma Inguinale

I. Definition
Granuloma inguinale (Donovanosis) is a chronic granulomatous bacterial infection usually involving the genitalia and surrounding tissues, and probably spread by sexual contact.

II. Etiology
A. Usually found in tropical and subtropical areas
B. Calymmato bacterium granulomatis (a difficult-to-grow encapsulated bacillus organism)
C. Incubation period, 5-6 weeks (some sources say 8-12 weeks)

III. History
A. What the client presents with
1. Female
   a. Painless papular or nodular ulcerative lesions arising on the vulva, in the vagina, urethra, anal area, inguinal region or on the perineum with proliferation of granulation tissue and local destruction with scar tissue formation
   b. Beefy red proliferative lesion of fourchette; bleeds easily
   c. Inguinal adenopathy (due to secondary infection)—bilateral
   d. Malodorous vaginal discharge
2. Male
   a. Lesion same as in the female and appearing on penis, scrotum, groin or thighs
   b. In homosexual males, lesions on anus and buttocks
B. Additional information to be obtained
1. History of sexually transmitted disease or pelvic inflammatory disease
2. History of chronic illness
3. Has client recently been out of country? Where? (Especially India, Papua New Guinea, central Australia, southern Africa.) Is client or client's partner from, or have they visited, southeastern U.S.?
4. Sexual preference; sexual practices (anal intercourse; sex toys)
5. Last sexual contact
6. Birth control method, current medications
7. Last menstrual period

IV. Physical Examination
A. Vital signs
1. Temperature   2. Blood pressure
3. Pulse   4. Respirations
B. External examination
   Observe vulva for lesions (papular, nodular, or vesicular), beefy red nodules which develop into a rounded, elevated,

velvety granulomatous mass; sharply defined borders; signs of secondary infection
C. Vaginal examination (speculum)
 1. Inspect vaginal walls for lesions
 2. Inspect cervix for lesions
D. Bimanual examination

V. Laboratory Diagnosis
A. Giemsa-stained smears of ulcer (diagnosis is confirmed by identifying Donovan bodies, large mononuclear cells with intracytoplasmic vacuoles containing the organism)—scrape at base of ulcer to get some fluid
B. Syphilis serology
C. HSV culture

VI. Differential Diagnosis
A. Syphilis1   C. Lymphogranuloma venereum
B. Herpes simplex   D. Chancroid

VII. Treatment
A. Medication
 1. Trimethoprim-sulfamethoxazole one double-strength tablet orally BID for a minimum of 3 weeks *OR*
 2. Doxycycline 100 mg orally BID for minimum of 3 weeks
B. Alternative regimes
 1. Ciprofloxacin 750 mg BID for a minimum of 3 weeks *OR*
 2. Erythromycin base 500 mg orally BID for minimum of 3 weeks
C. In pregnancy
 1. Erythromycin base 500 mg orally BID for minimum of 3 weeks plus strongly consider gentamicin parenterally (or other parenteral aminoglycoside)
D. Additional therapy for all adults
 1. Gentamicin 1 mg/kg IV every 8 hours if lesions do not respond within first few days of therapy (or other parenteral aminoglycoside)
E. General measures
 1. No sexual contact until treatment is completed

2. Stress importance of completing course of medication
3. Stress importance of examination of sexual contacts (within 60 days preceding onset of symptoms)

VIII. Complications
A. Scar tissue secondary to slow healing formation
B. Secondary infection, a common occurrence that results in gross tissue necrosis of genitalia
C. Deformity of genitalia
D. Dyspareunia
E. Systemic infection
F. Massive edema of vulva; penis (may be chronic)

IX. Consultation/Referral
A. With physician prior to treatment if disease is suspected
B. No response to treatment as discussed above in 7 days—contact CDC or state health department

X. Follow-up
A. After completion of 2 to 5 days of medication
B. Recheck every 2 weeks until healed
C. Check-up in 6 months and regularly thereafter; there is a possibility of scar carcinoma

See Bibliography 14.

Molluscum Contagiosum

Molluscum contagiosum is an infectious disease of the skin affecting the face, arms, genitals, abdomen, and thighs. It is caused by a virus (pox virus) and is seen in all age groups and in both sexes.

II. Etiology
A. Unknown
B. Probably transmitted through direct skin contact
C. Incubation 1 week-6 months (usual 14-40 days)

III. History
A. What the client may present with
1. Fleshy growths (1-20), primarily in genital area, but may be found on other body surfaces; may be 2-5 mm in diameter (but up to 15 mm), may be pedunculated
2. No other symptoms or complaints but occasional pruritus, tenderness and/or pain
B. Additional information to be considered
1. Previous episode of similar lesions
2. History of sexually transmitted disease
3. Sexual activity, last intercourse
4. Known contact
5. Method of birth control; other medications
6. Any drug allergies
7. HIV risk/exposure, especially with widespread lesions=to or >100

IV. Physical Examination
A. External examination
1. Observe perineum for fleshy, usually papular, skin-colored lesions with indented centers that contain white, curd-like material
2. Observe any other involved body area

V. Laboratory Examination
A. Visual examination
B. Pathology report on crushed excised lesion using Papanicolaou smear, Wright's, Giemsa's, or Gram's stain
C. Serology test for syphilis
D. Gonococcus culture/Chlamydia test
E. Further laboratory work as indicated by history
F. Consider HIV screen especially with 100 or more lesions

VI. Differential Diagnosis
A. Genital warts (condylomata acuminata)
B. Herpes simplex
C. Pyogenic granuloma
D. Folliculitis

VII. Treatment
A. Removal of lesion
   1. Cytotoxic agents—TCA (trichloracetic acid), BCA (bichloracetic acid), podophyllin
   2. Excision of lesions by curettage with cryanesthesia followed by application of silver nitrate
   3. Destruction of lesions by cryotherapy (MD consult)
B. General measures
   1. Return for weekly or biweekly evaluation and treatment until lesions have healed
   2. Avoid sex or use condom until partner(s) are cured and to prevent further infections
   3. Refer sexual partner(s) for evaluation

VIII. Complications
A. Secondary staphylococcus infection

IX. Consultation/Referral
A. For treatment stated above
B. Patients with extensive molluscum, lesions on face, or repeated recurrence after treatment should be reevaluated for HIV infection

X. Follow-up
A. Return for reevaluation if lesions persist/recur after treatment

See Bibliography 14.

Hepatitis

I. Definition
Hepatitis is an acute or chronic inflammation of the liver with or without permanent tissue damage and can be caused by many viruses including influenza viruses, mononucleosis and CMV; there are also hepatitis viruses whose only target is the liver. At least 6 are known at present and are designated by the letters A, B, C, D, E and G.

II. Etiology

Causative organisms include hepatitis viruses A to E and G, mononucleosis virus, CMV, and various influenza viruses

A. Hepatitis A (HAV) is transmitted enterically (rarely parenterally) with an incubation of 15-60 days, 28 day average
B. Hepatitis B (HBV) is transmitted parenterally, sexually via body fluids, perinatally, or from saliva from human bites; incubation 45-150 days, 120 day average
C. Hepatitis C (HCV) is transmitted parenterally only, with an incubation of 2-52 weeks; major cause of post-transfusion hepatitis. It is thought that sexual and perinatal transmission may be possible
D. Hepatitis D (HDV), known as Delta virus, only affects persons who have hepatitis B already; transmitted parenterally and sexually. Incubation 3-13 weeks.
E. Hepatitis E (HEV) is transmitted enterically (rarely parenterally) with 3-9 weeks incubation
F. Hepatitis G. Percutaneous route

III. History

A. What the client may present with
    1. Right upper quadrant pain (may be intermittent)
    2. Loss of appetite
    3. Malaise, fatigue (increased sleep, ↓ activity level, ↓ libido)
    4. Fever, often low grade
    5. Flu-like symptoms, including headache
    6. Adenopathy
    7. Jaundice
    8. Nausea and vomiting
    9. Rash, hives
    10. Joint pain
    11. Darkened urine
    12. Light-colored stools
    13. Taste and smell peculiarities
    14. Intolerance of fatty foods, cigarettes
B. Additional information to consider
    1. Use of recreational drugs

2. Alcohol use, quantity and frequency
3. Medication use (including nontraditional remedies, herbal preparations
4. Partner an injectable drug user
5. Recent transfusion of blood or blood products
6. Recent surgery
7. Eating raw or undercooked shellfish
8. Daycare worker or has child/children in day care
9. Occupational risks including exposure to body fluids, excrement; blood, blood products
10. Sexual history and habits, especially anal intercourse; number of partners; use of sex toys
11. History of sexually transmitted diseases
12. Sexual partner and/or household member with symptoms
13. Known exposure to someone with hepatitis
14. Military or civilian service in the Middle East
15. History of hepatitis B
16. Visited or from disease-endemic areas of world
17. Hemodialysis patient; transplant recipient
18. Inmate of correctional institution
19. Contraceptive history
20. History of needlestick injury, tattoos, body piercing
21. Infants of HBV + mothers

IV. Physical Examination
A. Vital signs
    1. Temperature   2. Pulse
    3. Respirations   4. Blood pressure
B. Abdomen
    1. Liver percussion, palpation
    2. Observation of skin color, turgor
    3. Organomegaly, tenderness
    4. Masses
    5. Adenopathy
C. Complete physical examination with careful attention to
    1. Skin: rash, hives, color, turgor
    2. Joints: joint pain on range of motion
    3. Adenopathy

V. Laboratory Examination
A. Feces for virus
B. Liver function tests
C. Mononucleosis screen
D. Serology to determine type of hepatitis

HAV: IgM anti-HAV in serum with acute or convalescent phase

HBV: several including HBsAg (HBV surface antigen); IgM Anti-HBc

HCV: test for antibody with ELISA followed by the RIBA (recombinant immunoblot assay); for ambiguous results PCR assay is used

HDV: HBsAg, Anti-HDV

HEV: no commercial tests; diagnosis by history and negative testing for HAV, HBV, HCV; testing available through CDC.

HGV: PCR testing

E. CMV
F. HIV testing
G. In severe hepatitis, serum albumin, prothrombin, and partial thromboplastin times, electrolytes, glucose, CBC, platelets

VI. Differential Diagnosis
Infectious mononucleosis, primary or secondary hepatic malignancy, ischemic hepatitis, drug-induced hepatitis, alcoholic hepatitis, acute fatty liver (acute fatty metamorphosis) of pregnancy

VII. Treatment
A. As needed according to laboratory report and etiology; generally referral for medical management and follow-up
B. Supportive for symptoms
   1. No alcohol during acute phase of hepatitis and for 6-12 months thereafter
   2. Adequate calories; balanced diet
C. Interferon is being used for HBV, HCV*

---

*Research on Hepatitis C with combination treatment Rebetron®, Rebetrol® (ribavirin) and Introl® (interferton alfa-26, recombinant)

D. Gamma globulin to household and daycare center contacts for hepatitis A within 2 weeks of exposure
E. Prevention for hepatitis B: for exposed persons HBV hyperimmune globulin and then hepatitis B vaccination after antibody testing
F. Prevention for hepatitis D: hepatitis B vaccination
G. HAV recovery not aided by activity limitation; isolate food handlers with HAV; prevention for HAV HAVRIX® or VAQTA® vaccine

VIII. Complications
A. Hepatitis A: rarely fatal, no chronic form
B. Hepatitis B: death; chronic disease in 5-10% of victims; of these, 50% get chronic liver disease leading to hepatocellular carcinoma in half of the cases; transmission to fetus likely
C. Hepatitis C: >50% of cases become chronic; cirrhosis; hepatocellular carcinoma
D. Hepatitis D: death, chronic disease; cirrhosis (70%)
E. Hepatitis E: high mortality in pregnancy (fetus and mother); no reported chronic cases
F. Hepatitis G: little information to date

IX. Consultation/Referral
A. For medical treatment and follow-up

X. Follow-up
A. As appropriate for type of hepatitis
B. Encourage hepatitis B vaccination (HBV) of those who have not had disease; schedule 3 dose administration; okay in pregnancy and lactation
C. Repeat laboratory work as indicated for monitoring liver function after illness
D. Test for chronic HBV with serum assay for HBsAg
E. Encourage HAV vaccination for persons at increased risk*

See Bibliography 14; http://www.cdc.gov

---

*One state now requires HAV vaccination for school children.

HIV/AIDS

PREFACE: Information on AIDS/HIV continues to increase and change. Since our role as practitioners in ambulatory settings is to identify, educate, and refer persons at high risk for the disease, the purpose of this protocol is to serve as a guide in those three areas only. Because AIDS has become the leading cause of death among young women, it has become increasingly important that women's health care providers keep abreast of current information by consulting professional journals and attending seminars on the subject.

I.   Definition
AIDS is the commonly used acronym for acquired immune deficiency syndrome, which is the name for a complex of health problems first reported in 1981.

II. Etiology
Caused by the human immune deficiency virus (HIV); infection mainly by sexual contact (anal, vaginal, oral), contaminated blood and blood products including needle and syringe sharing, contaminated semen used for artificial insemination, intrauterine acquisition (baby of woman with AIDS) and rarely breast milk.

III. History
A.   What the client may present with
1.   Rapid weight loss without known factor (>10%)
2.   Extreme fatigue; unexplained, increasing tiredness
3.   Chronic diarrhea (>1 month)
4.   Persistent dry cough, shortness of breath, dyspnea on exertion
5.   Prolonged fever, soaking night sweats, shaking chills
6.   Loss of appetite
7.   Purple or pink flat or raised lesions on skin or under skin, inside mouth, nose, eyelids, anus

8. Changes in neurological and/or cognitive function
9. Generalized adenopathy
10. Chronic herpes simplex
11. Recurrent herpes zoster
12. Generalized dermatitis pruritic
13. Oral and pharyngeal candidiasis; fungal infection of nails
14. Persistent muscle pain
15. Fear of exposure to AIDS through sexual partner or high-risk behavior or work-related accident (needle-stick, contact with infected blood)
16. Chronic sinusitis
17. History of abnormal Papanicolaou smears
18. Persistent vulvar, vaginal and anal condyloma

B. Additional information to be considered
1. Sexual history
   a. Homosexual encounters
   b. Use of condoms, other methods of contraception, anal intercourse as contraception
   c. High-risk partners
   d. High-risk sexual practices
   e. History of previous sexually transmitted disease
   f. Contact with prostitute
   g. Multiple partners or partner with multiple partners
2. Use of intravenous drugs by self or partner
3. High-risk occupation
4. History of blood transfusions or recipient of blood products
5. Duration and frequency of any presenting symptoms
6. Reason for fear of exposure to AIDS
7. Gynecological history
   a. Recurrent sexually transmitted diseases, vaginitis, vaginosis
   b. Widespread molluscum contagiosum =>100 lesions
   c. Infected with several sexually transmitted diseases

concurrently (may include gonorrhea, syphilis, Chlamydia)
d. Rapidly progressing cervical dysplasia
e. Papillomavirus on Papanicolaou smear
f. Recurrent, recalcitrant vaginal candidiasis
g. External condyloma unresponsive to treatment
h. Existing pregnancy
i. Anal discharge
j. Pelvic, abdominal pain

IV. Physical Examination
A. As appropriate to presenting complaint

V. Laboratory Examination
A. Per protocol for presenting complaint and symptoms
B. HIV testing if indicated or requested; if setting offers testing, resources must be in place for both pre-test and post-test counseling for positive or negative results and follow-up
C. All pregnant women should have HIV screen and encourage one for women planning a pregnancy
D. Work place exposures
E. Information on home test for HIV; follow-up counseling if test is positive

VI. Differential Diagnosis
A. Widely different depending on presenting complaint

VII. Treatment
A. General measures
  1. Counseling to avoid or minimize high-risk behaviors
    a. Instruction and counseling regarding safer sexual practices to protect self and partner from exchange of body fluids (e.g., by using latex condoms, female condoms, dental dams and/or spermicide (Nonoxynol-9); by avoiding anal intercourse and oral-genital contact; avoiding sharing sex toys such as vibrators

and dildos (or clean them with bleach or alcohol)
  b. Decreased number of sexual partners; mutual monogamy; abstinence
  c. Discourage use of injectable drugs; if client is using injectable drugs, stress the need to avoid needle, works, or cooker sharing; offer resources on drug rehabilitation programs
  d. Avoid unsafe sexual contact with persons who are injectable drug users or fall into other high-risk groups
  e. Sexual activities with partner with AIDS that do not involve direct passage of body fluids, such as light kissing, caressing, mutual masturbation
  f. Empowering women to maintain equal decision-making power in their relationship(s)
B. Specific treatment
  1. Per protocol for specific presenting complaint
  2. Refer those clients falling into high-risk groups for further counseling and appropriate testing and follow-up if setting does not offer such services
  3. Referral for exposure so prophylactic therapy can be instituted

VIII. Complications
A. Opportunistic infections
B. AIDS may be fatal to some of its victims within two years of diagnosis
C. Transmission to unborn child (infant's true HIV status will not be accurate until 15-18 months)

IX. Consultations and Referral
A. All clients falling into high-risk groups in need of testing for presence of HIV virus unless setting offers testing and counseling
B. Referral for all patients testing positive to HIV antibody for appropriate treatment

X. Follow-up

A. Per referral

B. Contraceptive and gynecological services for women with AIDS

See Appendix DD for self-assessment of AIDS (HIV) risk list which can be photocopied or adapted for your clients.
See bibliography 15.

Safe Practices for Practitioners*

1. Dispose of all needles, scalpels, capillary tubes, glass slides, lancets, and other sharp items in puncture-resistant containers. Handle as little as possible (i.e., do not recap needles).

2. Wear gloves** when anticipating exposure to body fluids, including for phlebotomy and for handling specimens (urine, blood, stool, sputum, vaginal secretions), and for contact with any mucus membranes (vaginal, oral, nasal, rectal) and open wounds. Don't substitute gloves for handwashing, however.

3. Wear gloves, gowns, masks, goggles as appropriate when there is to be extensive contact with body fluids as during surgery or delivery; wear double gloves for surgical procedures when possible. Change any blood-stained clothing as soon as

---

*Adapted from Bennett, B. & Duff, P. (1991). The effect of double gloving on frequency of glove perforations. *Obstetrics & Gynecology, 78,* 1019-1022; Gritter, M. (1998). The latex threat. *American Journal of Nursing, 98,* 26-32; Nenstiel, R.O., White, G.L. & Aikens, T. (1997). Handwashing: A century of evidence ignored. *Clinical Reviews, 7(1),* 55-62; Yeargin, P. (1998). An important risk group: Managing occupational HIV exposure. *ADVANCE for Nurse Practitioners, 6(11),* 55-93; Youngkin, E.Q. (1988). Keeping pelvic examination technique safe. The Nurse Practitioner, 13(1), 40-42. See also bibliography 15.

**Latex gloves are the best protection. However, be aware of the possibility of latex allergy. Symptoms can be mild to severe and are typical of anaphylactic reactions: watery eyes, itching rash, shortness of breath, decrease in blood pressure, and even death. Latex-free gloves are available. One can also wear vinyl gloves under latex gloves, or wear nylon or cloth glove liners.

possible.

4.   Wash thoroughly (with copious amounts of soap and water) following any skin contact with patient's body fluids.

5.   Wear gloves on both hands for vaginal and rectal exams; use careful technique to keep one hand clean when handling clean materials such as fixative spray for Pap smears or examination lights; wash after examination is completed. Goggles are now recommended for vaginal examinations and phlebotomy in ambulatory as well as inpatient settings.

6.   Change gloves for rectal examination after vaginal examination or for fitting a diaphragm or cervical cap after pelvic examination.

7.   Avoid contamination of surfaces in the examining room or laboratory with body fluids from clients.

8.   Use chlorine bleach solution 1:10* in a spray bottle to clean examining table and other surfaces and items contaminated with body fluids. Several other commercial products are available for this use. Wear gloves for clean-up.

9.   Keep hands from becoming dry and cracked.

10.   Follow Centers for Disease Control (CDC) and OSHA recommendations and updates for protection of self and clients. (CDC http://www.cdc.gov;   OSHA http://www.osha.gov)

11.   Assume every client has the potential to be infected with AIDS or to be HIV positive and protect him/her and yourself with good technique.

12.   Educate staff and clients about modes of infection, protection, and address myths to dispel unwarranted fears.

See Bibliography 15.

---

* Due to instability with exposure to oxygen, this must be prepared daily. Commercial products are also available in single-use packets. These maintain chemical stability.

Miscellaneous Gynecological Aberrations

Bartholin's Cyst

I. Definition
Bartholin's cyst is a post-inflammatory pseudocyst that forms proximally to the obstructed duct of a Bartholin's gland

II. Etiology
A. Gonococcus is the most common cause of cases of abscess
B. Other responsible organisms include
    1. Staphylococcus aureus
    2. Streptococcus fecalis
    3. Escherichia coli (E. coli)
    4. Pseudomonas may also be cultured from abscess

III. History
A. What the client may present with
    1. Painful, swollen lump in vaginal area
    2. Difficulty sitting and walking due to severe pain and swelling
B. Additional information to be considered
    1. Previous infection of a Bartholin's gland; if yes, how was it treated?
    2. History of sexually transmitted disease

IV. Physical Examination
A. Vital signs
    1. Temperature   2. Blood pressure
B. Visual examination of external genitalia
    1. Cyst is characteristically located in the lower half of the labia with its inner wall immediately adjacent to the lower vaginal canal

2. Lesions may vary in size from 1-10 cm
3. The involved area may be painfully tender
4. There may be no subjective symptoms

V. Laboratory Examination
A. Culture lesion at time of incision and drainage
B. Consider cervical cultures for Chlamydia and gonorrhea

VI. Differential Diagnosis
A. Lipoma
B. Fibroma
C. Hydrocele
D. Carcinoma of Bartholin's gland (extremely rare)
E. Inclusion cysts, sebaceous cysts
F. Congenital anomaly

VII. Treatment
A. Sitz baths QID x 2-3 days, then reexamine. If size has increased or there is no change, perform incision and drainage or refer to physician for possible marsupialization. If cyst is extremely painful or large, immediate physician referral
B. Antibiotics as appropriate to organism; most common ampicillin 500 mg QID x 7 days or cephalexin 250 mg QID x 7 days or 500 mg BID x 7 days

VIII. Complications
Recurrence

IX. Consultation/Referral
See VII. A. and B. above

X. Follow-up
At clinician's discretion after incision and drainage or marsupialization

See Bibliography 14.

Vulvar Conditions*

I. Definition

Primary vulvar conditions are those that arise from abnormal epithelial growth that can be inflammatory, dermatologic, or congenital in origin or from neoplastic alterations. Since the vulva include the labia majora and minora, the mons veneris, fourchette, and vestibule, and encompass the urethral and vaginal orifices and the ducts of the Skene's and Bartholin's glands, vulvar conditions are varied both in origin and in clinical manifestations. Please refer to separate protocols for sexually transmitted diseases that can cause clinical signs and symptoms on the vulva, and protocols for Bartholin's cyst, molluscum contagiosum, herpes, and condyloma.

II. Etiology

A. Allergy
B. Inflammatory response
C. Bacterial
   1. Staphylococci
   2. Streptococci
   3. Corynebacterium minutissimum
D. Viral
   1. HPV   2. Herpex simplex
E. Fungal
   1. Epidermophyton floccosum
   2. Trichophyton mentagrophytes
   3. Trichophyton rubrum
F. Pigmentation disorders
G. Benign epithelial changes
H. Neoplasms

III. History

A. What the client may present with
   1. Pruritus, rash

*The authors are indebted to Luisa Fertitta, MS, RNC, for her work in this area.

2. Hypopigmentation
3. Bullae
4. Weeping, scaling, crusting
5. Excoriation
6. Maceration
7. Thickening
8. Hyperkeratosis
9. Fissures
10. Abscesses
11. Lesions: macules, papules, vesicles, warty, pedunculated, domed, flat, plaques
12. Lichenification
13. Change in color of vulva
14. Dyspareunia
15. Burning

B. Additional information to be considered
1. Type of clothing commonly worn
2. Type of underwear: cotton, synthetic
3. Use of feminine deodorant products
4. Use of scented, deodorant tampons, pads, panty liners
5. Douching
6. Detergents, bathing soap, fabric softeners
7. Bubble bath or oils
8. Family or personal history of diabetes
9. Sexual partners, activity; contraception; STD history
10. Fungal infection of hands and feet, self or partner; oral candidiasis
11. Last menstrual period
12. Perimenopausal symptoms
13. History of dermatologic conditions including HPV anywhere on body
14. Fever, malaise, flu-like symptoms
15. Character and changes in lesions
16. Partner with symptoms
17. History of Crohn's disease
18. Genital HPV history, history of Papanicolaou smear with HPV; any abnormal Papanicolaou history

IV. Physical Examination
A. Vulva
1. Skin appearance: inflammation, edema, dry or moist, thickening hyperkeratosis
2. Lesions present
3. Weeping, scaling, crusting
4. Fissuring
5. Lichenification
6. Excoriation
7. Hypopigmentation
8. Hyperpigmentation
B. Adenopathy
C. Groin, inner thighs, buttocks
1. Lesions
D. Other systems as indicated by history and drugs

V. Laboratory Examination as Indicated by History and Appearance of Lesions
A. Bacterial cultures and sensitivities
B. Wood's lamp examination
C. Gram-stain scraping from lesions
D. Scrapings in KOH
E. Punch biopsy of lesions
F. Colposcopic examination
G. Staining with 1% toluidine blue
H. Fasting blood sugar
I. HPV testing

VI. Differential Diagnosis
A. Contact dermatitis: allergic or irritant
B. Inflammatory conditions and reactions
C. Bacterial infections
D. Viral infections
E. Fungal infections
1. Tinea cruris
F. Pigmentation disorders
1. Hyperpigmentation
2. Congenital hypopigmentation

    G.   Benign epithelial changes
    H.   Neoplasms
    I.   Lesions from Crohn's disease

VII. Treatment
A. Medication
    1.   Contact dermatitis: Burow's compresses; 1% cortisone cream
    2.   Bacterial infections: Erythromycin 250 mg QID x 14 days; tetracycline 250 mg QID x 10-14 days or until resolved
    3.   Tinea: topical antifungals such as GyneLotrimin, Mycelex, or Monistat Derm
    4.   Analgesics for pain
    5.   Topical antibiotics
B. Lifestyle changes and self-care measures
    1.   Loose cotton underwear; no underwear in bed
    2.   Keep area dry and clean
    3.   Discontinue use of irritant or allergen
    4.   Hot packs
    5.   Sitz baths
C. Teaching and reassurance

VIII. Complications
A. Secondary infection
B. Progressive disease
C. Masking more serious disease

IX. Consultation/Referral
A. Unable to identify lesion or condition
B. No response to treatment
C. Progression of disease
D. For biopsy, diagnostic work-up
E. For surgical excision or other surgical intervention
F. To specialist for systemic disease or dermatoses beyond the vulva

X. Follow-up
As indicated by therapy or for further diagnostic work.

Appendix FF gives directions for vulvar self-examination which you may want to distribute to your clients.
See Bibliography 21.

Acute Pelvic Pain

I. Definition
Acute pelvic pain can be defined as sudden onset of severe lower abdominal pain assessed to be gynecologic in nature

II. Etiology
A. Physiologic causes
   1. Infection from a variety of organisms resulting in pelvic inflammatory disease
   2. Extrauterine pregnancy
   3. Ovarian pathology
   4. Uterine perforation
   5. Ruptured pelvic abscess in a variety of sites
   6. Aberrant uterine leiomyomata
   7. Bladder pathology; bowel pathology
   8. Ureteral pathology
   9. Proliferate endometrium beyond the uterine corpus
   10. Post-surgical sequelae
   11. Mittelschmerz
   12. Trauma, abuse, sexual assault
B. Psychologic causes
   1. Secondary to pelvic surgery
   2. Secondary to pregnancy whatever the outcome
   3. Secondary to resolved pelvic pathology
   4. Primary or secondary as a focal site for stress; post-traumatic stress disorder 2° sexual abuse, assault

III. History
A. What the client may present with

1. Sudden onset of symptoms
2. Chills, fever
3. May have nausea, vomiting, and/or diarrhea
4. May have constipation
5. Increased vaginal discharge
6. Acute, continuous or intermittent cramping
7. Urinary symptoms including frequency and pain
8. Missed menses
9. Menses at time of onset
10. History of pelvic surgery
11. History of ovarian cysts
12. History of extrauterine pregnancy
13. History of PID
14. History of urinary tract infection
15. History of endometriosis
16. History of gonorrhea or Chlamydia infection
17. History of rape, sexual assault, incest

B. Additional information to be considered
1. Location of pain: stay in any one place or variable; ever have this pain before
2. Description of pain: sharp, dull, throbbing; rate pain
3. When does pain occur; does it wake client up
4. Does anything induce the pain such as eating, defecating, urinating, sexual intercourse, sexual stimulation; beliefs about cause of pain
5. What if anything relieves the pain
6. Any weight gain or loss
7. Associated symptoms such as diarrhea, blood in stool or urine, increase in vaginal discharge, vaginal bleeding
8. Timing in relation to menses, if any association
9. Duration of symptoms: days, weeks, months; regularity of symptoms
10. Sexual history: exposure to sexually transmitted disease, unprotected intercourse, new partner, change in contraception methods used in recent past and currently; use of sex toys
11. Psychosocial history: unusual stressors at time of onset of when pain occurs; life changes such as moving, new job, new relationship, end of relationship

12. Pelvic surgery in the past 12-24 months such as hysterectomy, laparotomy, tubal ligation
13. Diagnostic pelvic work-up such as laparoscopy, endometrial biopsy, colonoscopy, infertility work-up
14. Change in character of menses: heavier, lighter, more or less frequent

IV. Physical Examination

A. Vital signs as appropriate
   a. Temperature
   b. Blood pressure
   c. Pulse
   d. Respirations
B. Abdominal examination
   1. Bowel sounds: normal, hyperactive, sluggish, absent, any adventitious sounds, any bruits
   2. Generalized or localized lower abdominal tenderness
   3. Any guarding, pulsations observed
   4. Any rebound tenderness
   5. Any old scars
   6. Any distention
   7. Client's perception of location of pain
   8. On percussion, are liver or spleen enlarged or is bladder distended
   9. Any pain elicited with light touch; with deep palpation
   10. Any organomegaly or masses
C. Vaginal examination
   1. Examine cervix for discharge
   2. Examine vagina for lesions, discharge, and any unusual odor
D. Bimanual examination
   1. Examine cervix for cervical motion tenderness
   2. Examine uterus for tenderness
   3. Examine adnexa for ovarian tenderness, masses, or tenderness in rest of adnexa
E. Rectal examination
   1. Pain or tenderness   2. Masses   3. Melena
F. Elicit psoas sign; perform obturator maneuver

V. Laboratory Examination
A. Cultures as indicated might include gonococcus culture, Chlamydia smear; wet mount; pH of vaginal fluids
B. Complete blood count/differential
C. Sedimentation rate; C-Reactive protein
D. Urinary tract infection screen
E. Pregnancy test—urine, UCG quantitative
F. Ultrasound
G. Flat plate of abdomen
H. Other tests as symptoms and/or history indicate
I. Consider CA125 if age, history, and/or physical findings indicate

VI. Differential Diagnosis
A. Septic abortion
B. Ectopic pregnancy
C. Uterine leiomyomas with hemorrhage or infarction
D. Ovarian cyst with rupture extruding blood, cyst fluid, and dermoid contents into pelvic cavity
E. Uterine perforation
F. Ruptured abscess from ovary, uterus, bowel
G. Urinary tract infection: cystitis or pyelonephritis; kidney stones
H. Appendicitis
I. Adhesions
J. Solid ovarian tumor
K. Irritable bowel syndrome; diverticulitis, acute bowel
L. Primary dysmenorrhea, especially in women over 35
M. Pelvic inflammatory disease
N. Mittelschmerz, especially in women under 35
O. Endometriosis
P. Adenomatosis
Q. Complications of intrauterine device
R. Post-tubal ligation syndrome
S. Constipation
T. Lower bowel tumor

VII. Treatment
A. Medication as indicated for diagnosis

B. Physician consult for suspected ectopic pregnancy, appendicitis, ovarian pathology, abscess, complications of uterine leiomyomas, suspected pelvic adhesions, irritable bowel syndrome, suspected bowel or other tumors
C. Treatment for primary dysmenorrhea per protocol
D. Removal of IUD; consult as needed for complications
E. Teaching, interventions as indicated for post-tubal ligation syndrome
F. Teaching and comfort measures for Mittelschmerz

VIII. Complications
A. Generalized sepsis
B. Hemorrhage
C. Perforation of bowel
D. Rupture of abscess
E. Rupture of site of extrauterine pregnancy
F. Shock
G. Bowel obstruction
H. Interference with activities of daily living with mittelschmerz, dysmenorrhea, irritable bowel syndrome

IX. Consultation/Referral
A. Unable to find cause
B. Physician consult for medical or surgical intervention
C. For hospitalization if no admitting privileges
D. If symptoms worsen or recur after treatment
E. No response to treatment
F. Unable to remove IUD or find IUD or differentiate cause of problem with method

X. Follow-up
A. Consider reevaluation in 48 hours as warranted by clinical findings
B. Consider repeating bimanual and/or abdominal examination in one week and review status
C. Seek immediate clinical consultation if symptoms worsen
D. Follow up as appropriate for specific conditions such as PID

See Bibliography 17.

Chronic Pelvic Pain

I. Definition
Pain in any region of the pelvis that is long-term and unresponsive to treatment of symptoms and/or undiagnosed.

II. Etiology
A. 50% enigmatic
B. 25% endometriosis
C. 25% other pathology including subacute and chronic salpingitis

III. History
A. What the client may present with
  1. Chronic pelvic pain with or without menstrual exacerbation
  2. Dysmenorrhea
  3. Dyspareunia
  4. Dyschezia
  5. Chronicity of symptoms
  6. Absence of chills, fever associated with pain
  7. Nausea, vomiting, and/or diarrhea associated with pain
  8. Chronic constipation
  9. Chronic intermittent cramping

IV. Additional Information to Be Considered
A. Any symptoms of chronic bowel disease; any previous assessments for such and results
B. Any symptoms of chronic urinary tract infection, urinary tract anomaly, kidney disease
C. Location of pain, duration, exacerbation, and what precedes increased symptoms
D. Description of pain: sharp, dull, aching, cramping, intermittent, continuous
E. Pain relief measures; what helps
F. Any weight gain or loss
G. Symptoms that accompany pain

H. Sexual history including sexual responsiveness; STDs, PID; contraceptive history including IUD
I. Surgical history
J. Medical history
K. Pelvic surgery including laparoscopy, laparotomy, tubal ligation, hysterectomy, repair of cystocele, rectocele, urethrocele, appendectomy, myomectomy, cervical cone biopsy
L. Menstrual history
M. Pregnancy history including extrauterine pregnancy(ies), infertility assessments and/or treatments
N. Psychosocial history including life stressors, major life changes and timing in relation to onset of symptoms
O. History of incest, other sexual assault or abuse

V. Physical Examination
A. Vital signs as appropriate
B. Abdominal examination
    1. Bowel sounds: normal, hypo- or hyperactive, sluggish, absent, adventitious sounds, bruits
    2. Lower abdominal tenderness, sites of acute, dull pain elicited on superficial and/or deep palpation
    3. Any guarding
    4. Any rebound tenderness
    5. Scars
    6. Distention, asymmetry
    7. Client's perception of pain location
    8. On percussion, liver, spleen enlarged, bladder distended
    9. Organomegaly, masses
C. Vaginal examination
    1. Examine cervix for discharge
    2. Examine vagina for masses, lesions, discharge, unusual odor, color
D. Bimanual examination
    1. Examine cervix for cervical motion tenderness
    2. Examine uterus for tenderness, masses, shape, size, consistency
    3. Examine adnexa for ovarian shape, size, tenderness, masses, other adnexal masses or tenderness

E. Rectal examination
   1. Pain, tenderness
   2. Masses
   3. Melena
   4. Rectovaginal masses, fistulas, adhesions
   5. Rectocele
F. Elicit psoas sign; perform obturator maneuver

VI. Laboratory Examination
A. Cultures as indicated by history, physical findings
B. Complete blood count/differential
C. Sedimentation rate, C-reactive protein
D. Urinary tract infection screen
E. Pregnancy test
F. Ultrasound evaluation based on pelvic examination
G. Consider confutation for CAT scan and/or MRI if pelvic examination is abnormal
H. Consider psychological testing

VII. Differential Diagnosis
A. Consider possible causes under acute pelvic pain and rule out:
   1. GI and GU pathology including appendicitis, pancreatitis, bowel obstruction, ulcers, cholecystitis, cholelithiasis, biliary colic, rupture of spleen, diverticulitis, ileitis, carcinoma, irritable bowel syndrome, ulcerative colitis, pyelonephritis, hepatitis, hiatal hernia, urinary calculus, mesenteric thrombosis
   2. Endometriosis demonstrated by diagnostic laparoscopy, not by clinical diagnosis alone
   3. Psychogenic causes including those related to rape, sexual assault, incest
   4. Enigmatic pelvic pain
   5. Pelvic congestion syndrome in women who do not have orgasmic relief
   6. Pelvic congestion syndrome—following precipitous delivery, often includes varicosities of the uterine ligaments

7. Old injuries from childbirth, rape, and/or incest
8. Somatization disorders
9. Musculoskeletal factors

VIII. Consultation/Referral
A. For laparoscopic diagnostic examination
B. For medical evaluation of suspected GI, GU conditions as indicated by history and physical examination
C. For pelvic venography
D. To confirm a suspected diagnosis and initiate treatment as co-managers of care
E. For psychological evaluation
F. For ultrasound, MRI

IX. Treatment
A. Endometriosis
   1. Create a pseudomenopause with Danocrine 200-800 mg. bid p.o. for 6 months; or GnRH analogues for 6 months (Nafarelin nasal spray 400-800 gm daily) or Leuprolide acetate (Lupron depot) 1 mg IM daily for 6 months, Zoladex® (Goserlin Acetate) implant 3.6 mg administered subcutaneously g 28 days x 6 months
B. Other pathological causes
   1. Diagnose and treat cause according to established protocols (such as salpingitis, trauma from sexual assault, incest or rape, childbirth)
C. Enigmatic pelvic pain
   1. Follow-up to diagnostic laparoscopy as appropriate to any findings
   2. Multidisciplinary approach to pain management
D. Consideration of empiric therapy
   1. Antidepressant
   2. GnRH agonist
   3. Musculoskeletal relaxant

X. Follow-up
A. As appropriate for diagnosis and treatment
B. As desired by patient if no definitive cause is found and

palliative treatments are suggested
C. If symptoms continue, introduce the team approach
  1. Mental health care specialist
  2. Physical therapist
  3. Nutritionist
  4. Urogynecologist
  5. Gastroenterologist

See Bibliography 17.

Abdominal Pain

I. Definition
Pain (mild to severe) in any region of the abdomen as differentiated from the pelvic area, including the area from the costal margins to the beginning of the mons pubis including but not limited to the abdominal organs and anatomical structure.

II. Etiology
A. Inflammation, ulceration, infection
B. Space occupying lesion
C. Response to injury: intra-abdominal or extra-abdominal
D. Sequelae of surgery: adhesions, presence of foreign body, unrepaired perforation
E. Functional

III. History
A. What the client may present with
  1. Anorexia
  2. Vomiting
  3. Nausea
  4. Change in bowel habits
  5. Urinary symptoms
  6. Gynecological symptoms and history (see acute and chronic pelvic pain protocols)
  7. Diaphoresis
  8. Fainting

    9. Distention of the abdomen
  10. Dyspnea, tachycardia, bradycardia
  11. Fever
  12. Chills
B. Additional information to be considered (client will generally complain only of abdominal pain; history must be very thorough). Specific questioning is needed to elicit information about:
    1. Onset (sudden, gradual, chronic, and so on)
    2. Character, e.g., throbbing, aching, burning, knife-like
    3. Intensity: difficult to define, but can be likened to other pain such as toothache, cramps, labor pain
    4. Location—where did pain originate
    5. Radiation: does it travel elsewhere
    6. Pain relief measures: what helps
    7. Any weight gain or loss
    8. Pregnancy history; infertility diagnostics or treatments
    9. Psychosocial history including life stressors, major life changes and timing in relation to onset of symptoms
  10. History of incest, other sexual assault or abuse, violence or battering in relationships
  11. History of bowel obstruction, polyps
  12. History of abdominal tumors benign or malignant
  13. Use of GI irritants
  14. Possible contaminated drinking water source here and/ or abroad
  15. History of pelvic and/or abdominal surgery
  16. History of extrauterine pregnancy
  17. History of ovarian cysts, rupture of cysts
  18. History of chronic bowel syndrome, any bowel disease
  19. History of gall bladder disease
  20. History of hepatitis, jaundice, liver disease, mononucleosis, abnormal liver function
  21. History of trauma to the abdomen: accident, battering
  22. History of travel abroad, recent immigrant and from where
  23. History of exposure to industrial toxins, pesticides
  24. History of kidney anomaly or disease
  25. History of appendicitis chronic or acute

26. History of ulcers
27. Previous care for abdominal pain

IV. Physical Examination
A. Vital signs as appropriate
B. Cardiovascular, respiratory examinations
C. Abdominal examination
   1. Bowel sounds; normal, hypo- or hyperactive, sluggish, absent, adventitious sounds, bruits
   2. Abdominal tenderness, sites of acute, dull pain elicited on superficial and/or deep palpation
   3. Any guarding
   4. Any rebound tenderness
   5. Scars
   6. Distension, symmetry or asymmetry
   7. Client's perception of pain location
   8. On percussion liver or spleen enlarged, other abdominal organs enlarged
   9. Organomegaly, masses
D. Vaginal and bimanual examination
   1. Examine cervix for discharge
   2. Examine vagina for masses, lesions, discharge, unusual odor, color
   3. Examine cervix for cervical motion tenderness
   4. Examine uterus for tenderness, masses, shape, size, consistency
   5. Examine adnexa for ovarian shape, size, tenderness, masses; other adnexal masses or tenderness
E. Rectal examination
   1. Pain, tenderness
   2. Masses
   3. Melena
   4. Rectovaginal masses, fistulas, adhesions
   5. Rectocele

V. Laboratory Examination
A. Cultures as indicated by history, physical findings
B. Complete blood count/differential

C. Liver function studies, enzymes
D. Urinary tract infection screen
E. Pregnancy test
F. Ultrasound evaluation based on examination
G. Flat plate of abdomen if indicated
H. May consider consultation for CAT scan and/or MRI if abdominal or pelvic examination is abnormal
I. Sickle cell prep if indicated
J. ESR

VI. Differential Diagnosis

A. Consider possible causes under acute and chronic pelvic pain and rule out:
   1. GI and GU pathology including appendicitis, pancreatitis, bowel obstruction, ulcers, cholecystitis, cholelithiasis, biliary colic, rupture of spleen, diverticulitis, ileitis, carcinoma, irritable bowel syndrome, ulcerative colitis, pyelonephritis, hepatitis, hiatal hernia, urinary calculus, mesenteric thrombosis, urethral syndrome
   2. Acute or chronic constipation
   3. Dissecting aneurysm
   4. Ectopic pregnancy
   5. Acute gastritis
   6. Drug or toxin reaction
   7. Injury secondary to accident, violence including organ rupture
   8. Abdominal pain, undetermined etiology
   9. Referred pain from thoracic pathology: coronary thrombosis, pleural pneumonia, pleurisy, herpes zoster
   10. Gastritis, coronitis, ileitis secondary to parasitic infection, cholera, water-borne diseases

VII. Consultation/Referral

A. For laparoscopic diagnostic examination
B. For medical evaluation of suspected GI, GU conditions as indicated by history and physical examination
C. To confirm a suspected diagnosis and initiate treatment as co-managers of care

D. For surgical consultation as indicated by history and findings
E. For CAT scan, MRI

VIII. Treatment
A. As indicated by findings and history
B. Etiology undetermined, pain persists
   1. Follow-up to any diagnostic work-up
   2. Multidisciplinary approach to pain or symptom management

X. Follow-up
A. As appropriate for diagnosis and treatment
B. As desired by patient if no definitive cause is found and palliative treatments are suggested

See Bibliography 17.

Pelvic Inflammatory Disease (PID)

I. Definition
Pelvic inflammatory disease comprises a spectrum of inflammatory disorders of the upper genital tract. This may include any combination of endometritis, salpingitis, tuboovarian abscess, and pelvic peritonitis.

II. Etiology
Causative organisms include
A. Neisseria gonorrhoeae
B. Streptococcus; Streptococcus agalactiae
C. Peptostreptococcus
D. Bacteroides
E. Chlamydia trachomatis
F. Escherichia coli
G. Mycoplasma hominis
H. H. influenzae
I. U. urealyticum
J. Gardnerella vaginalis

III. History

A. What the client may present with (wide variation in symptomatology, making diagnosis difficult)
1. Lower abdominal pain, usually bilateral
2. Chills, fever
3. May have anorexia
4. May have nausea
5. May have vomiting
6. Increased vaginal discharge
7. Heavier than usual period
8. Urinary symptoms: frequency, pain
9. May complain of right upper quadrant pain; also Fitz-Hugh Curtis syndrome
10. Dyspareunia

B. Additional information to be considered
1. Known exposure to sexually transmitted disease
2. Previous sexually transmitted disease
3. Previous diagnosis of pelvic inflammatory disease
4. Previously diagnosed endometriosis
5. History of abdominal surgery
6. Chronic illness
7. Sexual activity (present and recent past)
8. Last menstrual period; birth control method; is there an intrauterine device in place; recent pregnancy
9. Medication allergy
10. Currently taking any medication
11. Recent pelvic surgery, i.e., therapeutic abortion or dilatation and curettage
12. Smoking cigarettes has recently been implicated as a risk factor for PID

IV. Physical Examination

A. Vital signs
1. Temperature   2. Blood pressure
3. Pulse   4. Respiration
B. Abdominal examination
1. Bowel sounds: normal, hyperactive, sluggish, absent
2. Generalized lower abdominal tenderness

    3. Guarding
    4. Rebound tenderness
C. External genitalia
    1. Lesions
    2. Observe and palpate Skene's and Bartholin's glands
D. Vaginal examination (speculum)
    1. Examine cervix for
      a. Erosion, ectropion
      b. Friability
      c. Discharge in os
E. Bimanual examination
    1. Examine cervix for cervical motion tenderness
    2. Examine uterus for tenderness
    3. Examine adnexa for
      a. Tenderness   b. Mass
    4. Rectovaginal examination for tenderness; if present, describe location, i.e., cervix, uterus, adnexa

V. Laboratory Examination
A. Gonococcus culture
B. Chlamydia smear
C. Complete blood count/differential, C-reactive protein
D. Sedimentation rate
E. Urinary tract infection screen
F. Serology test for syphilis
G. Human chorionic gonadotropin if history indicates

VI. Criteria for Clinical Diagnosis
A. Criteria for ambulatory treatment
    1. The three minimum criteria for diagnosis of PID are:
      a. History of lower abdominal pain and presence of lower abdominal tenderness
      b. Cervical motion tenderness
      c. Adnexal tenderness
    2. Additional criteria that will increase the specificity of diagnosis
      a. Temperature above 100.9°F (> 38.3C)
      b. Elevated white blood count > 10,500

    c. Culdocentesis yielding peritoneal fluid which contains bacteria, white blood cells

    d. Presence of adnexal mass noted on bimanual examination; tubo-ovarian abscess on sonography

    e. Elevated sedimentation rate

    f. Positive gonococcal culture from cervix

    g. Positive Chlamydia smear from cervix

    h. Abnormal cervical or vaginal discharge

B. Criteria for hospitalization (CDC Guidelines 1998)

    1. Surgical emergencies such as appendicitis cannot be excluded

    2. The patient is pregnant

    3. The patient does not respond clinically to oral antimicrobial therapy

    4. The patient is unable to follow or tolerate an outpatient oral regimen

    5. The patient has severe illness, nausea and vomiting or high fever

    6. The patient has a tubo-ovarian abscess

    7. The patient is immunodeficient (i.e., has HIV infection with low counts, is taking immunosuppressant therapy), or has another disease

VII. Differential Diagnosis

A. Septic abortion	B. Ectopic gestation
C. Ovarian cyst	D. Ruptured ovarian cyst
E. Cystitis	F. Pyelonephritis
G. Peptic ulcer disease	I. Hepatitis
J. Appendicitis	K. Adhesions
L. Endometriosis	M. Diverticular disease
N. Pelvic neoplasms	O. Irritable bowel syndrome

VIII. Treatment (CDC Recommendations) for Uncomplicated Pelvic Inflammatory Disease

A. Medication

    1. Ofloxacin 400 mg orally BID x 14 days **PLUS** Metronidazole 500 mg orally BID for 14 days

    2. Alternative regimens

    a. Ceftriaxone 250 mg IM once *O R*

    b. Cefoxitin 2 gm IM plus Probenecid 1 gram orally once *OR*

    c. Other parenteral 3rd generation cephalosporin (e.g., ceftizoxime or cefotaxime *PLUS* Doxycycline 100 mg orally BID for 14 days (for a, b, or c)

  3. Pregnant women: Hospitalize and treat with parenteral antibiotics per CDC guidelines for hospitalization

  4. Refer to CDC guidelines if patient meets hospitalization criteria

B. General measures
1. Bed rest
2. Increased fluid intake
3. General diet
4. Stress importance of partner being examined and treated
5. Stress use of condoms to prevent reinfection or future infections
6. No douching

C. Management of sex partners
1. Examine and treat if sexual contact with patient during 60 days prior to onset of symptoms

IX. Complications
A. Sterility
B. Generalized sepsis
C. Chronic pelvic pain
D. Tubal pregnancy
E. Surgical interventions
F. Dyspareunia

X. Consultation/Referral
A. If failure to improve 48 hours after starting above treatment
B. For hospitalization

XI. Follow-up
A. Reevaluate in 48-72 hours or sooner if symptoms worsen or do not improve
B. After completion of medication course (no sooner than 7 days)
1. Bimanual
2. Cultures if indicated (i.e., positive lab results prior to

treatment); some recommend rescreening for gonorrhea and Chlamydia trachomatis regardless of prior culture results 4-6 weeks after completion of therapy

See Bibliography 18.

Pelvic Mass

I. Definition
Mass found in adnexa, cul de sac, or uterus during bimanual examination

II. Etiology
A pelvic mass may be caused by any number of factors. This protocol is meant to assist the clinician in the screening and referral process.

III. History
A. What the client may present with
  1. May be asymptomatic
  2. Bloating
  3. Abdominal pain (generalized or localized)
  4. Flatulence
  5. Dysfunctional bleeding
  6. Amenorrhea
  7. Vaginal discharge
  8. Low back pain and/or pressure
  9. Dyspareunia
  10. Bowel or bladder dysfunction
  11. Prior abdominal surgery
  12. Prior pelvic surgery
  13. Endometriosis
  14. Pregnancy history
B. Additional information to be obtained
  1. LMP
  2. Contraception used
  3. Menstruation, pregnancy, and infertility history

    4. Any change in bowel habits; last bowel movement
    5. History of ovarian cysts
    6. History of uterine fibroids
    7. History of pelvic inflammatory disease (PID)
    8. History of Chlamydia or gonorrhea
    9. History of IUD use

IV. Physical Examination

A. Vaginal examination
    1. Examine cervix for discharge
    2. Examine vagina for masses, lesions, discharge
B. Bimanual examination
    1. Examine cervix for cervical motion tenderness
    2. Examine uterus for tenderness, masses, shape, size, and consistency
    3. Examine adnexa for masses, attempting to differentiate between ovaries and bowel
    4. Evaluate mass for shape, consistency, size, mobility and tenderness
    5. Examine bladder
    6. Cul de sac for mass
    7. Thickening or tenderness at or near utero sacral ligaments
C. Rectal examination
    1. Pain, tenderness   2. Masses
    3. Melena   4. Rectovaginal masses,
    5. Rectocele/occult blood   fistulas

V. Laboratory Examination

    1. Cultures as indicated
    2. Wet prep as indicated
    3. Serum pregnancy test as indicated
    4. CBC with sed rate; C-reactive protein
    5. Ultrasound; transvaginal and transabdominal or with doppler as indicated
    6. CA 125, ovarian cancer tumor marker as indicated

VI. Treatment

A. Adnexal masses

    1. If thought to be retained stool or intestinal gas, client should have bowel prep and be reexamined

    2. If thought to be ovarian in origin, the following differentiation must be made

       a. Age of patient (ovulation or using ovulation inhibitor, perimenopausal or menopausal)

       b. Menstrual history

       c. Indication of infection

       d. Is pregnancy test positive

    3. If ovulation is presumed, assess size of mass if:

       a. Greater than 5 cm, M.D. referral is indicated

       b. Less than 5 cm and asymptomatic, reexamine after next menses; if unchanged may recommend ovulatory inhibitor x 3 months and reexamine. If remaining after 3 months, refer to M.D.

    4. If on ovulatory inhibitor, do appropriate work-up (i.e., ultrasound) and refer or refer immediately depending on setting

    5. Perimenopausal/menopausal

       a. Do appropriate work-up; refer for M.D. evaluation as indicated

B. Uterine mass

    1. Do ultrasound—small, non-symptomatic fibroids may be followed and assessed on a 6-month to 12-month basis as appropriate to setting. Large fibroids or other finding refer immediately to M.D.

VII. Differential Diagnosis

A. Adnexal mass

    1. Retained stool

    2. Inflammatory bowel process

    3. Functional cysts

    4. Neoplasms

       a. Benign (i.e., dermoid, endometrioma)

       b. Malignant (i.e., epithelial and nonepithelial)

    5. Abscess

B. Uterine mass

    1. Fibroid tumors or leiomyomatas

2. Intrauterine pregnancy
3. Intrauterine pregnancy in a bicornuate uterus
4. Neoplasm
C. Miscellaneous
   1. Distended bladder   2. Pelvic kidney
   3. Urachal cyst   4. Abdominal wall hematoma or
   5. Retroperitoneal neoplasm   abscess

VIII. Complications
A. Complication of individual entity as listed in differential diagnosis

IX. Consultation and Referral
A. As indicated by laboratory work-up and physical findings indicated in VI treatment

X. Follow-up
A. As indicated by diagnosis

See Bibliography 17.

Uterine Leiomyomata

I. Definition
Often referred to as uterine fibroids, fibromyomas, myomas, or fibromas, leiomyomas are benign uterine tumors arising from the smooth muscle and having some connective tissue elements as well.

II. Etiology
A. Physiology
   1. Appear to arise from single neoplastic smooth muscle cells (4th and 5th decades) within the myometrium
   2. May be single or multiple
   3. May range in size from a few millimeters to more than 20 cm
   4. May occur within the uterine wall (intramural) or extend

externally from the serosal surface (subserosal) internally into endometrial cavity (submucous)
5. Occur most commonly during a woman's fertile years
6. Usually undergo regression with menopause
7. Sometimes increase in size with oral contraceptives or pregnancy

III. History
A. What the client may present with
1. Pelvic pain (acute or chronic)
2. Abnormal vaginal bleeding
3. Urinary frequency and/or retention
4. Constipation
5. Pelvic pressure
6. Dyspareunia
B. Additional information to be considered
1. Menstrual history
2. History of infertility
3. Habitual spontaneous abortions
4. Menopausal symptoms
5. Last menstrual period; methods of birth control; intrauterine device in place; ever use intrauterine device
6. Any pelvic surgery
7. Pregnancy history
8. Use of hormones: oral contraceptives, hormone therapy, infertility drugs

IV. Physical Examination
A. Vital signs as indicated
B. Abdominal examination
1. Any abdominal guarding or tenderness
2. Location of any pain
3. Bladder palpable or distended
C. Vaginal examination
1. Examine cervix for any extraneous tissue, distortion of configuration
2. Palpate vagina for any masses
3. Examine any bleeding or discharge

D. Bimanual examination
    1. Examine uterus for tenderness, masses
    2. Examine adnexa for masses, tenderness
    3. Locate any pain if possible
E. Rectovaginal examination for tenderness, masses

V. Laboratory Examination
A. Ultrasound
B. Pregnancy test if pre- or perimenopausal
C. CBC

VI. Differential Diagnosis
A. Uterine pregnancy
B. Malignant uterine tumor
C. Ovarian cyst or tumor
D. Extrauterine pelvic mass
E. Bowel tumor

F. Bladder tumor
G. Tumor of ureter
H. Pelvic abscess
I. Extrauterine pregnancy

VII. Treatment
A. As indicated by ultrasound
    1. Watch size of leiomyomata with bimanual examination
       and repeat ultrasound
    2. Consultation for medical management: progestins, gonad-
       otropin releasing hormone (GnRH)
    3. Consultation for surgical management: hysterectomy,
       myomectomy, hysteroscope, resectoscope, laser ablation;
       myolysis or myoma coagulation

VIII. Complications
A. Torsion of pedunculated leiomyomata resulting in necrosis
B. Uterine abscess
C. Infarction
D. Hemorrhage
E. Degeneration: hyalinization, cystic, calcification, fatty

IX. Consultation/Referral
A. Rapid change in size
B. Signs of complications

C. Menorrhagia
D. Compromise of adjacent organs
E. Intractable pelvic pressure or pain

X. Follow-up
A. Reevaluate every 6-12 months or as indicated
B. As indicated under medical management with medication

See Bibliography 17.

Scabies

I. Definition
A highly contagious papulofollicular skin rash whose chief symptom is pruritus. Rash and itching are thought to be hypersensitivity reactions to the mites and are not confined to the locations of mite burrows. Scabies among adults may be sexually transmitted.

II. Etiology
Sarcoptes scabiel mite. The mite burrows into skin, deposits eggs along a tunnel. Larvae hatch in 3-5 days and gather around hair follicles. Newly hatched female burrows into the skin, maturing in 10-19 days, then mates and starts a new cycle.

III. History
A. What the client may present with:
   1. Pruritus—worse at night or at times when body temperature is raised, i.e., after exercise. Pruritus exists prior to physical manifestations
   2. Lesions are usually on interdigital webs of hands, flexor aspects of wrists, extensor surfaces of the elbows, areas surrounding the nipples, anterior axillary folds, umbilicus, belt line, lower abdomen, genitalia and gluteal cleft
B. Additional information to be considered
   1. Known contact with scabies. Incubation period in persons

without previous exposure is usually 4-6 weeks. Persons who were previously infected develop symptoms 1-4 days after repeat exposure to the mite. These reinfections are usually milder

2. Lifestyle. Persons living in close proximity with others, dormitories, crowded living conditions, shared clothing, shelters, are at increased risk for non-sexual exposures
3. History of atopic dermatitis, +HIV, or other immunosuppressed condition

IV. Physical Examination
A. Skin: Thorough examination of lesions and of those areas most frequently involved
1. Linear burrows about 1.5 to 2 cm. in length terminating in a papule or vesicle
2. Lesions: papules or vesicles
3. Scaling, crustation lesions, furuncles, excoriations may be present with secondary infection

V. Labóratory
A. KOH prep of scraping from several of the excoriated lesions, examined under low power. It may be difficult to find mite. Application of water, alcohol, or mineral oil to the skin facilitates collection of the scraping
B. Diagnosis is usually made on the basis of clinical presentation

VI. Differential Diagnosis
A. Atopic dermatitis   B. Impetigo   C. Urticaria

VII. Treatment
A. Medication
1. 5% permethrin cream (Elimite®), applied to all areas of the body from neck down and washed off after 8-14 hours,
2. OR 1% lindane (Kwell®, Scabene®), applied to the entire body, left on for 6-8 hours, and washed off thoroughly. Lindane applications should not be in excess of these recommendations to avoid the possibility of neurotoxicity

from absorption through the skin. Lindane should not be used during pregnancy,

3. *OR* sulfur 6% precipitated in ointment to all areas of the body q noc x 3 nights
4. In pregnancy and lactation and for children under 2 use only permethrin or sulfa. Do not use lindane.

B. Symptomatic treatment
1. Antihistamines may be given to relieve pruritus
2. Client should be informed that pruritus may persist for several weeks. If client does not respond to therapy and itching is still persistent after one week, she/he should be instructed to contact health care provider to decide if further therapy is necessary

C. General measures
1. Clothing, towels, bed linens should be laundered (hot cycle) or dry cleaned on the day of treatment
2. If clothing items can't be washed or dry cleaned, these should be separated from washed clothes and not worn for at least 72 hours. Mites cannot exist for more than 2-3 days away from the body
3. Sexual partners and close personal or household contacts within the past month should be informed, examined, and treated if necessary
4. Client should be instructed to follow treatment regime carefully
5. Although fumigation of living areas is not necessary, some clients may wish to decontaminate mattresses, sofas, and other inanimate objects that cannot be washed. OTC sprays are available for this purpose

VIII. Complications
A. Secondary infection
B. Reaction to lindane (Kwell®, Scabene®)
  1. Dermatitis   2. CNS toxicity

IX. Consultation and Referral
A. Secondary infection
B. Generalized widespread inflammatory response

C. Failure to respond to therapy
D. Reaction to lindane (Kwell®, Scabene®)
E. Clients with coexisting dermatitis or other dermatologic condition
F. Clients with coexisting HIV infection or who are otherwise immunosuppressed

X. Follow-up
A. Failure to respond to therapy. Some experts recommend retreatment after 1 week for clients who are still symptomatic; others recommend retreatment only if live mites can be observed. Retreatment should be with an alternative regimen
B. Recurrence

Appendix LL may be copied/adapted for your clients.

Pediculosis

I. Definition
Pediculosis is the state of being infested with lice that may be found on the skin, particularly the hairy areas such as the scalp and pubis, and may cause intense pruritus.

II. Etiology
A. Two species that look like each other but have different feeding habits are:
   1. Pediculus humanus: inhabits the skin of the head or body; transmitted by shared clothing, towels, brushes, bedding, headphones, hats
   2. Phthirius pubis ("crab louse", pubic louse); inhabits the genital area; transmitted by close personal contact, bedding
B. Nits hatch in 5-10 days incubation; adult pubic lice probably survive no more than 24 hours off their host; nits can survive in hot and humid climates up to 10 days

III. History
A. What the client may present with
   1. Pruritus
   2. Visual identification of the parasite
   3. Known exposure to household member or intimate partner with head, body, or pubic lice
B. Additional information to be considered
   Lifestyle: shared clothing, towels, beds, pillows; shag rugs or carpets, upholstered furniture

IV. Physical Examination
A. Pediculosis capitis (infestation with head lice); examine for
   1. The parasite
   2. Greenish-white oval attachments to hair shaft (nits)
   3. Secondary impetigo and furunculosis
   4. Cervical lymphadenopathy
B. Pediculosis corporis (infestation with body lice): examine for
   1. Parallel linear scratch marks on back, shoulders, trunk, buttocks (areas easily reached for scratching)
   2. Impetigo lesions and furuncles associated with scratch marks secondary to scratching
   3. Lice on clothing, especially the seams, as lice are very rarely found on the body
C. Pediculosis pubis (infestation with pubic (crab) lice): examine for
   1. The parasite (rarely found)
   2. Oval attachments on pubic hair (nits)
   3. Black dots (representing excreta) on surrounding skin and underclothing
   4. Nits in eyebrows, eyelashes, scalp hair, axillary hair, and other body hair
   5. Crusts or scabs in pubic area

V. Laboratory Examination
None

VI. Differential Diagnosis
See Etiology

VII. Treatment

A. General measures
   1. Wash with hot water, dry clean, or run through a dryer all contaminated clothing, hats, towels, bedclothes, etc., to destroy nits and lice; wash combs and hairbrushes in hot soapy water letting them soak for at least 15 minutes
   2. Spray couches, chairs, car seats and items that can't be washed or dry cleaned with over-the-counter product (A-200 Pyrinate® (pyrethrin), Triplex®, or RID (permethrin); alternative is to vacuum carefully to pick up living lice and nits

B. Specific treatment
   1. Pediculosis capitis (infestation with head lice)
      a. Thoroughly wet hair with Kwell®* (lindane) shampoo (1% gamma benzene hexachloride) or Triplex Kit (pyrethrins + piperonyl butoxide); Pronto (piperonyl), RID (permethrin) shampoo or R&C shampoo (pyrethrins and piperonyl butoxide) or End Lice (pyrethins and piperonyl); work up lather, adding water as necessary; shampoo thoroughly leaving shampoo on head for 5 minutes; rinse, or use Nix® (permethrin 1% cream rinse), leave on 10 minutes and rinse thoroughly; or use Pronto shampoo/conditioner (piperonyl butoxide)
      b. Rinse thoroughly, towel dry
      c. Remove remaining nits with fine-tooth metal comb or tweezers (use of vinegar solution and hair conditioner or olive oil make combing easier)
   2. Pediculosis corporis (infestation with body lice)
      a. Bathe with soap and water if no lice are found
      b. Wash with hot water and dry in dryer all clothing, bedclothes, towels, etc.
      c. Dry clean items that cannot be washed; for items that cannot be washed or dry cleaned, seal in a plastic bag for 1 week: lice will suffocate; (in cold climates put

---

*Kwell is not recommended for use in pregnancy or lactation or for children under 2. Pregnant and lactating women should be treated only with 1% permethrin (Nix) or with pyrethrins with piperonyl betoxide. All products are OTC except Kwell; permethrin is available as a generic product. In a large review of efficacy, permethrin was the only product to show sufficient efficacy (cure rate measured as nit free after 14 days)

bags outside for 10 days; temperature change kills lice)
- d. If evidence of lice is found or patient is not relieved by a. and b. above, Kwell (lindane) Lotion® may be applied, allowed to remain 8-10 hours, and thoroughly rinsed off
3. Pediculosis pubis (infestation with pubic lice)
    - a. Kwell® shampoo (lindane) (left on 4 minutes); apply to hair and skin of pubic hair, or A.200 Pyrinate Gel® (pyrethrin) as directed
    - b. Rinse thoroughly
    - c. Repeat application in 7-10 days
    - d. Treat sexual partner simultaneously
    - e. Wash in hot water and thoroughly dry all clothing, bed linen, towels, etc.
C. Stress importance of careful checking of family and household members and close contacts; no treatment is needed unless there is evidence of contamination
D. Put nonwashable items in hot dryer; or spray with permethrin (RID, NIX)—check safety with children and pets

VIII. Complications
A. Secondary infection
B. Sensitivity reactions to treatment
C. Excoriations

IX. Consultation/Referral
A. Lice found in eyelashes: since shampoo cannot be used, Vaseline or ophthalmic ointment is applied to the eyelashes
B. Treatment failures
C. Co-existing dermatologic conditions

X. Follow-up
Instruct patient to return for repeat treatment if parasites are still present or if symptoms persist or recur

See Appendix KK and Bibiography 14.

Breast Conditions

Breast Mass

I. Definition

A breast mass is a thickening or lump which is felt in a woman's breast which may or may not have the following characteristics:

A. Nipple retraction
B. Dimpling
C. Inflammation
D. Palpable axillary or supraclavicular nodes
E. Tenderness
F. Discharge from nipple

II. Etiology

A. "Fibrocystic disease"—catch-all term for non-malignant conditions
B. Fibroadenoma
C. Carcinoma
D. Mammary duct ectasia
E. Intraductal papilloma
F. Normal premenstrual breast tissue, i.e., with tenderness and prominent breast tissue secondary to hormone levels
G. Mastalgia
H. Mastitis: cellulitis, skin boils, abscess

III. History

A. What woman may present with
1. Lump
2. Pain
3. Swelling
4. Redness; bruised area that doesn't resolve
5. Discharge from nipple
6. Nipple retraction
7. Change in appearance of skin

B. Additional information to be considered
1. Family history of breast disease
2. History of previous breast lumps or breast disease; biopsy (type) or aspiration; breast surgery including reduction, enlargement; implants and type

3. Last menstrual period (has patient noticed a relationship to menses?)
4. Birth control method(s) used
5. Diet
6. Adolescents' most common complaint
   a. Trauma (sports or sexual activity)
7. Recent pregnancy, lactation
8. Risk factors
   a. Hormonal
      1) Early menarche (11 or younger) or late menopause (55 or older)
      2) First full-term pregnancy after 30; nullipara
      3) Obesity in postmenopausal women (produce more estrogen)
      4) Breast feeding—may be protective but data are not conclusive
   b. Genetic (70% of breast cancer = no known family history)
      1) Risk increases with 1st or 2nd degree relatives — maternal or paternal—with breast cancer—mother, daughter, sister, aunt, grandmother
      2) BRCA1 or BRCA2 gene mutation
   c. External
      1) Diet (areas under investigation): fat—low fat diet may be beneficial;   increased risk with high animal fat diet
      2) Low vitamin A intake may increase breast cancer risk
      3) Alcohol even in moderate amounts (3-9 drinks a week) may increase risk
      4) Radiation—risk in moderate doses (10-500 rads) (level of radiation in an up-to-date mammogram = 1/4 rad)
      5) Exogenous hormones
         ☐ DES exposure in utero or as a DES mother
         ☐ Postmenopausal hormone therapy: estrogen 10 or more years possibly increases relative risk
         ☐ possibility that organochlorines (pesticides) can act like estrogen in the body
      6) Exercise—strenuous exercise in adolescence and

continued exercise in adulthood may have a protective effect
7) Other: Previous diagnosis of breast cancer or atypical hyperplasia

IV. Physical Examination
A. Breast Physical Examination
1. Examine in both upright and supine positions
2. Measurement, location, consistency of any lesion
3. Note any skin changes such as dimpling, retraction, erythema, nipple scaling
4. Examine for spontaneous breast discharge
5. Examine regional lymph nodes (axillary and supra-infraclavicular)
B. Palpation for the following:
1. Accurate location of any detected lesion
2. Solitary or multiple lesion(s)
3. Consistency and extent of any mass
4. Tenderness of mass
5. Movable or fixed on chest wall
6. Displacement or retraction of nipple
7. Retraction or dimpling of skin overlying mass
8. Palpability of regional lymph nodes (axillary or supra/infraclavicular)
9. Discharge expressed; color, amount, uni- or bilateral, consistency
C. Express breast for any discharge if none noted on palpation

V. Laboratory Examination
If discharge present, microscopic examination to identify fat globules

VI. Differential
See Etiology

VII. Treatment
A. Medication
1. Appropriate antibiotic for mastitis, abscess

B. General measures
1. If mass does not fit criteria for physician referral, have patient return 1 week after next menses for reevaluation and possible referral
2. Dietary; discuss use of caffeine, chocolate, and salt; low fat diet
3. Consider homeopathic remedies: evening primrose oil, ginseng tea, vitamins A and B for cyclical mastalgia

VIII. Complications
May be grave and extensive if misdiagnosed

IX. Consultation/Referral
A. Any of the following lesions should be referred immediately to physician
1. Fixed mass
2. Mass associated with nipple retraction
3. Dimpling of skin; orange peel appearance to skin
4. Inflammation
5. Palpable axillary or supra/infraclavicular nodes
6. Discrete mass
7. Discharge that it is not fat globules: green = infection; red or brown = possible tumor
8. Cystic mass; for possible aspiration
B. Refer to physician
1. Women who do not fit above criteria but in whom mass is still found one week past next menses
2. Women in whom mass is palpable despite negative mammogram
3. Consider referral to breast center, specialist

X. Follow-up
Appropriate to VII. B. 1. and VII. B. 2.

XI. Mammogram Screening
A. All women with a breast mass (although ultrasound may be more useful for women under 35)
B. Baseline between 35 and 40

C. Earlier if family history of breast cancer in mother, sister, daughter, aunt, grandmother
D. Annually 40 and older

See Appendix X and Bibliography 19.

Abnormal Breast Discharge

I. Definition
Under certain conditions an abnormal fluid may be expressed from the breast(s) or flow spontaneously.

II. Etiology
A. Physiological cause
  1. Pregnancy puerperium
  2. Intercourse
  3. Stimulation of the breast
  4. Chest wall surgery or trauma
  5. Exercise
  6. Emotional stress
  7. Sleep (affects measurable amounts of prolactin)
B. Pharmacological causes
  1. Numerous psychotropic drugs
  2. Cimetidine
  3. Some antihypertensives
  4. Opiates
  5. Estrogens/oral contraceptives/progestins
  6. Antiemetics
  7. Alcohol (chronic abuse)
  8. Marijuana
  9. Danazol
  10. Isoniazid (INH)
C. Pathological causes
  1. Breast tumor   5. Empty sella syndrome
  2. Pituitary tumor   6. Hypothyroidism
  3. Hypothalamic tumor   7. Polycystic ovaries
  4. Infections   8. Benign intraductal papilloma

III. History

A. What the client may present with
   1. Breast discharge
   2. Amenorrhea
   3. Possibly pain
   4. Possibly localized heat and swelling
   5. Possibly, no symptoms (discharge can be an incidental finding of breast exam)
B. Additional information to be considered
   1. Last menstrual period
   2. Sexual activity
   3. Birth control method
   4. Medications or illegal drugs currently being used
   5. Medications recently taken
   6. Recent pregnancy (within 1 year), regardless of outcome
   7. Exercise program, e.g., jogging
   8. Nipple stimulation, e.g., fondling, sucking
   9. Recent trauma to chest or surgery
   10. Description of discharge
   11. Chronic illness, e.g., thyroid disease, psychiatric illness
   12. Lifestyle changes, e.g., increased stress
   13. Alcohol consumption (chronic abuse)
   14. Family history of breast disease
   15. Breast pain or tenderness
   16. Breast surgery: biopsy, reduction, augmentation, implants
   17. Duration of discharge

IV. Physical Examination*

A. Complete examination
   1. Palpate nipple by compressing nipple areola with thumb and index finger, gently milking the subareolar ducts from just outside the apex of the papilla. Repeat in 3 or 4 different directions, noting number of droplets that appear
   2. If discharge is expressed, is it unilateral, bilateral, clear, cloudy, dark, light, milky, bloody, thick, thin

---

* Per breast mass protocol

B. Thyroid: palpate for nodes, size
C. Bimanual examination
1. Ovarian irregularity or enlargement

V. Laboratory Examination
A. Initially on all patients
1. Microscopic examination for fat globules
2. Prolactin level; sample should be drawn between 8 and 10 a.m. (literature indicates prolactin level is lowest between 8 and 10 a.m. but not directly after gynecological examination, intercourse, exercise, or breast stimulation including breast examination)
2. Uterine enlargement
3. Thyroid panel
4. Consider mammogram, ultrasound, MRI with consultation
5. Serum pregnancy test if indicated

VI. Differential Diagnosis
See Etiology

VII. Treatment
As needed according to laboratory report and etiology

VIII. Complications
Individual, according to diagnosis

IX. Consultation/Referral
A. Abnormal lab results
B. Lack of definitive diagnosis
C. Consider referral to breast center, specialist

X. Follow-up
A. If first visit was a consult visit, encourage complete physical
B. Repeat laboratory work as indicated in V.

See Appendix X, Breast Self-examination
See Bibliography 19.

Cervical Aberrations

Papanicolaou (Pap) Smear and Colposcopy

I. Definition

The Papanicolaou (Pap) test examines exfoliated cells from the endocervix to detect pre-invasive lesions (e.g., dysplasia, carcinoma-in-situ) as well as invasive lesions.

II. Screening

A. History
1. DES exposure in utero
2. Smoking: exposure to passive smoke
3. Previous abnormal Papanicolaou smear
4. HPV, other sexually transmitted diseases
5. Sexual practices, partners (number, partner with previous partner with abnormal Pap, partner's sexual history)
6. Family history of cervical cancer
7. Age of beginning sexual activity
8. Immunosuppressive therapy
9. HIV/AIDS or risk

III. Technique

A. Cytologic specimens may be obtained prior to the bimanual pelvic exam; a non-lubricated speculum must be used (speculum can be warmed with water)
B. May do a palpation of the vagina and cervix to locate the cervix and identify the position of the os
C. The cervix and vagina must be fully visible when the smear is obtained in order to see entire squamo columnar junction
D. Vaginal discharge, when present in large amounts, should be carefully removed with a large swab prior to obtaining the smear. The presence of small amount of blood should not preclude cytologic sampling

E. The spatula is applied to the entire cervix to include the entire squamocolumnar junction. In some settings, the handle of the spatula is used to sample the vaginal pool prior to sampling the cervix. A cytobrush is inserted into the endocervix, rotated 1/2 turn, removed, and the material is rolled on a slide. If woman is pregnant, use a cotton-tipped applicator moistened with saline instead of cytobrush. Uniform application of the material to the slide, without clumping, and with immediate fixation (within 10 seconds) to prevent drying, is required

F. For DES-exposed women, additional slides are prepared using smear taken from the upper two-thirds of the vagina at its circumferences. Gentle wiping of the vaginal wall mucosa initially to remove discharge increases the diagnostic accuracy

G. With the Thin Prep Pap Test^{TM}, the sample is collected on a broom-type cervical sampling device. This device then is rinsed in a vial of preserving solution and discarded. The vial is capped, labeled, and sent to the lab. A plastic spatula to sample the portio and cytobrush for the endocervix can be substituted for the broom

IV. Basic Terminology in Reporting Laboratory Findings
Since 1991, a cytology reporting system for cervical/vaginal smears, based on the Bethesda Reporting System developed at the National Cancer Institute, has been used by an increasing number of laboratories. This is the nationally accepted reporting system

A. The 1991 Bethesda System*
  1. Adequacy of the specimen
     Satisfactory for evaluation
     Satisfactory for evaluation but limited by (specify reason)
     Unsatisfactory for evaluation (specify reason)
     General categorization (optional)
  2. Within normal limits
     Benign cellular changes: see descriptive diagnoses
     Epithelial cell abnormalities: see descriptive diagnoses

---

*The next revision will be Bethesda System 2000.
HPV indicates human papillomavirus; CIN, cervical intraepithelial neoplasia; CIS, carcinoma in situ; and NOS, non-organic specific.

Descriptive diagnoses

3. Benign cellular changes
   Infection
   Trichomonas vaginalis
   Fungal organisms morphologically consistent with Candida species
   Predominance of coccobacilli consistent with shift in vaginal flora
   Bacteria morphologically consistent with Actinomyces species
   Cellular changes associated with herpes simplex virus
   Other*

4. Reactive changes
   Reactive cellular changes associated with inflammation (includes typical repair)
   Atrophy with inflammation ("atrophic vaginitis")
   Radiation
   Intrauterine contraceptive device
   Other

5. Epithelial cell abnormalities
   a. Squamous cell
      Atypical squamous cells of undetermined significance (ASCUS): Qualify**
   b. Low-grade squamous intraepithelial lesion (LSIL) encompassing
      HPV*; mild dysplasia/CIN 1
   c. High-grade squamous intraepithelial lesion (HSIL) encompassing moderate and severe dysplasia, CIS/CIN 2 and CIN 3
   d. Squamous cell carcinoma

6. Glandular cell
   a. Endometrial cells, cytologically benign, in a pre-

---

*Cellular changes of HPV previously termed koilocytosis, koilocytotic atypia, or condylomatous atypia are included in the category of low-grade squamous intraepithelial lesion.

**Atypical squamous or glandular cells of undetermined significance should be further qualified, if possible, as to whether a reactive or a premalignant/malignant process is favored.

menopausal woman
   b. Atypical glandular cells of undetermined significance (AGCUS): Qualify (**, page 195)
   c. Endocervical adenocarcinoma
   d. Endometrial adenocarcinoma
   e. Extrauterine adenocarcinoma
   f. Adenocarcinoma, not otherwise specified
7. Other malignant neoplasms: Specify
8. Hormonal evaluation (applies to vaginal smears only) only
   a. Hormonal pattern compatible with age and history.
   b. Hormonal pattern incompatible with age and history: Specify
   c. Hormonal evaluation not possible due to: Specify

V. Guidelines for Further Evaluation

These guidelines are continually evolving. Therefore, they must be viewed as interim and the clinician needs to remain current as changes occur. The following guidelines must be adapted to each clinical practice.

A. Interim guidelines from the National Cancer Institute, (Kurman et al., 1994, see Bibliography 21)

Papanicolaou Smear Diagnosis	Clinical Management
1. Satisfactory for evaluation	No action; repeat Pap smear in 1 year
2. Satisfactory, but limited by:	Test may or may not be repeated based on the clinical situation as determined by clinician
3. Unsatisfactory for diagnosis a. Benign cellular changes	Treat as follows
i. With no specific organism identified	Treat according to individual's history and clinical data
ii. Specific organism identified	Offer testing or treat on Pap diagnosis

b. Reactive and reparative
  i. Inflammation

Evaluate history and cervical data and if no signs and symptoms, use clincal judgement. If cervical data indicate and STD and bacterial vaginosis work-up not done at time of Pap, do now. If cervical data indicate and/or treatment is initiated, then repeat Pap in 6 months. If findings persist, consult with MD or refer

  ii. Atrophy with inflammation

Offer ET/HT (see HT protocol)

  iii. Hyperkeratosis

With cervical abnormality, refer for colposcopy

Epithelial Changes

  i. Atypical squamous cells of undetermined significance (ASCUS)
    ASCUS favors reactive/reparative

Repeat Pap in 4-6 months x 2. If 2 subsequent Paps show ASCUS, then refer for colposcopy

    ASCUS favors
      SIL
      LSIL
      HSIL
      Squamous cell carcinoma

Colposcopy
Colposcopy
Colposcopy
Colposcopy

Glandular Changes

  i. Atypical glandular cells of undetermined etiology (AGCUS)

Colposcopy

  ii. Adenocarcinoma

Refer for evaluation

  iii. Endometrial cells in a post-menopausal woman

Refer for evaluation

B. Guidelines for ASCUS management (American Society for Colposcopy and Cervical Pathology, 1996; Rubin, 1999, see Bibliography 21)

1. Repeat Pap and refer for colposcopy when repeat Pap smear is abnormal (repeat every 4-6 months over 1-2 years until 3 successive completely normal Paps); consider colposcopy when concern for compliance with recommendation for Pap smears, *OR*

2. Colposcopy for all women with ASCUS—consider cost, access to colposcopy, *OR*

3. Manage ASCUS with adjunctive test
   a. HPV test for high-risk types, repeat Pap
      1) HPV positive or repeat abnormal Pap (ASCUS or LGSIL) → colposcopy; if negative repeat Pap q 6 months for 2 years, following appropriately for abnormal Paps
      2) HPV negative, repeat Pap WNL → repeat Pap in 6 months; if repeat Pap ASCUS or LGSIL → colposcopy; negative repeat Pap → annual Paps
   b. Cervigram
      1) Positive cervigram or repeat abnormal Pap → colposcopy → negative → repeat Pap q 6 months x 2 years (only for ASCUS or LGSIL)
      2) Negative cervigram, repeat Pap normal → repeat Pap in 6 months; if normal → annual Pap; if abnormal → colposcopy *OR*

4. Manage ASCUS by subdivision
   a. ASCUS favoring neoplasia → colposcopy → normal, return to annual Pap
   b. ASCUS unqualified → repeat Pap q 4-6 months x 3; if any not normal, colposcopy, and if normal colposcopy, return to annual Pap
   c. ASCUS favoring reactive → repeat Pap of 4-6 months x 3; if not normal, colposcopy, and if normal colposcopy, return to annual Pap
      1) If all 3 normal, return to annual Pap

C. Automated screening systems (Rubin, 1999; see Bibliography 21)

1. AutoPap®—computer driven cytosmear evaluation technique approved by FDA for selection of 10% of Pap smears to be manually rescreened; selects 10% most likely to exhibit abnormalities
   a. Consider offering to patients when available in lab used; can increase cost
2. PAPNET®—computerized system programmed to recognize cellular abnormalities on Pap slides prepared in the conventional way
   a. Consider offering to patients when available; can add to cost of Pap smear

D. Adjunctive screening
   1. Speculoscopy; combines with conventional Pap smear
      a. Pap smear is obtained
      b. Cervix is washed with vinegar solution and then illuminated with a chemiluminescent light attached to the upper blade of the speculum (Speculite®)—assists clinician in visualizing aceto-white areas of cervix

VI. Follow-up for Any Abnormal Papanicolaou Test Finding

A. Follow-up as indicated in V
B. Procedures for follow-up (one example)
   1. If report recommends repeat test or treatment, the client is notified by letter and perhaps by telephone as well; also it may be useful to have a stamp with "Pap letter sent" on it to stamp the lab result sheet, and the nurse practitioner can also sign and date this sheet
   2. A file card is filled out with the client's name and ID number, the nurse practitioner's initials, and the date and results of the test. (File the card under the months of requested repeat). In some settings, a Papanicolaou book is also kept cross-referenced to the card file.*
   3. At the end of each month, the cards are pulled, attached to the client's chart, and given to the nurse practitioner who performed the Papanicolaou smear originally and who is

---

*Increasingly, computers are being used for this function. We recommend that a card system be continued for back-up.

responsible for sending a letter to the client reminding her of the need to repeat the test. (The card should be refiled for the next month.) If the client still has not had a repeat test by the end of the second month, another letter is sent. If the results are less than LSIL, the nurse practitioner's responsibility ends. If results are LSIL or greater at this time, a registered letter with this information is sent to the client. All letters and visits should be documented on charts and file cards.

4. If test results show no abnormal cells but indicate reactive and reparative changes: inflammation, a letter should be sent to the client stating that the laboratory findings for malignancy were negative but that there is evidence of a possible infection, and that an infection check is recommended if no check was done at the time of the Pap. No follow-up letters are necessary; no entries on cards are necessary.

5. Some settings mark the record in some way and indicate that an annual Papanicolaou was done.

VII. Indications for Colposcopy
A. As indicated by Papanicolaou test; algorithm with ASCCP guidelines for ASCUS
B. History of physical examination that revealed possible diethylstilbestrol exposure
C. Any obvious lesions of the cervix
D. Lesions in vagina or vulva that are a diagnostic problem
E. If deemed necessary by physician or nurse practitioner

VIII. Colposcopy Referral Procedure
A. Refer woman to physician of her choice or one available at same setting or to nurse practitioner or nurse midwife (increasingly being trained in colposcopy)
B. Instruct woman that she will probably be billed for procedure, which is generally covered by insurance; make any arrangements possible if she has no insurance
C. When client chooses an outside physician or nurse practitioner or nurse midwife, a signed release form will be sent

with referral sheet so a copy of the referral visit report can be returned to the original facility

IX. Use of Colposcope by Nurse Practitioner
A. Use of colposcopy examination with HPV treatment
   1. A colposcopy examination of vulva, vagina, cervix done on all women found to have vulvar HPV lesions prior to beginning treatment
      a. Vulvar warts: treat according to protocol
      b. Cervical warts: refer to gynecologist or treat per nurse practitioner preparation
   2. Colposcopy examination may be done at each visit. If warts are still present after 8-12 treatments, consult with gynecologist
   3. Colposcopy examination when warts appear to have resolved to verify treatment
B. Use of colposcope as diagnostic tool
   1. Used at discretion of nurse practitioner for closer inspection of vulva, vagina, and/or cervix
C. Procedure for colposcopy examination
   1. Explain procedure to woman
   2. Complete all necessary lab work
   3. Prepare area
      a. Swab entire vulva and vagina with acetic acid (white vinegar), applying generously
   4. Examine with colposcope
   5. Perform any biopsies indicated based on Pap findings

X. Follow-up
Per protocol of setting, based on Papanicolaou findings, colposcopy follow-up protocol; follow-up protocols for other evaluation methods.

AHCPR report on cervical cytology: www.ahcpr.gov/clinic/

Appendix Y contains information about colposcopy which you may wish photocopy or adapt for your clients.

See Bibliographies 20 and 21.

Cervicitis

I. Definition
A. Chronic or acute inflammation of the cervix that is visible to the examiner. Causes symptoms observed by the woman and/or by cytologic examination
B. Mucopurulent cervicitis: characterized by mucopurulent exudate and easily induced cervical bleeding (CDC criteria) for diagnosing indicated below by an asterisk (*)

II. Etiology
A. Bacterial
   1. Neisseria gonorrhoea
   2. Mycoplasmas
   3. Ureaplasmas
   4. Chlamydia trachomatis
B. Viral
   1. Herpes simplex
   2. Human papilloma virus (HPV)
C. Parasitic
   1. Trichomonas vaginalis

III. History
A. What the client may present with
   1. No symptoms
   2. Friable cervix
   3. Post-coital bleeding
   4. Erythema of cervix (*if friable with first pass of swab)
   5. Edematous cervix
   6. Ulcerated or eroded cervix
   7. Hypertrophied cervix
   8. Ectropion
   9. Cervical discharge; may be purulent endocervical exudate on exam*
   10. Vaginal discharge
   11. Leukoplakia on cervix

B. Additional information to be considered
1. Onset of symptoms
2. Partner with symptoms
3. History of sexually transmitted disease
4. Sexual lifestyle; use of sex toys
5. Last Papanicolaou smear and results; any history of abnormal Papanicolaou
6. Contraception past and present
7. Colposcopy, cone biopsy, cauterization of cervix
8. Laceration of cervix
9. Pregnancy history, infertility
10. Dyspareunia, pelvic pain
11. Urinary symptoms: frequency, urgency, dysuria
12. Menstrual history: last menstrual period
13. DES exposure

IV. Physical Examination
A. Cervix
1. Color
2. Character of any discharge: green, yellow, opaque, white, clear, cloudy, purulent, serous, pH
3. Size
4. Lesions
5. Friability
6. Hood
7. Any polyps noted
B. Vagina
1. Color
2. Erythema
3. Lesions
4. Discharge
C. Bimanual exam
1. Masses
2. Tenderness
3. Cervical motion tenderness

    4. Uterine enlargement

    5. Position of organs

D. Adenopathy

V. Laboratory Examination

A. As indicated by findings

    1. Gonorrhea culture

    2. Chlamydia smear

    3. Wet prep: saline, KOH

    4. Papanicolaou smear

    5. Culture for bacteria

    6. Gram stain * > 30 PMN leukocytes

    7. Serology test for syphilis

    8. Herpes culture

    9. Viratyping (usually only available in research settings)

VI. Differential Diagnosis

A. Condyloma acuminata

B. Chlamydia

C. Gonorrhea

D. Cervical cancer

E. Cervical infection: bacterial including mycoplasma, urea-plasma

F. Ectropion

G. Leukoplakia

H. Herpetic exocervicitis

I. Trichomonas

J. Cervical ulceration (erosion) due to trauma: fingernail, cervical biopsy, postpartum, sex toys

K. Pelvic inflammatory disease (PID)

L. Infection secondary to trauma with sex toy

M. Cervical polyp

VII. Treatment

A. Medication

    1. As indicated by organism (see protocols for gonorrhea,

Chlamydia, herpes, condyloma, trichomonas, PID)
2. Bacterial (mycoplasma, ureaplasma): see PID protocol
3. Mucopurulent cervicitis (all women meeting CDC criteria should be treated with: Ceftriaxone 125-150 mg IM single dose plus Doxycycline 100 mg p.o. BID x 7 days)

B. Other measures
 1. Ectropion: evaluate Papanicolaou results and follow-up as indicated; document with diagram and description for later follow-up; with persistent friability: refer or evaluate with colposcopy and biopsy
 2. Leukoplakia: refer or evaluate with colposcopy and biopsy
 3. Cervical cancer: refer for medical evaluation and intervention; in suspected cases in spite of negative Papanicolaou smear, refer or evaluate with colposcopy and biopsy
 4. Cervical ulceration, erosion: follow-up as indicated by extent and nature of trauma; consider referral for medical evaluation and intervention
 5. Consider colposcopy for all women who do not meet CDC guidelines for mucopurulent cervicitis, have a negative STD screen, and negative Papanicolaou

VII. Complications
Progression of condition to secondary or systemic infection (depending on organism) or PID; to metastatic disease; infertility; cervical stenosis

IX. Consultation/Referral
A. Unable to evaluate and diagnose
B. No response to treatment
C. For colposcopy, biopsy

X. Follow-up
A. As indicated by condition and treatment

See Bibliography 14.

Menstrual Disorders

Dysmenorrhea

I. Definition
A. Primary dysmenorrhea is the occurrence of painful menses beginning within several years of menarche and in the absence of any pelvic pathology.
B. Secondary dysmenorrhea is painful menstruation due to an identifiable pathologic or iatrogenic condition, which may be readily identifiable on the basis of the history and the findings in a physical examination.

II. Etiology
A. Primary dysmenorrhea
   1. Caused by prostaglandins produced in the uterine lining and released into the bloodstream as the lining is shed, causing smooth muscle contraction, nausea, and/or diarrhea
B. Secondary dysmenorrhea
   1. Extrauterine causes
      a. Endometriosis
      b. Tumors
         1) Subserosal leiomyomata
         2) Malignancies
         3) Pelvic tumors
      c. Ovarian cysts
      d. Pelvic inflammatory disease
   2. Intrauterine causes
      a. Adenomyosis
      b. Endometriosis
      c. Intramural leiomyomata

   d. Polyps
     1) Endometrial   2) Cervical
   e. Presence of an intrauterine device
   f. Cervical stenosis

III. History
A. What the client may present with
  1. Recurrent pain monthly, prior to menses, sometimes with menses
    a. Abdominal pain
    b. Pelvic pain
    c. Severe backache
  2. Nausea; diarrhea or constipation
  3. Weakness
  4. Dizziness
  5. Weight gain
  6. Breast tenderness
  7. Backache
  8. Tension and nervousness
  9. Irritability and depression
B. Additional information to be obtained by asking the following questions:
  1. Relationship to menarche
  2. When does pain begin
  3. How long does it last
  4. Does anything make it feel better
  5. Last menstrual period
  6. Birth control method used
  7. Any relationship to intercourse
  8. Any vaginal discharge
  9. Any fever related to pain
  10. What is menstrual flow like
  11. Is this new; is this a change in pattern
  12. Sensitivity to aspirin
  13. History of chronic illness (kidney disease)
  14. Current medications (prescription and over-the-counter)
  15. Postcoital bleeding
  16. Home remedies and/or folk remedies tried

IV. Physical Examination

A. Vital signs
   1. Blood pressure
   2. Pulse
   3. Temperature, if symptoms are present at time of visit
   4. Weight
B. Vaginal examination (speculum): cervix, cervical pathology
C. Bimanual examination

V. Laboratory Examination

   1. Chlamydia (if not done within 1 year or woman has a new sexual partner), or cervical picture indicates, or if severity of symptoms has increased
   2. Gonorrhea culture (same as Chlamydia)

VI. Differential Diagnosis

See Etiology

VII. Treatment

A. Medication
   1. Ibuprofen (Motrin®) 400 mg, 1 QID
   2. Mefenamic acid (Ponstel®) 250 mg, 2 stat and 1 q 6○
   3. Naproxen (Anaprox®) 275 mg, 2 stat and 1 q 6-8○ (no more than 5 tabs per day)
   4. Anaprox DS® 550 mg =1 q 12 hours
   5. Aspirin with codeine gr ½ 1-2 tabs q 4○ prn
   6. Ibuprofen (Advil®) 200 mg, 2 tabs QID (OTC), or
   7. Flurbiprofen (Ansaid) 100 mg p.o. bid or tid
   8. Meclofenamate (Meclomen®) 1 tab (100 mg) q 6° prn
   9. Other OTC analogue
   10. Oral contraceptive (to produce anovulatory state)
B. Other measures
   1. Reassurance
   2. Refer to premenstrual syndrome protocols for diet, exercise, and vitamin recommendations
   3. Heating pad

VIII. Complications
May occur with failure to recognize presence of entity as described in differential diagnosis which results in lack of appropriate treatment

IX. Consultation/Referral
A. Diagnosis of secondary dysmenorrhea
B. Failure to improve after treatment as in VII. above

X. Follow-up
A. Yearly health examination and Papanicolaou smear
B. Serology test for syphilis as symptoms indicate
C. Secondary dysmenorrhea follow-up as indicated by physician or with consult

See Bibliography 22.

Amenorrhea

I. Definition
A. Primary amenorrhea: failure of the menses to occur at puberty
B. Secondary amenorrhea: cessation of the menses for a woman who has established menses for at least 3 cycles

II. Etiology for Secondary Amenorrhea
A. Pregnancy
B. Pituitary tumor
C. Menopause
D. Too little body fat (about 22% required for menses)
E. Excessive exercise (e.g., long-distance running or ballet dancing)
F. Rapid weight loss
G. Cessation of menstruation following use of oral contraceptives, Depo-Provera, Norplant
H. Recent change in lifestyle (e.g., increase in stress)
I. Thyroid disease
J. Polycystic ovary syndrome

K. Anorexia nervosa or other eating disorders
L. Premature ovarian failure, ovarian dysgenesis, infection, hemorrhage, necrosis, neoplasm
M. Asherman's syndrome
N. Absence of hypothalamic hormones
O. Cervical stenosis

III. History
A. What the client presents with
1. Absence of menstruation
2. Possible breast discharge
3. Other symptoms secondary to underlying etiology
B. Additional information to be considered
1. Careful menstrual history; pregnancy history
2. Sexual history
3. Contraceptive history
4. Medications—OTC, prescription, homeopathic
5. Sources of emotional stress
6. Symptoms of climacteric
7. Any current acute illness
8. History of chronic illness
9. Present weight, weight 1 year ago
10. Amount of daily exercise
11. Recent D&C or abortion
12. History of tuberculosis

IV. Physical Examination
A. Weigh patient
B. Neck: thyroid gland (look for nodes: palpable, enlarged)
C. Breast: discharge
1. Check both breasts
2. Milky, clear, dark, light, bloody, thick, thin
D. Vaginal examination (speculum): vagina may be atrophic and there may be no cervical mucus
E. Bimanual examination
1. Uterus: may be enlarged
2. Cervix—scarring, stenosis
3. Adnexa: ovaries may be enlarged—cystic

4. Recto-vaginal examination
F. Measure ratio of body far to lean mass

V. Laboratory Examination
A. Human chorionic gonadotropin (HCG) qualitative, quantitative
B. Prolactin level
C. Thyroid stimulating hormone
D. Follicle stimulating hormone, luteinizing hormone, Dehydroepiandrosterone sulfate (DHEAS), and serum testosterone (if patient is hirsute)
E. Papanicolaou smear
F. Microscopic examination of cervical mucus
G. TB test if no history
H. Consider pituitary function assessment, CAT scan, MRI after consultation with a physician
I. GnRH stimulation test

VI. Differential Diagnosis
See Etiology

VII. Treatment
A. If breast discharge is present, do not wait: do work-up as per breast discharge protocol
B. If human chorionic gonadotropin (HCG) and prolactin levels are within normal limits, pregnancy test is negative and cervical mucus positive (ferning), the nurse practitioner may give: Medroxyprogesterone acetate (Provera®) 10 mg x 5-10 days
   1. If no withdrawal bleed in 3-7 days after progestin, do follicle stimulating hormone and luteinizing hormone assays 2 weeks after Provera. Try oral estrogen to prime the endometrium (estropipate) for 21 days; if no bleeding, add progestin during third week of estrogen. If no withdrawal bleed, refer to physician
   2. If woman wishes to start oral contraceptives and has no withdrawal bleed from Provera, repeat HCG if indicated and start oral contraceptives the following Sunday regard-

less of brand of oral contraceptive used. If no withdrawal bleed after first cycle, consult with physician
3. If woman wishes to start oral contraceptives and has withdrawal bleed from Provera, start oral contraceptives after start of bleed; if Provera is not completed by that time, discontinue and discard remainder (some providers have woman complete Provera)
4. If withdrawal bleed occurs with Provera, then no menses for 2 months following the bleed, possible consult with physician, then give Provera 10 mg x 10 days every 2 months. If sexually active, an HCG must be run prior to taking medication each time
5. If woman has a history of uterine infection or trauma to the uterus through multiple curettages (postpartum or postabortion), or if the work-up is negative and there is no response to Provera, referral for further evaluation (hysterosalpingography; hysteroscopy to lyse adhesions; estrogen to restore endometrium)
6. Instruct woman to complete 10 days of Provera even if withdrawal bleed begins, unless starting oral contraceptives as 3 above

VIII. Complications
Inability to conceive
Sequelae of underlying cause

IX. Consultation/Referral
A. As outlined under Treatment VII.B.5
B. After work-up for hirsutism is completed (see V.D.)
C. For all primary amenorrhea cases

X. Follow-up
A. As deemed necessary with physician consult
B. Yearly
C. Every 6 months; if taking Provera, every 2 months

See Bibliography 22.

Abnormal Vaginal Bleeding

I. Definition
Any variation from a woman's usual menstrual pattern

II. Etiology
A. Systemic illnesses, i.e., thyroid disease, blood dyscrasias, adrenal imbalance
B. Submucous leiomyomata in uterus; polyps, liver disease, clotting disorders, kidney disease, leukemia
C. Tumor in vagina, uterus
D. Trauma to vagina, cervix; scar tissue
E. Cervical lesions
   1. Polyps
   2. Carcinoma
F. Abnormal hormone secretion (with anovulatory bleeding)
G. Change in ovarian function (peri-menopause)
H. Endometrial polyps or leiomyomata in cervix, uterus
I. Pelvic malignancy—nodes, uterus, bladder, rectum, vagina
J. Ectopic pregnancy
K. Abortion
L. Placental accidents
M. Hyperplasia
N. Stress
O. Postmenopausal bleed
P. Pharmacotherapeutics
Q. STDs, PID
R. Endometriosis/adenomyosis

III. History
A. What the client may present with
   1. Mid-cycle bleeding
   2. Spotting
   3. Pain
   4. Sudden onset of heavy bleeding
   5. Postmenopausal bleeding

B. Additional information to be considered
   1. Is bleeding recent or since menarche
   2. Onset of bleeding
   3. Amount of flow (pads per hour); clots and size of clots
   4. Normal bleeding pattern: how does this episode differ from normal menstruation
   5. Current or recent use of medication
   6. Last menstrual period; previous menstrual period
   7. Last sexual contact, if sexually active
   8. Birth control method(s)
   9. Recent trauma to pelvic area or any other part of body
   10. Characteristics of present bleeding: clots, tissue
   11. Any related pain
   12. Any fever
   13. Any dizziness; syncope
   14. Symptoms of changing ovarian function (menopausal)

IV. Physical Examination
A. Vital signs
   1. Blood pressure
   2. Pulse
   3. Temperature
B. Skin: examine for evidence of bleeding disorder, e.g., petechiae or ecchymosis; pallor; fine, thinning hair
C. Neck—thyroid: examine for enlargement, palpate nodes
D. Breasts
   1. Development
   2. Masses
   3. Tenderness
E. Abdomen
   1. Tenderness
   2. Guarding
   3. Bowel sounds
   4. Distension
   5. Hepatosplenomegaly
F. Genital examination: Observe perineum for trauma
G. Vaginal examination (speculum)
   1. Observe vaginal walls for lesions or evidence of trauma

    2. Observe cervix for
       a. Polyps
       b. Lesions (evidence of trauma)
       c. Erosion or ectropion
       d. Whether os is closed or dilated; discharge in os
    3. Evaluate amount and type of bleeding
  H. Bimanual examination
    1. Uterus: evaluate size, shape, position, any pain
    2. Adnexa: evaluate for possible mass, pain
    3. Recto-vaginal exam
       a. Fullness (fluid)
       b. Pain
       c. Bleeding

V. Laboratory Examination (will depend on history and assessment of bleeding)
A. Complete blood count, differential with hematocrit or hemoglobin; platelet count
B. Serum pregnancy test
C. Gonococcal culture
D. Chlamydia smear
E. Thyroid studies if indicated
F. Hormone levels
G. Urinalysis
H. STD screen

VI. Differential Diagnosis
See Etiology

VII. Treatment
A. For light flow/regular/irregular bleeding (e.g., mid-cycle)
    1. Lab work as history demands
    2. May observe 2-3 months as indicated by history and physical findings. Woman should be instructed to keep record of days that bleeding occurs.
    3. After 2-3 cycles, after normal physical exam and Papanicolaou smear with appropriate lab work, consider
       a. Provera 10 mg qd x 10 days or

  b. Monophasic OC x 1-3 months or 6-12 months
B. For heavy bleeding
 1. Consult/refer to physician after appropriate work-up
C. For bleeding with IUD in place see IUD protocol
D. For bleeding associated with Norplant®, consider addition of low dose oral contraceptive x 3 cycles or Premarin 1.25 mg qd until bleeding stops
E. For heavy bleeding with Depo-Provera*, consider same regimen as in D. above
F. If bleeding persists with a positive HCG
 1. Physician consultation
 2. Referral as indicated
G. If bleeding postmenopausal will need an endometrial biopsy (see Endometrial Biopsy protocol)

VIII. Complications
A. Severe hemorrhage
B. Shock
C. Of underlying systemic illnesses

IX. Consultation/Referral
A. After completion of all laboratory work and physical examination, nurse practitioner may consult with physician
B. Immediate referral to physician if excessive bleeding after laboratory work and work-up by nurse practitioner

X. Follow-up
As indicated by diagnosis and treatment

 See Bibliography 22.

---

 * Approach this regimen with caution remembering that menstrual changes are recognized as an early phenomenon with progestin-only contraception, decreasing with prolonged use. Also, if client is a long-term user, the onset of new bleeding may indicate underlying pathology.

Endometrial Biopsy

I. Definition
Endometrial biopsy is a method of obtaining a sample of the nonpregnant uterine lining for purposes of cytologic and histologic examination. The procedure can be done in an ambulatory setting with or without local anesthesia. The specimen obtained is glandular epithelium.

II. Etiology
Reasons for performing this diagnostic procedure may include:
A. Unexplained abnormal vaginal bleeding in the premenstrual, perimenstrual, or postmenstrual woman
B. Rule out endometrial pathology prior to initiation of hormone therapy (HT) in the postmenopausal woman and periodically monitor endometrial status with unopposed estrogen use
C. Determine response of the endometrium to hormonal intervention in women experiencing infertility
D. Evaluate endometrial response during tamoxifen therapy to rule out pathologic response

III. History
A. What the client may present with
   1. Postmenopausal bleeding
   2. Unexplained abnormal vaginal bleeding in a premenopausal woman
   3. Desire for hormone therapy
   4. Currently taking hormone therapy with intact uterus
   5. Unsuccessful attempts at pregnancy
   6. Current tamoxifen therapy for breast disease
B. Additional information to be considered
   1. Hormone therapy: type, purpose, duration, dosage, side effects, bleeding history
   2. Gynecologic and pregnancy including STD and PID episodes; elective abortions
   3. Gynecologic surgery including previous endometrial biopsies and results

4. Medical conditions: cardiac, bleeding disorders, hypo-glycemia
5. Current medications including over-the-counter and botanical preparations
6. Allergies to pharmacologics including local anesthetic agents and povidone-iodine (Betadine, similar products)
7. Vasovagal episodes especially with pelvic examinations, uterine sounding, IUD insertion, elective abortion
8. Symptoms of vaginitis, cervicitis, STD, PID
9. Contraceptive methods including current method and consistency of use; any recent exposure to pregnancy risk and date
10. Menstrual cycles, peri- and postmenopausal bleeding; LMP, PMP

IV. Physical Examination

A. Bimanual examination: uterine position, pain, flexion, size, shape; adnexal or uterine masses, cervical motion tenderness, adnexal exam; any pelvic pain, determine involution if woman is postpartum, postabortion
B. Recto-vaginal examination to determine uterine size, position, rule out pregnancy
C. Vital signs: blood pressure, temperature (rule out fever)
D. General status: last meal or snack, fluids (rule out hypoglycemia); offer juice, snack
E. Administer mild prostaglandin inhibitor 20 minutes before biopsy
F. Teach woman about the procedure and possible complications, and obtain her consent to proceed

V. Reasons to Defer Procedure

A. Pregnancy or possible pregnancy
B. PID, STD with PID as complication, cervicitis
C. Poor involution of uterus postpartum or postabortion
D. Heart murmur, rheumatic heart disease (may consult prior to procedure, prophylactic antibiotics, usually oral ampicillin 2 grams 1 hour before procedure. Consult if penicillin allergic)
E. Fever

F. Blood dyscrasias, especially bleeding disorders, severe anemia
G. Extremely anteflexed or retroflexed uterus or cervical stenosis—may need to do biopsy under general anesthesia
H. Vaginitis—defer procedure until diagnosis and treatment regimen completed

VI. Laboratory
A. Pregnancy test
B. Hematocrit as indicated
C. Post-procedure biopsy specimen(s) for histologic screening

VII. Biopsy Technique
A. Collect any routine specimens, cultures as indicated; bimanual exam to determine position of uterus
B. Visualize the cervix and inspect for any mucopurulent discharge, visual signs of cervicitis; if found, defer procedure to collect any additional specimens and treat
C. Cleanse cervix and vagina with antiseptic, considering any sensitivities, allergies
D. Administer local anesthetic agent to the cervix (lidocaine gels, other topical gel or spray products, or paracervical block) if necessary/desired depending on sampling technique and equipment to be used
E. Sound the uterus (if using curette for sampling); prior to this, grasping the cervix with a fine tenaculum is necessary (using local anesthetic gel at the site for tenaculum placement reduces pain for the woman). Having the patient cough when applying and removing the tenaculum often reduces discomfort
F. Insert the sampling device* in the os, taking care not to force the device through a resistant os; if the os is stenotic, cervical dilators may be used. Use one of the following techniques:
   1. Pipelle device (flexible sampler with a piston to create suction for sampling): insert up to fundus, pull back completely on the piston to create suction and rotate the pipelle continuously moving it from the fundus and back again

---

*These include Pipelle®, Gyno Sampler®, Novak Curette®, Tis-u-trap®, Vabra aspirator®.

several times to collect the sample completely filling the plastic tube; withdraw the pipelle and push in the piston to deposit sample into the preservative. Some devices require cutting off the tip to expel the specimen

2. Pipelle device attached to suction pump: insert as above and collect specimen by connecting the external pump, continuing suction until the device is filled
3. Suction curette that is steel and reusable or plastic and disposable: sound the uterus stabilizing the cervix with a tenaculum and then insert the curette and gently sample in a manner similar to using the pipelle devices (some are attached to a 10 cc syringe to provide the suction and some to an external pump); withdraw the curette, deposit the specimen in the preservative

G. Monitor woman's condition during and after the procedure to assess for vasovagal response, signs and symptoms of uterine perforation
H. Allow woman to rest briefly with her legs flat before getting off the examination table. Assure that she is not feeling faint and is able to get dressed safely
I. Instruct woman regarding post-procedure care
   1. Signs and symptoms of complications: severe cramping or pelvic pain; bright red bleeding with or without clots; fever, chills, foul-smelling vaginal discharge—call provider and/or go to urgent care setting
   2. Expect spotting for 1-2 days after the biopsy; define spotting and the difference between spotting and bleeding
   3. Patient may resume vaginal intercourse in 3 days or whenever she desires
   4. Prophylactic antibiotic regimen if necessary
   5. Prostaglandin inhibitor for mild cramping
   6. Resumption of menses if premenopausal and having menstrual cycles

VIII. Referral//Consultation for Procedure

A. Women with severe cervical stenosis to consider procedure under general anesthesia
B. Women with a heart murmur and/or history of rheumatic fever

for possible antibiotic prophylaxis
C. Women with contraindications for procedure

IX. Follow-up
A. Arrange for an opportunity to review laboratory findings
B. Care based on reason for endometrial biopsy and laboratory results

X. Referral/Consultation for Results
A. Endometrial carcinoma—referral for treatment or co-management
B. Hyperplasia without atypia—usually means atrophic changes
   1. Secretory: follow but no need for treatment unless bleeding persists and consider Provera
   2. Proliferative may benefit from Provera
C. Complex hyperplasia without atypia
   1. Desires pregnancy: consider risks and co-manage with physician
   2. Does not desire pregnancy: to remove unopposed estrogen, cycle with progestins and repeat endometrial biopsy in 3-6 months
D. Complex hyperplasia with atypia—referral for D&C
   1. Co-management for pregnancy if desired and no malignancy or for surgical high risk
   2. Surgery and/or treatment per staging if malignant
   3. Hysterectomy if nonmalignant and no pregnancy desired

See Bibliography 22.

Premenstrual Syndrome (PMS)*

I. Definition
PMS (premenstrual syndrome, also known as premenstrual tension, PMT) is a cluster of physical, emotional, and behavioral symptoms related to the menstrual cycle, developing or worsen-

---

* Known as periluteal phase dysphoric disorder in DSM-IV diagnosis

ing during the luteal phase and clearing with the onset of the menstrual flow.

II. Etiology
No single etiology explains the various symptoms associated with PMS. A multifactorial cause is probable, involving psychosocial, genetic, hormonal, and neurotransmitter components (serotonergic dysfunction)

III. History
A. What the client presents with (may include some or all of the following symptoms, in varying degrees)
   1. Headache, backache, migraine, syncope
   2. Edema
   3. Breast tenderness, engorgement, enlargement, heaviness
   4. Hot flashes
   5. Paresthesia of hands or feet, aggravation of epilepsy
   6. Weight gain
   7. Fluid retention
   8. Abdominal bloating
   9. Increase in appetite and/or impulsive eating; craving for sweets and/or salt; food cravings in general
   10. Nausea, vomiting, constipation
   11. Decreased urine output, cystitis, urethritis, enuresis
   12. Exacerbation or recurrence of acne, boils, urticaria, easy bruising, herpes, rhinitis, colds, hoarseness, increased asthma, sore throat, sinusitis
   13. Emotional lability (anxiety, depression, crying, fatigue, aggression, irritability), difficulty in concentrating
   14. Changes in libido
   15. Lethargy, fatigue
   16. Sleep disturbances
   17. Palpitations
   18. Any symptoms, physical or emotional, that cluster during the same phase of menstrual cycle
B. Additional information to be considered
   1. When did these symptoms first occur in relationship to menarche

2. When do they begin and end in relationship to menses
3. Has there been a recent change in symptoms
4. Do you have cramps with your period
5. Has there been any change in your lifestyle (work, personal, family)
6. What is your diet like
7. How much exercise do you get
8. Are you or have you ever been in counseling
9. What medications are you taking
10. Do you have a history of chronic illness; if so, which
11. When was your last menstrual period
12. When was your last sexual contact (if sexually active)
13. What birth control method do you use
14. Have you had tubal ligation and if so, when
15. Have you ever thought about suicide or harm to others
16. Have you experienced depression or agitation at other times in your life

IV. Physical Examination
A. Vital signs
B. Complete physical examination
C. Mental status examination

V. Laboratory Examination
A. Only as indicated medically   B. Papanicolaou smear

VI. Treatment
A. Treatment is multifaceted and diverse, aimed at symptoms which client finds most debilitating. To aid in diagnosis and treatment, 2 months of retrospective daily logs help to confirm diagnosis and guide selection of appropriate treatment
1. Vitamin B_6 (pyridoxine). Begin with 50 mg to 100 mg total daily dose. Do not exceed recommended dosage. This vitamin has been shown to be toxic in large doses.
2. Vitamin E 400 mg daily or twice a day
3. Evening Primrose Oil. Begin with 2 capsules twice a day. May increase to 4 capsules twice a day. Improvement will occur slowly over 3-9 months. Contains vita-

min E, so client should not take both

4. Prostaglandin inhibitors may provide relief taken during the second half of the menstrual cycle
5. May consider:
   a. Ovulation blockers (birth control pills)
   b. Diuretics
   c. Antidepressants
   d. Antianxiety drugs
   e. Progesterone (synthesized, natural)
6. Calcium 1000 mg daily; magnesium 360 mg daily

B. General measures*
   1. Lifestyle changes including stress reduction, i.e., meditation yoga, or other relaxation techniques
   2. Diet recommendations
      a. Limit consumption of refined sugar (e.g., cookies, cakes, jelly, honey) to 5 tbs/day
      b. Limit salt intake to 3 gm or less per day (e.g., avoid using salt shaker)
      c. Limit intake of alcohol and nicotine
      d. Avoid caffeine (e.g., coffee, tea, chocolate, soft drinks)
      e. Increase intake of complex carbohydrates (e.g., fresh fruits, vegetables, whole grains, pasta, rice, potatoes)
      f. Consume moderate amounts of protein and fat (decease animal fats and increase vegetable oils)
      g. Limit red meat consumption to 2 x weekly or less
      These dietary changes should be ongoing. It is not enough to modify one's diet only on the days prior to menstruation
   3. Exercise plan recommendations: exercise three times per week for 30-40 minutes (brisk walking, jogging, aerobic dancing, swimming)
   4. Consider other complementary therapies including botanicals, aroma and music therapy, acupuncture, and

---

*A number of commercial products for PMS exist including: Ultravite PMS™, Lydia's Secret, PMS Escape, Aphrodite, the LightMask, Pro-Gest, and the His and Hers PMS Calendar. Evaluating these is helpful in answering patients' questions.

energy healing
5. Keep a diary of daily symptoms, diet, body temperature

VII. Differential Diagnosis
A. Sexual dysfunction
B. Chronic pelvic pain
C. Endometriosis
D. Primary dysmenorrhea
E. Post-tubal ligation syndrome
F. Prolactin-producing tumors
G. Perimenopausal symptoms
H. Fibrocystic breast disease
I. Depression
J. Psychopathology
K. Somatization of stress
L. Life stressors
M. Systemic lupus erythematosus
N. Hypertension
O. Meningioma
P. Attention-deficit disorder (residual type)

VIII. Complications
A. Serious psychological problem misdiagnosed as PMS
B. Systemic disease misdiagnosed as premenstrual syndrome

IX. Consultation/Referral
A. Referral to physician at discretion of nurse practitioner, after review of history and physical examination
B. Mental health referral if appropriate
C. Referral to nutritionist if needed/desired by woman
D. Support group referral if desired

X. Follow-up
A. Monthly x 3 checks
B. Yearly if improvement in relief of symptoms
C. If symptoms increase or change

See Appendix Z and Bibliography 22.

Post-Abortion Care

Examination after Normal Abortion

I. Definition
An examination two weeks after uncomplicated therapeutic abortion to assess the client's physical and mental status.

II. Etiology
Therapeutic abortion

III. History
A. What the client may present with
   No unusual complaints
B. Additional information to be considered
   1. Date of abortion; type of procedure
   2. Date of last menstrual period
   3. Are pregnancy symptoms gone
   4. How long after procedure did bleeding continue; any pain associated with bleeding; how much bleeding; any clots; fever
   5. Results of pathological examination of products of conception (if available)
   6. Any change in relationship with partner
   7. Present emotional status
   8. Birth control method
   9. Intercourse since procedure
   10. Medications taken including antibiotics, oxytocins

IV. Physical Examination
A. Vital signs: blood pressure, pulse
B. Abdominal examination
C. Vaginal examination (speculum)
   1. Observe for bleeding or other discharge

   2. Cervix
       a. Os closed   b. Any lesions   c.   Any discharge
D. Bimanual exam
   1. Uterus
       a. Size   b. Consistency   c.   Tenderness
       d. Cervix: positive Chandelier's sign (cervical motion
          tenderness)
   2. Adnexa
       a. Tenderness
       b. Masses
   3. Rectovaginal: any abnormal findings

V. Treatment
A. Birth control
   1. Birth control pill, Depo-Provera®
   2. Diaphragm, cap
   3. Intrauterine device, hormonal (Norplant®) implants
   4. Other methods (OTC): condoms, spermicides
   5. Sterilization (if desired)
B. General measures: review use and sign informed consent
   form for birth control method (see Appendixes E, F, G, and
   H)

VI. Laboratory Examination
A. Pregnancy test as indicated
B. Wet mount as indicated

VII. Differential Diagnosis
None

VIII. Complications
See Post-Abortion with Complications, pages 228-230

IX. Consultation/Referral
A. See Post-Abortion with Complications, pages 228-230
B. If unresolved issues are apparent, follow-up counseling will
   be recommended

X. Follow-up
A. Yearly for health examination, Papanicolaou smear, reevaluation of family planning needs
B. As per protocol for contraceptive of woman's choice

See Appendix AA and Bibliography 24.

Post-Abortion with Complications

I. Definition
Any sequelae or unexpected/untoward events or conditions following a therapeutic abortion.

II. Etiology
Therapeutic abortion

III. History
A. What the client may present with
 1. Fever, body aches, chills
 2. Pelvic main, severe cramps
 3. Bleeding; more than 1 pad an hour
 4. Passing clots larger than a quarter
 5. Abdominal pain: R or L side or bilateral; onset, duration, how relieved
 6. Nausea, vomiting
 7. Breast tenderness, discharge
 8. Foul vaginal discharge
 9. Vertigo
B. Additional information to be considered
 1. Where and when was the procedure done; has the woman spoken to that facility regarding her symptoms or follow-up care; what procedure was done
 2. How much physical activity since procedure, type
 3. Any intercourse since procedure
 4. Anything used in vagina since procedure: contraceptive device; tampons; sex toy; douche product
 5. Any exposure to flu or anyone with similar symptoms

6. Any medications taken such as analgesics, ergotrate, antibiotics, over-the-counter or prescription drugs
7. Urinary tract symptoms
8. Bowel symptoms
9. Still feels pregnant; symptoms of pregnancy

IV. Physical Examination
A. Vital signs
1. Temperature   2. Pulse
3. Blood pressure   4. Respirations
B. Breast examination: tender/more/less/same as before procedure (if indicated); discharge
C. Abdomen
1. Bowel signs
2. Guarding
3. Rebound tenderness
4. Referred pain (shoulder pain)
D. Vaginal examination (sterile if within 1 week after procedure):
1. Os dilated
2. Any tissue in os
3. Amount of bleeding; character
4. Any discharge present; odor
E. Bimanual examination
1. Cervical motion tenderness: positive Chandelier's sign
2. Uterine tenderness, enlargement; note consistency
3. Adnexa
   a. Tenderness   b. Mass   c. Fullness
4. Rectovaginal examination: tenderness; if present, describe location

V. Laboratory Examination
A. Serum pregnancy test—quantitative
B. Gonococcal culture
C. Chlamydia smear
D. Cervical culture
E. Complete blood count with differential, sedimentation rate
F. Urinalysis and urine culture

G. Call laboratory of referring facility to get results of pathology report

VI. Differential Diagnosis
A. Retained secundae; continuation of pregnancy
B. Uterine infection, endometritis
C. Delayed involution
D. Pelvic inflammatory disease
E. Urinary tract infection
F. Uterine perforation, bowel perforation
G. Ectopic pregnancy
H. See Acute Pelvic Pain and Abdominal Pain protocols

VII. Treatment
As indicated by symptoms and diagnosis; may include appropriate antibiotics, treatment of any urinary infection, ergotrate product to promote involution; re-evacuation; referral for evaluation of possible ectopic pregnancy (see Pelvic Inflammatory Disease protocol and Genitourinary Tract [Urinary Tract Infection] protocol)

VIII. Complications
A. Sepsis
B. Ruptured ectopic pregnancy
C. Hemorrhage
D. Uterine perforation, bowel perforation
E. Ascherman's syndrome

IX. Consultation/Referral
Call facility or provider that performed the abortion for a consult and arrangement for return visit and further evaluation

X. Follow-up
Follow routine post-abortion protocol

See Appendix AA and Bibliography 24.

Abuse, Battering, Violence, and Sexual Assault

Abuse Assessment Screen*,**

CONDUCT THIS SCREENING WITH THE WOMAN ALONE IN A PRIVATE SETTING

Inform her that
Since 1 in 6 pregnant women are abused, all women are being asked about risks at home
This information will not be shared without her permission

1. Have you EVER been emotionally or physically abused by
your partner or someone important to you?   YES NO

2. WITHIN THE LAST YEAR, have you been pushed, shoved,
hit, slapped, kicked or otherwise physically hurt by someone?   YES NO

    If YES, by whom? _____
    Total number of times _____

3. SINCE YOU'VE BEEN PREGNANT, were you pushed, shoved,
hit, slapped, kicked or otherwise physically hurt by someone?   YES NO

    If YES, by whom? _____
    Total number of times _____

Mark the areas of injury on the body map.
Score each incident according to the following scale:
1 = Threats of abuse, including use of a weapon
2 = Slapping, pushing; no injuries and/or lasting pain
3 = Punching, kicking, bruises, cuts, and/or continuing pain
4 = Beaten up, severe contusions, burns, broken bones
5 = Head injury, internal injury, permanent injury
6 = Use of weapon; wound from weapon

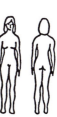

(If any of the descriptions for the higher number apply, use the higher number)

4. WITHIN THE LAST YEAR, has anyone forced you to have
sexual activities?   YES NO

    IF YES, who? _____
    Total number of times _____

5. ARE YOU AFRAID of your partner or anyone in your life?   YES NO

---

    *You can use the Abuse Assessment Screen with all women by deleting the pregnancy question.
    **Developed by the Nursing Research Consortium on Violence and Abuse. Readers are encouraged to reproduce and use this assessment tool. Adapted by Pregnancy Support Project, Boston College School of Nursing.

Assessment for Abuse and/or Violence*

I. Definition

Abuse and/or violence in a relationship is said to occur when one person physically, sexually, verbally and/or emotionally abuses another and/or destroys the property of the person. Experiencing fear for one's person in a relationship is characteristic of an abusive situation, regardless of whether or not there is physical violence. Fearing physical harm is enough to consider the relationship abusive. Power or control by one person over another in a relationship can constitute abuse; power and control in a relationship are hallmarks of abuse. Dating violence affects an estimated 1.8 adolescents and domestic violence, 1:4 to 1:10 women.

II. History: Consider each woman in any setting abused until proven otherwise

A. What the client may present with
1. Description of abuse or violence in the relationship
2. Unexplained symptoms inconsistent with any disease pathology
3. Numerous psychosomatic complaints with no physical evidence
4. Vague physical complaints
5. The woman's partner gives history and answers questions directed toward woman
6. Delay between presenting injury or problem and seeking care
7. Woman seems embarrassed or evasive in giving history
8. Woman seems fearful, withdrawn, does not name friends, family members as resources

---

*Kathleen K. Furniss, RNC, MSN, a consultant for this protocol, suggests asking 2 or 3 simple questions and varying the query for the clinical situation, e.g., "Is someone physically hurting you?" Kathleen is author of many articles on abuse and is a founder of the Jersey Battered Women's Service and a principal in the Domestic Violence Prevention Project, St. Barnabas Medical Center, Livingston, NJ

B. Additional information to be considered (see questions on previous protocol)
   1. Psychiatric, alcohol, and/or drug abuse by patient and/or partner
   2. Suicide gestures or attempts; suicidal ideation
   3. Many "accidents" in record, visits to emergency department
   4. Any gynecologic or gastrointestinal complaints
   5. Level of anxiety the woman demonstrates over the visit or the physical exam

III. Physical Examination

A. Unexplained bruises; whip-like injuries consistent with shaking; erythematous areas consistent with slapping; lacerations, burn marks, fractures, and/or multiple injuries in various stages of healing
B. Injuries on body hidden by clothing and injuries inconsistent with common accidents such as on the genitals, breasts, chest, head, face, and abdomen
C. Evidence of sexual abuse—lacerations on breasts, labia, urethra, perineum, anal area
D. Healed fractures or scars
E. Fractures inconsistent with story of accident
F. Apprehensive during examination and injuries and other findings are inappropriate to her story or inexplicable

IV. Laboratory Examination

A. As indicated by physical findings
B. May include x-rays for evidence of new, healing, or old fractures

V. Interviewing the Woman

A. Provide a safe place alone and private where partner/spouse/abuser cannot hear
B. Assure her of confidentiality and safety
C. Phrase questions in a non-threatening way conveying empathy such as: "I notice you have some bruises. Can you tell me how they happened? Have you been hit by someone?" (see

also questions on Abuse Assessment Screen on page *231*

D.   Assess for current danger and for emotional and/or physical injuries (see Danger Assessment tool in Appendix N)

E.   Ask what the woman's assessment is of her current danger

VI. Documenting Evidence

A.   Data from medical records and those of other health care providers

B.   Record most recent, as well as past incidents

C.   Record any witnesses to abuse

D.   Quote the woman's statements of abuse with, "Patient states . . ."

E.   Protect patient by deleting any statements such as, "He hurt me so much I wanted to kill him"

F.   If woman denies any abuse, record your assessment and suspicions for possible future use

G.   Record any injuries or symptoms in detail as to size, location, duration, onset, age, pattern. Make a body map and locate injuries in as much detail as you can. Indicate any evidence of sexual abuse, restraint marks on skin

H.   Collect physical evidence of injuries and label after obtaining with the woman's written permission to do so

I.   Photograph all evidence of injuries with the woman's written permission

VII. Treatment

A.   Assure the woman she is not alone

B.   Assure the woman of confidentiality and that only she can authorize the release of evidence to the police, the release of her records, and your verbal testimony

C.   Provide support that she does not deserve abuse and that no person should perpetrate any kind of abuse or violence on her

D.   Show her the documentation in her record and indicate that its purpose is to protect her

E.   Provide resources for her safety and for escape if she decides to do so; empower her to make her own plans and choices

F.   Teach her about the patterns of violence and the laws in your state concerning abuse and violence in relationships; have copies of the state laws available

G. If she chooses to remain in the relationship, you can offer her emergency numbers of police, any domestic violence units or special forces, local emergency room(s) and shelters; help make a safety plan (money, car keys, important documents, where to go); for undocumented immigrant women who need counseling, give phone numbers of culturally sensitive programs

VIII. Referrals/Consultation

A. Medical consultation as appropriate for treatment of injuries
B. Police if woman chooses to file a complaint or police report
C. Shelters, special services for women in abusing/violent relationships
D. Mental health consultation if you believe woman is suicidal
E. Substance abuse, alcohol abuse treatment programs as appropriate and desired by the woman

X. Follow-up

A. Plan return visit so woman has another opportunity for contact with you
B. As appropriate for care of injuries, presenting concerns, contraceptive needs, treatment of STDs, vaginitis, gynecologic conditions

Appendix N on danger assessment may be photocopied or adapted for your clients.

See Bibliography 25 on abuse, battering, and violence.

Form for Report of Alleged Sexual Assault*

Victim's Complaint _____

Date_____ Time_____

Victim's Name _____
                          Last   First   Middle

Address _____

Mode of Transportation to Facility _____

PART 1

Date and time of alleged assault _____
                                              Month   Day   Year   Time

Date and time of presentation for care _____
                                              Month   Day   Year   Time

History of Alleged Assault

   1. History as related to nurse practitioner by patient:

_____

_____

_____

_____

_____

_____

by_____RNC,NP. Date:_/_/___

Witnessed by_____Date:_/_/___

---

*You may want to develop a consent form for any or all of the following: consent for treatment by nurse practitioner and/or other member of the assault crisis team to perform physical examinations, laboratory tests, evidence collection, appropriate intervention, appropriate photographs.

Make note of any comments that may be of help such as perpetrator's techniques, hang-ups, perversions, conversation, preoccupation with certain body parts and slang names for same.

2. Patient's report of pain (note location and bleeding, if any):

    ____Abdominal   ____Pelvic   ____Muscle

    ____Dysuria   ____Tenesmus   ____Skeletal

    ____Bleeding (indicate source) _____

    Other (explain) _____

3. Since the incident,

has the patient changed clothing?	____Yes	____ No
douched?	____Yes	____ No
urinated?	____Yes	____ No
bathed?	____Yes	____ No
had B.M.?	____Yes	____ No

Explain _____

4. Was there penetration of the:

	Yes	No	Not Known
a. vulva			
b. vagina			
c. mouth			
d. anus			
e. ear			
f. other			

5. Did the alleged assailant

	Yes	No	Not Known
a. bind or tie the victim			
b. threaten the patient			
c. strike the patient			
d. threaten the victim's family, friends, others			
e. wear a condom			
f. ejaculate			
g. use a foreign object in any manner sexually			

h. use a lubricant   _____ _____ _____

6. Whom has the patient notified _____
7. Does patient wish anyone notified _____
8. Have police been notified. _____
   Date _____ Time _____ a.m./p.m.
9. Does patient wish to have police notified _____

Medical History

1. Birthdate, _____
2. Race: White___ Black___ Hispanic___ Asian ___Other___
3. Marital status:
   Single___Married___ Separated___ Divorced___ Widowed___
4. Menstrual history
   a. Last menstrual period ____/____/____
   b. Last vaginal intercourse with permission within
      last 72 hours. Date:____/____/____ Time:____
5. Contraceptive history
   Method of birth control (if any):
   a. Birth control pill _____
   b. IUD _____
   c. Other _____
   d. Tubal ligation _____
   e. Hysterectomy _____
6. Significant allergies _____
7. Medications taken by patient, including alcohol and street
   drugs _____
8. Recent injury or illness _____
9. Other relevant history _____
   _____

History obtained
by_____RNC,NP. Date:_/_/___
Witnessed by_____Date:_/_/___

PART 2

Physical Examination (Please note bruising, lacerations, or any other physical trauma sustained by patient.)

Vital signs: B/P_____ P_____ T_____ R_____

1. HEENT (taking careful note of pupils and nostrils):

2. Chest-lungs:

3. Breast:

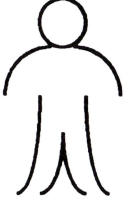

4. Heart:

5. Abdomen:

6. Extremities:

7. Neurologic:

8. Pelvic Examination:

    a. vulva
    b. mons veneris , perineum
    c. urethra
    d. clitoris
    e. vagina
    f. cervix
    g. uterus
    h. adnexa, right
              left

i. anus/rectum
j. rectum/vagina

Other comments (describe evidence of trauma in detail)

_____
_____
_____
_____
_____
_____
_____
_____
_____

Impression: _____
_____
_____
_____
_____
_____

_____ , RNC, NP

PART 3

Laboratory Evaluation
1. Slides
2. Pubic hair specimens
3. GC culture (note origin):
   Cervix_____ Urethra_____ Rectum_____ Pharynx_____
4. Serology test for syphilis
5. HCG
6. Urinalysis
7. Other(specify):_____

8. Wet mount
9. Chlamydia

Treatment Plan
1. Prophylactic antibiotic, 1998 CDC guidelines: Since not all experts agree with this regimen, individual clinical judgment must be exercised:
   a. Ceftriaxone 125 mg in a single IM dose plus Metronidazole 2 gm p.o. single dose plus Doxycycline 100 mg p.o. BID x 7 days
   b. HBV vaccine started (if not previously vaccinated)
2. Emergency contraception (see protocol)
   a. Review options with patient
3. Tetanus toxoid
   Given____Refused____(date of last TT)_____
4. Other medications (specify): _____

   _____
5. Laceration repair (specify):_____

   _____
6. Other:_____

   _____

History obtained by: _____ RN,NP. Date__/__/__
Witnessed by: _____ Date__/__/__

Follow-up (describe, give dates and times of appointments. Give patient this information in writing)
1. Medical
2. Gynecological: including syphilis, HIV screen 12 weeks after assault; STD screen 2 weeks after assault
3. Mental health counseling
4. Legal
5. Clergy
6. Other (depending on lab findings, emergency contraception); for HBV vaccine #2,3

Facility Follow-up
1. Appointment should be made for 14 days for repeat STD screening and pregnancy testing at 30 days.
2. Pregnancy testing may be done before 30 days if menses is delayed.
3. If pregnancy test is positive, appropriate counseling will be done.
4. All patients should be contacted (whenever possible) one month after alleged assault for follow-up.
5. HIV screen and serology for syphilis 12 weeks after assault.

History obtained by:

_____ RN,NP. Date:__/__/__
Witnessed by:_____Date:__/__/__

PART 4
Photographs
All bruises,* lacerations, and other wounds, particularly in the pubic area, thigh, knees, breasts, and neck. Make notes on all photos.
Photo #:____
Description and remarks: _____

_____
_____
_____
_____
_____
_____
_____
_____
_____
_____
_____
_____
_____
_____

---

*Bruises may not show up well until a day or two after alleged assault. Victim may be asked to come back if bruises appear.

PART 5

Victim Property and Clothing List

Victim_____ Date_____ Time_____

Item   Number of
Number   Articles   Description

_____

_____

_____

_____

_____

_____

_____

_____

_____

_____

_____

Clothing: If any clothing is submitted as evidence, it should be labeled and placed in a paper *(not plastic)* bag. If submitted as evidence, clothing in bag should be included with rape kit in large bag or envelope and signed again by nurse and attending officer.

The disposition of patient's clothing (sent home with family, friends, remaining with patient, or sent to police) should be noted on patient's chart and co-signed by police officer (if indicated).

The Above Listed Items Were Turned Over to _____

Of_____ On_____ At_____ (Hrs)

Signed _____

Received by_____ (Police Officer)

(Family member, friend)

(Patient)

See Appendix N on danger assessment.

See Bibliography 25 on abuse, sexual assault, and battering.

Patient Information Sheet

Name of Patient: _____ Date: _____

We understand that this experience has been a traumatic one and your initial response may be a wish to forget. However, follow-up care, both physical and emotional, is of utmost importance.

The following is information that will be important to you during the next days and weeks.

We recommend a pregnancy test if your menstrual period is delayed one week beyond its due date. Please call to make arrangements.

Although we have tested you for sexually transmitted diseases, *repeat testing is necessary at 2 weeks and at 12 weeks.* Please help yourself by returning for repeat testing.

Listed below are the procedures that were performed during this visit plus special instructions (if any) for you.

Procedures Performed	Special Instructions

Please feel free to contact us at any time if you need further support._____, RN, NP

Telephone Number: _____

Sexual Dysfunction

I. Definition

Diminished libido or lack of libido, diminished sexual response or lack of response to sexual stimulation. Vaginismus, involuntary spasm or constriction of the distal third of the vaginal musculature around the introitus on one or more occasions.

II. Etiology

A. Organic and physiologic disorders
1. Hormonal imbalance
2. Injuries or anomalies of the genital tract
3. Infection of the genitalia
4. Lesions
5. Nerve impairment
6. Substance abuse: alcohol, recreational drugs
7. Recent pregnancy
8. Effects of medications—prescription or over-the-counter
9. Chronic illness

B. Relationship disorders
1. Partner's and/or client's lack of desire for sex
2. Medical conditions
3. Lack of privacy
4. Fear of failure in the sexual act; lack of knowledge re: sexual response(s)
5. Shame, guilt
6. Expectations different from those of partner; miscommunication
7. Rape trauma; sexual assault or abuse at any age; domestic violence
8. Improper use of barrier or chemical contraceptives
9. Recent event affecting sexuality, such as sterilization

    10. Difficulties in sexual orientation
    11. Clinical depression of client and/or partner
    12. Recent pregnancy, abortion, hysterectomy, tubal ligation

III. History
A. What the client may present with
    1. Lack of sexual desire
    2. Lack of response to stimulation
    3. Inability to have an orgasm
    4. Vaginal or vulvar irritation, bleeding, soreness
    5. Lack of vaginal lubrication
    6. Inability to have vaginal intercourse
    7. Dyspareunia
B. Other signs and symptoms
    1. Rectal or perineal pain
    2. Perineal lesions
    3. Abdominal pain
    4. Fever
    5. Bladder, urethral pain
C. Additional information to be considered
    1. Sexual history: ever had intercourse; ever experienced orgasm
    2. Contraceptive history and method presently using
    3. Any gynecological/obstetrical history, diethylstilbestrol exposure, peri-menopausal problems
    4. Any recent contributing events: change of partner or new relationship, marriage, divorce, separation, sterilization, pregnancy, infection, surgery, or sexual assault
    5. Any cultural or religious beliefs that relate to sexual activity
    6. Alcohol, drug use; any changes
    7. Expectations of self and partner
    8. Any problems with privacy, time together, living arrangements
    9. Use of sex toys
    10. Pattern of sexual expression
    11. You might ask, "What do you do, how do you do it, and how does it make you feel?"

12. Sexual fantasies, preoccupations
13. Difficulties focusing on tactile or other sensations previously erotic

IV. Physical Examination
A. Vital signs
    1. Pulse   3. Temperature
    2. Blood pressure   4. Weight
B. General physical examination including thyroid, breasts, CVA tenderness, neurological
C. Abdominal examination with special attention to
    1. Guarding
    2. Pain
    3. Masses
D. External examination
    1. Anomalies   4. Status of hyman
    2. Skene's glands,   5. Perineum
       Bartholin's glands   6. Urethra
    3. Clitoris   7. Lesions, signs of infection, injury
E. Vaginal examination (speculum)
    1. Vaginal walls: infection, anomalies, atrophy, injuries
    2. Discharge, lesions
    3. Cervix: lesions, signs of infection, anomalies, scarring
    4. Tolerance of speculum and size accommodated, length of vagina
F. Bimanual examination
    1. Pain on cervical manipulation
    2. Uterus: tenderness
    3. Adnexa: mass, tenderness
    4. Vaginal lesions

V. Laboratory Examination
A. Appropriate cultures when evidence of infection; wet mount; urinalysis
B. Consider thyroid panel, FBS, liver, renal function tests, serum

corticosteroids if history and/or clinical findings warrant
C. Hormone assays as indicated

VI. Differential Diagnosis
A. Hormonal imbalance: estrogen, androgens
B. Anomaly, injury
C. Infection
D. Substance abuse: drugs, alcohol
E. Nerve impairment: spinal cord injury, neurologic diseases
F. Changes due to aging: slower responses
G. Adrenal, thyroid, liver, kidney problems
H. Diabetes, diabetic neuropathy
I. Medication side effects
J. Depression
K. Psychosocial problems
L. Post-traumatic stress disorder (PTSD) secondary to incest, rape, sexual assault, domestic violence
M. Vestibulitis, vulvodynia

VII. Treatment
A. Medications: treat any infection present (see specific protocol); consider hormones especially if postmenopausal; new drugs for women—analogues to Sildennafil citrate (Viagra®) when available
B. General measures
   1. Education about changes in sexual response that accompany aging; need for privacy, making time for intimacy
   2. Education about a woman's sexual response, how it differs from that of a man; teach Kegel (pelvic floor) exercises; positions
   3. Explore partner relationship: changes, previous responsiveness, sexual preference, communication, expectations, guilt; screen for abuse
   4. Education on techniques for stretching hymen, vagina
   5. Education regarding techniques for learning about sexual response and excitation, self and partner

6. Emphasize role of self-care: diet, exercise, vitamins, hygiene, stress reduction
7. Education about lubricants, other sexual aids

VIII. Complications
A. Long-term disruption of relationships
B. Exploitation in relationships: abuse, violence

IX. Consultation/Referral
A. Physician for possible hormonal imbalance, genital anomaly, nerve impairment, medical conditions underlying problem
B. Counselor for rape trauma, PTSD, exploitative relationships, abuse, depression
C. Sex therapist—single or couples
D. Support group

X. Follow-up
A. Check if infection is present; reevaluate for further treatment
B. Arrange repeat visit as appropriate for discussion of relationship problems
C. Assess success of vaginal, hymenal stretching; stimulation techniques
D. For medical/medication problems, laboratory results as appropriate

See Bibliography 26.

Peri- and Postmenopause

General Care Measures

I. Definition
The menopause is the landmark event of the climacteric, the 10-to-15-year period, beginning at about age 35 to 40, when women's bodies are changing and preparing for cessation of menses. A woman cannot say that she has gone through menopause until at least one full year has passed without any menstrual period (uterine bleeding). The postmenopausal time begins when menopause is complete and menses no longer occur. For women today, the postmenopausal years may comprise as much as three-eighths of their lives or more, the age for menopause being about 50 in the U.S. (mean 50.4 years). A woman who has had a hysterectomy (removal of uterus only) is not considered menopausal with cessation of menses.

II.   Etiology
A.   Physiologic: The gradual diminution of estrogens, resulting in cessation of ovulation and thus of menstruation
B.   Anatomic: Surgical removal of the uterus and ovaries which results in surgical menopause, an abrupt end to ovulation and menstruation

III. History
A.   What the client presents with
    1.   Changes in character of the menstrual cycle
        a.   Menstrual periods that are more frequent, less frequent, of longer duration or shorter duration
        b.   Scanty flow
        c.   Flooding at onset of flow
        d.   Gradual or abrupt cessation of menses for one or

more months
    e. Irregular periods over a period of time or abrupt cessation of menstruation

2. Changes related to menopause and/or the aging process (these changes are the presenting complaint of women with previous surgical removal of the uterus and intact ovaries)
    a. Hot flashes, hot flushes
    b. Vaginal dryness, atrophy of vaginal tissues
    c. Night sweats
    d. Dry skin and hair; skeletal pain or stiffness
    e. Graying of hair
    f. Loss of skin elasticity
    g. Alterations in sleep patterns
    h. Developmental occurrences of aging: empty nest, caring for aging parents, changing roles, retirement
    i. Alterations in sexual response: longer time needed for arousal, lessened vaginal lubrication
    j. Mons and vulva flatten, less fatty tissue padding, thinning of pubic hair

3. Recent history of gynecologic surgery: hysterectomy, oophorectomy, salpingectomy, dilatation and curettage

B. Additional information to be considered
1. Menstrual history, past year; previous year
2. Contraceptive use to present
3. Obstetrical history: pregnancies, abortions, stillbirths
4. Gynecologic history: surgery, endometriosis, infertility, anomalies, last Papanicolaou smear, any breast problems, last mammogram, sexually transmitted disease, infections; does she do SBE; any stress incontinence
5. Sexual history: dysfunction, unresponsiveness, recent changes, use of sex toys (see sexual dysfunction protocol)
6. Life event changes: resumption of career, retirement, caring for older family members, adult children in or out of home, divorce, separation, marriage, new sexual relationship, caring for grandchildren
7. Lifestyle: exercise, diet, smoking, recreation, stressors,

    recreational drugs
8. Medical history: chronic disease, medications (OTC, prescription)
9. Use of complementary therapies (botanicals, homeopathics, acupuncture, Chinese medicine, aromatherapy, etc.)
10. Beliefs about menopause and expectations

IV. Physical Examination

A. Vital signs
1. Blood pressure
2. Pulse
3. Height
4. Weight

B. General health examination
1. Head
2. Neck
3. Heart
4. Lungs
5. Abdomen
6. Extremities, joints, spine

C. External examination for lesions, infection, atrophy, anomaly
1. Urethral orifice
2. Clitoris
3. Labia
4. Perineum

D. Vaginal examination (speculum)
1. Walls
2. Discharge
3. Lesions
4. Cervix
5. Careful inspection of vaginal vault noting if post-hysterectomy

E. Bimanual examination
1. Adnexa
   a. Tenderness
   b. Masses
   c. Palpable tubes or ovaries, if present
2. Uterus
   a. Size
   b. Mobility
   c. Tenderness
   d. Masses
3. Cystocle, rectocele, urethrocele

F. Rectal examination: fecal occult blood

V. Laboratory Examination

A. Appropriate cultures, smears if suspicion of infection
B. Papanicolaou smear if none done in past year
C. Mammogram per American Cancer Society guidelines

(baseline at 35, annually at 40 and after); may be altered with family history or personal risk factors for breast cancer and new recommendations from ACS or NCI

D. Consider serum FSH level to assess for menopause if no menses for 12 months or on OCs, age ≥ 50 and/or desire to consider HT [≥ 40 m IU/ml]. Discontinue hormones for the 2 weeks prior to blood work measuring FSH.

VI. Differential Diagnosis
A. Carcinoma of genital tract
B. Pregnancy
C. Endocrine disorders
D. ↓ nutritional state; obesity
E. Marked ↑ in exercise regimen

VII. Treatment
A. Medication
   1. Perimenopausal: consider low dose oral contraceptive for contraception after assessment for risks, desire for contraceptive protection; consider cycling with Provera 10 mg x 10 days monthly if intermenstrual time decreases and/or heavy bleeding/flooding characterize menses
   2. Postmenopausal: consider nonhormonal or hormone (see hormone therapy protocol) interventions per clinical picture and client's wishes
B. General measures
   1. Teaching about normal menopausal symptoms, changes with aging, need for more time for arousal, use of supplemental lubrication (saliva, water-soluble jelly, water soluble lubricants—these come as creams, jellies, and as vaginal inserts), non-hormonal agents to re-store/maintain vaginal mucosa and vaginal moisture such as Replens®, Comfrey ointment, vitamin E supplement + 100-600 mg/day or evening primrose oil 2-4 capsules/day (also helpful for hot flashes), changes in sexual response that accompany removal of the uterus/ovaries
   2. Teaching about self-care: diet, exercise, prevention of osteoporosis (calcium intake 1200-1500 grams/day and

400-800 IU [20 mg] vitamin D/day in foods or supplement); breast self-examination, need for Papanicolaou smear and pelvic examination yearly; regular mammograms; contraception until one full year without menses (some say 2 years); signs and symptoms of problems: post-menopausal bleeding; prevention of vaginal infections (see protocols)

3. Teaching re: urinary health: 6-8 glasses of water a day, ↓ caffeine, Kegel exercises; quit smoking
4. Teaching re: triggers for hot flashes—electric blanket, alcohol, spicy foods, overheating, constrictive clothing
5. Consider non-hormonal synthetic medication and bioflavonoid alternatives for symptom management; other botanicals, homeopathic medicines
6. Diet: low fat, avoid or ↓ caffeine, zinc 15 mg/day in foods and/or in supplements; vitamin C and B complex vitamins, ↑ fiber; ↑ phytoestrogens

VIII. Complications/Risks
A. Pregnancy
B. Carcinoma of reproductive tract
C. Breast cancer (risk is higher after menopausal years)
D. Incapacitating menopausal symptoms: hot flashes that disrupt normal life, night sweats, sleep disturbances
E. Osteoporosis
F. Possible increased risk for heart attacks

IX. Consultation/Referral
A. To physician or other health care professional as appropriate for complications listed above
B. Possible consultation for
   1. HT; ET   2. Pathology
C. Sex therapist for prolonged or severe disruption in sexual relationship
D. Counseling: stresses of the middle years, depression
E. Consider consultation for nonhormonal synthetic medication and/or bioflavonoid therapies; homeopath; herbalist, naturopath, Ayurvedic practitioner

X. Follow-up
A. Annual examination, Papanicolaou smear, pelvic exam
B. Mammograms as recommended
C. As needed if problems continue or become exacerbated

See Bibliography 27.

Hormone Therapy

I. Definition
Hormone therapy is the use of exogenous natural or synthetic estrogen or estrogen and progestin in combination by the postmenopausal woman (whether natural or surgical menopause has occurred) to alleviate the symptoms of lower amounts of natural estrogen. It is known as HT and was once known as estrogen replacement therapy (ERT) or estrogen therapy when unopposed estrogen was used for all women.

II. Etiology
A. The theca interna and granulosa cells of the ovarian follicles and the corpus luteum produce three naturally occurring estrogens: estradiol, estrone and estriol, in concert with precursors LH and FSH from the anterior pituitary and androstenedione from the adrenals. The corpus luteum and ovarian follicle produce progesterone. The stromal tissues of the ovaries produce insignificant amounts of androgens; the major sources of androgens in women are the adrenals. During the perimenopausal years, there is a gradual decrease of the production of these hormones.

III. History
A. What the client may present with
   1. Irregular menstrual cycles: longer than 35 days, shorter than 21 days
   2. Changes in character of cycles: scanty, brief duration, begin with flooding, clots, dysmenorrhea

3. Sleep disturbances, night sweats
4. Experiencing hot flashes and hot flushes
5. Dyspareunia
6. Changes in vaginal tissue: dryness, itching, burning of vulva
7. Urinary urgency or frequency; urethral pain; irritation at meatus
8. No vaginal bleeding for prior 12 months or more
9. Surgical menopause: hysterectomy with oophorectomy and salpingectomy

B. Additional information to be considered
1. Age of client and of her biological mother at menopause
2. Last Papanicolaou smear, breast self-examination, mammogram
3. Personal medical, surgical, and gynecologic/obstetric history; history of pelvic surgery
4. Family medical history, especially osteoporosis, heart disease, carcinoma, Alzheimers disease
5. Signs, symptoms of possible vaginitis, STD, cystitis
6. Lifestyle: diet, exercise
7. Change in mood or sense of wellbeing

IV. Physical Examination

A. Vital signs
B. Complete physical examination
C. Pelvic examination
1. Vulva and perineum, noting any signs of infection, atrophy, irritation; hair distribution and signs of thinning; loss of adipose tissue
2. Vagina: color, rugae, signs of atrophy, infection or irritation, length
3. Cervix: color, any lesions, ectropion
4. Urethral os: signs of irritation, atrophy, urethrocele
5. Pelvic floor integrity: cystocele, rectocele, uterine prolapse
6. Uterus: size, shape, position, contour, mobility, presence of masses, tenderness
7. Adnexa: masses, tenderness

8. Rectal exam: masses, rectocele, uterine anomalies, occult blood

V. Laboratory
A. Papanicolaou smear with maturation index
B. Mammogram
C. May consider endometrial biopsy with intact uterus
D. Vaginal and/or urine cultures: HIV, STD screen as appropriate
E. Serum FSH or testosterone assay as indicated
F. Lipid profiles
G. Hematocrit or hemoglobin as indicated
H. Bone assays if indicated and feasible
I. Pelvic ultrasound if pelvic examination is positive for masses (vaginal probe ultrasound)
J. May consider baseline EKG
K. Per findings of physical examination and from history

VI. Considering HT
A. Contraindications*
   1. Undiagnosed vaginal bleeding
   2. Known or suspected pregnancy
   3. History of nontraumatic pulmonary embolism (PE) or deep vein thrombosis (DVT) or PE or DVT in past 6 months
   4. Known or suspected cancer of the breast or reproductive tract (estrogen-dependent carcinomas); malignant melanoma at any stage
   5. Currently on anticoagulants or tamoxifen
B. Precautions: consider clinical data, risk and benefits
   1. Active gallbladder disease
   2. Family history of breast cancer
   3. Migraine headaches
   4. Elevated triglycerides, ↑LDL, ↓HDL

---

*From the Women's Health Initiative Criteria, NIH.

C. Weighing risks and benefits
1. Osteoporosis in family or personal history; risk factors for osteoporosis (see osteoporosis handout in appendix)
2. Personal and family medical history including heart and Alzheimers disease
3. Presence of indicators for benefits in absence of absolute contraindications and weighing of relative risks
4. The use of hormone therapy remains a highly individualized decision and controversial issues remain
5. Access to health care for follow-up: endometrial biopsy, mammography, monitoring for side effects, danger signs
6. Alternatives to HT: diet, exercise, calcium from exogenous source in addition to foods, botanicals, vitamins, non-hormonal vaginal lubricants (such as Astroglide®), naturalistic interventions, homeopathic preparations (see peri- and postmenopausal general care protocol)

VII. Hormone Regimens
A. Absence of uterus: estrogen only or estrogen and androgen
1. Conjugated equine estrogen (Premarin®) 0.3-1.25 mg/day p.o.q.d. (or days 1-25)
2. Modified estrone from plant compounds (Estratab®/ Menest®) 0.3-2.5 mg/day p.o.q.d. (or days 1-25)
3. Micronized plant estrogen, estradiol (Estrace®) 0.5-2 mg/day (or days 1-25)
4. Estropipate (synthesized from estrone) (Ogen®, Ortho-Est®) 0.625-1.25 mg/day p.o.q.d. (or days 1-25)
5. Estradiol natural plant compound transdermal patch (Alora®) 0.05-0.1 mg/day—apply patch twice/week Climara® 0.05-0.1 mg day—apply patch once/week Estraderm® 0.05-0.1 mg/day—apply patch twice/week FemPatch® 0.025 mg/day—apply patch weekly Vivelle® 0.0375 mg-0.1 mg/day—apply patch twice a week
6. Estrogen vaginal cream or suppository for dryness, atrophy: dienestrol 0.7 mg (DV) or diethylstilbestrol 0.1 mg, 0.2 mg suppositories 1 or 2   daily; conjugated

estrogens (Premarin) 0.625 mg/gm or dienestrol 0.01% (Ortho Dienestrol) or dienestrol 0.01% with lactose (DV, Estroguard) or estropipate 1.5 mg/gm (Ogen) cream 1-2 applicators full per day; estradiol cream (Estrace) 2-4 gm daily for 1-2 weeks; then 1-2 gm daily for 1-2 weeks; maintenance 1 gm 1-3x/week 3 weeks on, 1 off

7. Estradiol (Estring®) (2 mg) vaginal ring (rapid release for first 24 hours, then continuous low dose of 7.5 mg/24 hours). Replaced q 90 days. May be used by post-menopausal women both with and without a uterus who desire symptomatic relief from local symptoms of urogenital atrophy. Addition of progestin not necessary for woman with a uterus since adverse effects on endo-metrium unlikely with consistent low daily dose

8. Estratab/methyltestosterone (Estratest®) 1.25 mg estrogen estrogen/2.5 mg testosterone or Estratest HS® 1/2 strength

B. Presence of uterus: add progestin
   1. Medroxyprogesterone acetate (MPA) synthetic proges-terone (Provera®, Cycrin®) 2.3-10 mg p.o.
      a. 10 mg MPA p.o. taken in combination with estrogen for last 12 days (days 14-25)
      b. 2.5-5 mg MPA p.o. taken in combination with es-trogen on days 1-5 or q.d.
   2. Norethindrone or norethindrone acetate synthetic progesterone (Micronor®, Aygestin®) 0.35-2.5 mg/day p.o. taken as in B.1.a/b
   3. Micronized progesterone from plant sources (Prome-trium®) 200 mg/day p.o. taken as in B.1.a/b (capsules contain peanut oil; avoid for patients with peanut allergies)
   4. Micronized progesterone from plant sources timed release intrauterine device (IUD) Progestasert® provides continuous source of progestin for combination therapy
   5. Combination products
      a. Conjugated estrogens 0.62mg/2.5-5 mg daily p.o.

(Prempro®)
b. Conjugated estrogens 0.625 mg p.o. alone for 14 days (Premphase®); conjugated estrogens 0.625 mg MPA p.o. for 14 days
c. Estradiol/norethindrone acetate transdermal system (CombiPatch®). Two systems available: Continuous combined regimen 0.05 mg estradiol/0.14 mg nor-ethindrone acetate continuously, changed x 2/week; continuous sequential regimen 0.05 mg estradiol patch x 14 days (Vivelle®) (replaced x2 weekly) then 0.05 mg estradiol/0.14 mg norethinrone acetate (CombiPatch®) (replaced x2 weekly)
C. Other
1. Raloxifene hydrochloride (Evista®) synthetic selective estrogen-receptor modulator 60 mg p.o.q.d. Use daily for osteoporosis protection
D. Withdrawal bleeding
1. Will occur with sequential use of progestin
2. No bleeding will occur with continuous use

VIII. Clinical Management
A. Side effects
1. Bleeding with hormone use
   a. with sequential use (see VIII.D)
   b. With continuous use
      1) Consider change in dosage or medication
      2) If not effective, do endometrial biopsy
   c. Unopposed estrogen use (still prescribed by some providers)
      1) Encourage combination therapy; prior to changing therapy, consider using Provera® 10 mg for 10 days. If no bleeding, begin new regimen. If bleeding does occur, do endometrial biopsy or do an ultrasound to measure lining
2. Breast tenderness
3. Fluid retention
4. Weight gain (increased appetite)

    5. Dysmenorrhea with withdrawal bleed
    6. Depression
    7. Irritability or emotional lability
    8. Possible increase in size of uterine leiomyomata
    9. Allergic response to patch
  10. Virilization with androgens (rare)

B. Other clinic management strategies
    1. Short-term topical estrogen for vaginal dryness; discontinue after 6 months or oral estrogen (no longer necessary)
    2. Alternative non-hormonal vaginal lubricants such as Astroglide®, non-hormonal products such as Replens® to maintain or restore vaginal mucosa
    3. Complementary/alternative modalities to be considered, including many botanicals as well as acupuncture, massage, and relaxation, can increase a woman's feeling of well-being. Unfortunately, a limited body of scientific information about botanicals is available in English. We have included a list of resources in the bibliography
    4. Careful teaching about modalities utilized

C. Follow-up and lifestyle on HT
    1. Reinforce need for calcium intake both from food and supplementary sources. Will also need a consistent source of vitamin D and appropriate dose for adequate absorption
    2. Regular program of exercise, strength training
    3. Reinforce knowledge of risks and benefits
    4. Preventive health care: annual examination, Papanicolaou smear as indicated, mammography, breast and vulvar self-examination
    5. Consider periodic monitoring for bone density, lipid profile
    6. Vaginal lubricants, signs of vaginal infection or cystitis versus dryness, Kegel exercises, sexuality

See Appendix HH and Bibliography 27.

Osteoporosis

I. Definition
Osteoporosis is a skeletal disease characterized by low bone mass and microarchitectual deterioration of bone tissue, leading to enhanced bone fragility and a consequent increase in fracture risk.

II. Etiology
Three main factors are responsible for the fragility of bone:
A. Reduced bone mass
B. Impaired repair of microdamage caused by normal wear and tear of bone, with disruption in continuity of the plates in cancellous (trabecular) bone
C. Falls

III. Clinical Types
A. Primary or idiopathic osteoporosis
   1. Type I bone loss occurs primarily in the trabecular compartment and is closely related to postmenopausal loss of ovarian function
   2. Type II bone loss involves cortical bone and is thought to be an exaggeration of the physiologic aging process
B. Secondary osteoporosis
   1. Medical conditions
      a. Chronic renal failure
      b. Gastrectomy and intestinal bypass
      c. malabsorption syndrome
      d. metastic cancer
   2. Endocrinopathies
      a. Hyperprolactinemia
      b. Hyperthyroidism
      c. Hyperparathyroidism
      d. Adrenocortical over-activity
      e. Diabetes
      f. Tumer's syndrome
      g. Premature ovarian failure
      h. Hypogonadism
   3. Connective tissue disorder
      a. Osteogenesis imperfecta
      b. Ehlers-Danlos syndrome
      c. Homocystinuria
      d. Rheumatoid arthritis

4. Medications
    a. Anticonvulsants
    b. Antacids (with aluminum)
    c. Thyroid hormone therapy

IV. History

A. Woman's medical history, including but not limited to: refer to III.B
B. Medication history
    1. Current prescription medication
    2. Current over-the-counter medication
    3. Current vitamin and botanical use
C. Ob-gyn history
    1. Age at menarche
    2. Age at menopause
    3. Months (years) of oral contraceptive use
    4. Parity
    5. Estrogen use
    6. History of menstrual dysfunction
        a. Late menarche
        b. Oligohypomenorrhea
        c. Exercise-induced amenorrhea
        d. Previous hysterectomy
    7. History of extended breast feeding
D. Nutritional status
    1. Height and weight
    2. Eating habits
    3. Consumption of caffeine and alcoholic beverage
    4. History of an eating disorder
    5. Current and past exercise habits
    6. Smoker
E. Life style
    1. Excessive use of alcohol   2. Smoking
    3. Caffeine ingestion   4. Inactivity
F. Family history

V. Physical Examination. Including but Not Limited to:

A. Height (compare to previous measurement), (loss of 1½")

B. Weight
C. Observe back for dorsal kyphosis and cervical lordosis
D. Assess for physical abnormalities that interfere with mobility
E. Assess for bone pain
F. Assess for change of stature

VI. Laboratory

A. Consider one of the following screening tests
    1. X-ray densitometry (DEXA) gold standard
    2. Bone ultrasound
    3. Genotyping
    4. Bone turnover markers (Urinary N-Tetopeptide) (NTX)
    5. Single Energy X-ray absorptrometry (measures the bones of the wrist or heel)
    6. Quantitative Computed Tomography (measures the bone density of the spine). This test is expensive and exposes the woman to a higher dose of radiation than other screening tests
    7. Consider calcium and albumin (hyperparathyroidism)
    8. Consider 25 hydroxy, vitamin D (vitamin D deficiency)
    9. Consider Thyroid Stimulating Hormone (TSH) (hyperthyroidism)

VII. Treatment

A. Medication
    1. Estrogen (see Hormone Therapy protocol)
    2. Bisphosphonates (Alendronate, Fosamax)
    Regimen: An Alendronate regimen should include:
        a. 5 mg/10 mg a day with 6-8 ounces of water on arising, at least a half hour before breakfast
        b. Calcium supplements and antacids interfere with absorption of Alendronate; these should be taken at least a half hour later
        c. To prevent GI complications, the woman must remain in an upright position for one half hour after taking medication
    3. Calcitonin-Salmon

   a. Injection treatment: 100 IU subcutaneously or intramuscularly every other day
   b. Nasal spray treatment: 200 IU intranasally once a day
4. Selective estrogen receptor modulators: Raloxifene (Evista®), 60 mg daily
5. Calcium, 1200-1500 mg with vitamin D, 400-800 IU daily (20 mg), and a multivitamin with magnesium 600 mg daily

B. General measures
   1. Increase exercise
      a. Muscle strengthening exercises concentrating on large muscle groups
      b. Aerobic exercise: walking, walking on a treadmill, climbing a Stairmaster, riding a bicycle, using a cross-country ski-type apparatus
   2. Increase dietary intake of calcium, vitamin D, magnesium
   3. Decrease dietary intake of caffeine and alcohol
   4. Decrease or stop smoking (see smoking cessation protocol)

VIII. Differential Diagnosis
A. Osteopenia—reduced bone mass due to inadequate osteoid synthesis
B. Arthritis
C. Paget's disease
D. Fracture

IX. Complications
A. Fracture with associated complications   B. Physical deformity

Referral/Consultation
A. Lack of response to treatment
B. Fractures
C. Nutritional guidance
D. Exercise program (organizations providing moderate to low cost for physical fitness)

See Appendix II and Bibliography 28.

Smoking Cessation

I. Definition
Smoking is the leading cause of preventable illness and premature death in the United States. An estimated 40 million Americans smoke, and it is estimated that of this number 70% want to quit. Quitting involves the process of fighting both the physical and psychological dependence of smoking. It is believed that nicotine is as addictive as cocaine, opiates, amphetamines and alcohol.

II. Etiology
A. The nicotine contained in inhaled cigarette smoke reaches the brain in approximately 10 seconds. Once received in the brain, nicotine causes the brain to release dopamine and norepinephrine. When nicotine is inhaled in a regular fashion, the brain accepts the chemicals by increasing the number of nicotine receptor sites. This mechanism is believed to underlay nicotine dependence. When inhaled nicotine binds to these receptor sites, it causes arousal, stimulation, increased heart rate and increased blood pressure. These physical reactions cause the smoker to experience mood elevation, reduced anxiety and stimulation within seconds of inhalation. Signs and symptoms of withdrawal may begin within a few hours of the last cigarette, peak at 48-72 hours and return to baseline 3-4 weeks after quitting.

B. Problems associated with smoking
1. Pregnancy complications (low birth weight, miscarriages, preterm delivery)
2. Cervical dysplasia
3. Increased risk for cancer (esophageal, bladder, kidney, pancreatic, leukemia)
4. Gastric and duodenal ulcers
5. Premature wrinkling of the skin
6. Decreased bone density, osteoporosis, fractures
7. Impotence and fertility problems

8. Lung disease
9. Decreased HDL
10. Peripheral vascular disease
11. Periodontal and dental distress
12. Depression
13. Early menopause

III. Barriers to Smoking Cessation
A. Physical dependence
  1. Withdrawal symptoms
     a. Depressed mood
     b. Insomnia
     c. Irritability
     e. Difficulty concentrating
     f. Increased appetite—weight gain
     f. Anger
     g. Restlessness
     h. Frustration
     i. Decreased heart
B. Psychological dependence
  1. Behaviors associated with smoking become integrated into a person's routine
  2. Smoking once integrated into routine becomes associated with pleasure and enjoyment
  3. Smoking may also be used to cope with stress or lessen negative emotions

IV. History
A. Risk assessment
  1. Do you smoke
  2. How many cigarettes a day—for how long
  3. How soon after awakening do you smoke your first cigarette
  4. Do you waken at night to smoke
  5. Is it difficult for you to observe "no smoking" rules
  6. Which cigarette would be hardest to give up
  7. Do you smoke more cigarettes in the first hours of your days than at other times
  8. Have you ever attempted to stop smoking
  9. If yes, what got in your way
B. What the client may present with
  1. Nagging, chronic cough

2. Sinus congestion
3. Shortness of breath
4. Fatigue
5. Elevated blood pressure
6. Inability to meet physical challenges (run for a bus, play with young children)
7. Decreased fertility
8. Osteoporosis, decreased bone density
9. Premature wrinkling
10. Gum disease

C. Additional questions to be asked
   1. Pregnancy complications
   2. History of abnormal Pap smears
   3. History of or presently existing cancer
   4. Fractures
   5. Cataracts/glaucoma
   6. Problems with cold hands or feet or leg pain
   7. Diabetes
   8. Gastric or duodenal ulcer
   9. Current medicines

V. Physical Examination

A. Vital signs
   1. Temperature
   2. Pulse , repirations
   3. Blood pressure

B. Skin
   1. Observe for color, tone and premature wrinkling

C. ENT
   1. Thorough examination of oral cavity. Observe for dental cavities, stained teeth, tongue or buccal lesions, gum disease, foul breath

D. Lungs
   1. Listen for adventitious sounds (wheezes, rales, crackles)

E. Breast examination

F. Abdominal examination

G. Gynecologic examination (Pap, cultures, bimanual)

H. Extremities
1. Observe extremities for signs of circulatory, peripheral vessel involvement, pulses, pedal edema

V. Laboratory Examination
A. CBC (elevated hematocrit, WBC, platelets, decreased leukocytes)
B. Lipid level (decreased HDL)
C. Consider
1. Vitamin C level (decreased)
2. Serum uric acid (decreased)
3. Serum albumin (decreased)
4. Pulmonary function tests

VI. Differential Diagnosis
A. Per physical findings   B. Depression   C. Anxiety

VII. Treatment
A. Intervention needs to be multi-faceted and tailored to each client's needs
B. Any approach needs to include information regarding the following:
1. A clear, strong stop smoking message
2. Risks associated with smoking
3. Benefits of cessation
4. Addictive components of smoking
5. What to expect during withdrawal period
6. Potential risk of relapse
C. Personalize the risks to each individual. Relate her current health problems or findings on physical examination to the effects of smoking
D. Emphasize how smoking cessation can reward the individual
E. If the patient indicates a willingness to quit, form a contract for a quit date. This date should be within a short time frame (1-2 weeks). A notation of this date should be made and the clinician should reinforce the contract with a phone call
F. Factors involved in successful cessation efforts include:
1. Timely intervention and motivation by clinician

2. Individual's desire and motivation
3. Multifaceted program
4. Individualization of program to patient's situation
G. Methods (may be used individually or in conjunction with each other)
   1. Behavioral
      a. Draft list of reasons to quit smoking and the rewards of quitting. This list should be kept with the person and reviewed when the urge to smoke "hits" and he or she is in need of reinforcement
      b. Inform family and friends and ask for their support and encouragement
      c. Smoker should keep a journal. In pre-cessation stage the smoker can use the journal to record each cigarette smoked, the social cues experienced, the setting, the intensity of the craving and the time of day. This can help identify the individual's triggers and assist smoker to adapt strategies and coping skills to get past the triggers. Keeping a journal during cessation is helpful for expressing feelings and recording the steps of the journey.
      d. Client should avoid alcohol, which weakens resolve
      e. Client should throw out all cigarettes, ashtrays, etc.
      f. Client should avoid being around smokers
      g. If possible, client should establish a "no smoking" living space
      h. Client should increase exercise level (walking, weight lifting, yoga). Exercise assists in weight management, stress reduction, sense of well being
      i. Consider use of meditation or relaxation tapes
   2. Nicotine replacement. The theory behind nicotine replacement is that by replacing the nicotine, the smoker can deal with the emotional factors and utilize behavioral changes without having to deal with the full impact of physical withdrawal at the same time
      a. Gum—offers episodic satisfaction for nicotine craving as it arises

1) Nicotine Polacrilex (Nicorette^{TM} 2 mg per piece (maximum 30 pieces per day)
2) Nicotine Polacrilex (Nicorette D.S.$^{TM)}$ 4 mg per piece— maximum 20 pieces per day)
3) Adverse effects:
   - mouth sores
   - hiccups
   - dyspepsia
   - jaw ache
   - 10% of those who use gum may become dependent requiring long-term use (1-2 years) to re main abstinent

b. Transdermal patches. If a client chooses to use the patch, there should be a contract not to smoke during its use
   1) Nicotine transdermal therapeutic system (Habitrol^{TM}) 21 mg/day (24 hours) for 4-6 weeks, then 14 mg/day for 2-4 weeks, then 7 mg/day for 2-4 weeks
   2) Nicotine transdermal system (Nicoderm^{TM}) 21 mg/day (24 hours) for 4-6 weeks, then 14 mg/day for 2-4 weeks, then 7 mg/day for 4-6 weeks
   3) Nicotine transdermal system (Nicotrol^{TM}) 15 mg/day (16 hours) for 4-6 weeks
   4) Nicotine transdermal system (ProStep^{TM}) 22 mg/day (24 hours) for 4-8 weeks, then 11 mg/day for 2-4 weeks
   5) Adverse effects:
      - skin reactions
      - vivid dreams
      - insomnia
      - myalgia

      If vivid dreams and/or insomnia are a problem, the patient may remove the patch prior to retiring and apply new patch on arising
      NOTE: If waking during the night is a problem, the 24-hour patches may provide more relief

c. Nasal spray—has the advantage of being an accelerated delivery system, delivering nicotine on demand (within 10 seconds) as a cigarette does
   1) Nicotine nasal spray (Nicotrol NS^{TM}) 1 spray (0.5 mg) in each nostril (8-40 mg/day) to a maximum

of 5 times per hour or 40 times per 24 hours

2) Adverse effects:
- •higher incidence of dependence
- •rhinitis
- •watering eyes
- • nasal irritation
- •throat irritation
- • sneezing
- • coughing

d. Oral medication
1) Bupropion Hydrochloride (Zyban™ or Wellbutrin SR™) 150 mg every day for 2 days, then 150 mg b.i.d. for 7-12 weeks. Initiate medication one week prior to start date. This week allows the patient to initiate behavioral interventions and prepare psychologically for quitting. Bupropion Hydrochloride is an antidepressant which acts as an inhibitor of the neuronal uptake of norepinephrine, serotonin and dopamine. The mechanism of action in smoking cessation is unknown, but it may serve to mimic the neurochemical effects of nicotine that serve as the pathway to addiction

2) Contraindications
History of seizure disorder
Prior diagnosis of eating disorder
Concurrent use of monoamine oxidase inhibitor

3) Possible adverse reactions:
- •rash
- • nausea
- •agitation
- •migraine

NOTE: If a prescription is written for Zyban Advantage Plan™ the patient receives material providing a toll-free 800 number. A phone call will enroll the patient in an individualized program providing behavioral modification and patient support materials as well as information on smoking cessation and 3 months of personal support at no additional cost

e. Hypnosis
f. Plastic "cigarettes"

VII. Complications

A. Relapse—most people who return to smoking do so within a

month of quitting. The longer persons have abstained, the more likely they are to continue to do so

1. Patient may be doing well when a situation or stressor makes smoking too enticing to resist
2. Patient may experience side effects from product used and lose resolve

VIII. Consultation

A. Question regarding possible medical contraindication to use of nicotine replacement or Bupropion Hydrochloride
B. Referral to intensive group sessions such as those offered by Nicotine Anonymous, American Cancer Society, American Lung Association, or a local hospital

IV.   Follow-up

A. Telephone call to patient within 1-2 weeks of quit date
B. Office follow-up at 1 and 3 months
C. If relapse occurs
   1. Discuss and review problems and stressors that contributed to relapse
   2. Review and reinforce strategies that smoker can utilize to meet future challenges
   3. Renew smoker's commitment to total abstinence
   4. Review why patient wishes to quit; contract with patient to set another quit date
   5. Reassure patient that success is often achieved only after 5 to 6 repeated attempts; success may take several years

See Appendix PP for a client information sheet for photocopying or adapting.
See Bibliography 33.

Loss of Integrity of Pelvic Floor Structures

I. Definition
Loss of tone of pelvic floor soft tissues is often associated with childbirth and/or the general effects of aging, and may result in cystocele, rectocele, urethrocele, stress incontinence, and/or uterine prolapse. It can also result from sexual assault or abuse including incest.

II. Etiology
A. Childbirth trauma: precipitous delivery, especially of a very large baby, grandmultigravida, inadequate repair of episiotomy or of lacerations
B. Aging: loss of muscle tone, relaxation of muscles, ligaments
C. Trauma due to sexual assault, incest, abuse
D. Secondary to surgery, infection especially STDs with scarring

III. History
A. What the client may present with
   1. Stress incontinence; urge incontinence
   2. Feeling of pressure in pelvic area
   3. Pain on defecation, fecal incontinence
   4. Inability to empty bladder completely; frequency, urgency
   5. Dyspareunia
B. Additional information to be considered
   1. Menstrual and reproductive history; pregnancies, route of delivery, any laceration, episiotomy, pelvic surgery or repair
   2. Occurrence of present symptoms: onset, frequency, conditions under which they occur, relief measures tried
   3. Contraceptive history: methods used, present method
   4. History of sexual assault, abuse, incest

5. STDs, especially with tissue destruction and scarring
6. History of ritual circumcision
7. Caffeine intake; diet; alcohol; smoking
8. Medications including OTC

IV. Physical Examination
A. Abdominal examination
   1. Masses   2. Tenderness
B. External examination
   1. Urethra
   2. Perineum
   3. Vulva
      a. Cystocele   d. Prolapsed uterus
      b. Rectocele   e. Ritual circumcision
      c. Urethrocele
C. Vaginal examination
   1. Speculum
      a. Condition of vagina: lax, good tone, any lesions
      b. Presence of cervix
      c. Integrity of vaginal walls
      d. Visible cystocele, urethrocele, and/or rectocele; uterine prolapse
   2. Digital
      a. Palpate cystocele, urethrocele
      b. Palpate rectocele both vaginally and rectally
D. Bimanual examination
   1. Uterus
      a. Position   b. Tenderness   c. Masses
   2. Adnexa
      a. Masses   b. Tenderness
   3. Palpable cystocele, urethrocele, scars
   4. Rectal exam:rectocele
E. Standing evaluation: cough stress test to confirm urine loss from urethra
F. Use perineometer to measure strength of pelvic floor contractions

V. Laboratory Examination
Urinalysis for stress or urge incontinence, to rule out infection

VI. Differential Diagnosis
A. Urinary tract infection   B.   Genital tract mass/carcinoma

VII. Treatment
A. Medication
1. Prescription for urinary tract infection if indicated; see urinary tract infection protocol
2. Consider hormone therapy
3. Treat any vaginitis, STD
4. Non-hormonal vaginal moisturizers such as Replens®
5. Detrol® (Tolterodine tartrate) 2 mg BID for overactive bladder, urinary frequency, urgency, or urge incontinence
B. General measures
1. Teach Kegel (pelvic floor) exercises for stress incontinence (if there is no prolapse, cystocele, or urethrocele). (A commercial product of graduated weighted cones is available to assist in Kegel exercises; a cone is inserted in the vagina and Kegels are performed using the cones' feedback; when weight of cone can be maintained 15 minutes when walking or standing, move to next cone)
2. Keep diary of occurrence of stress or urge incontinence (see Appendix BB for teaching materials and diaries; bladder retraining techniques)
3. Suggestions for hygiene measures
4. Eliminate bladder irritants including caffeine, nicotine, alcohol, artificial sweeteners, spicy and acidic foods
5. Improve hydration
6. Relaxation training
7. Pessary for uterine prolapse (continence ring, Mar-Land)
8. Stress incontinence devices: bladder neck support prothesis (Introl®), the Reliance® urethral insert, the Softpatch®, FemAssist®, Impress®

VIII. Consultation/Referral
To physician for
1. Possible surgical repair, hysterectomy
2. Possible reconstruction 2° prior surgery, scarring

See Appendix BB, which can be photocopied or adapted for your clients. See Bibliography 29.

Genitourinary Tract

Urinary Tract Infection

I. Definition
An infection of the urethra, bladder (cystitis), ureters, or kidneys.

II. Etiology
A. Specific causes
   1. Bacteria
      a. E. coli—80% of all infections
      b. Staphylococcus saprophyticus, second most commonly isolated organism; formerly thought to be a contaminant; now thought to be of causative significance, especially in women aged 16-25
      c. Others: Klebsiella, Enterobacteriaceae, Serratia, Proteus, Providencia, Pseudomonas, Group D Streptococcus, Staphylococcus aureus, Staphylococcus epidermidis
   2. Fungi: especially in diabetes and patients with catheters; immunocompromised persons
   3. Viruses that cause viruria: measles, mumps, herpes simplex, cytomegalo-virus, adenovirus varicella zoster leading to hemorrhage in bladder, and cystitis
B. Mechanism: most commonly ascending infection
   1. In females: gastrointestinal flora (E. coli)
   2. In males: prostate plays a role in harboring infection, constricting urethra causing urine retention
C. Other predisposing factors
   1. Size of inoculum
   2. Virulence of organism
   3. Incomplete or infrequent bladder emptying
   4. Urinary tract abnormalities: obstruction, calculi, congen-

ital defects, prostatic hypertrophy
5. Use of catheters
6. Newly sexually active ("honeymoon cystitis)"
7. Chemical contamination secondary to spermicidal, barrier methods of contraception

III. History
A. What the client may present with
1. Dysuria
2. Frequency, urgency
3. Suprapubic pain
4. Back pain
5. No systemic symptoms except occasionally a low grade fever, < 101
6. Gross hematuria
7. Vague abdominal discomfort
B. Additional information to consider
1. Any previous cystitis or pyelonephritis: when, how treated, response to treatment
2. Previous urologic work-up
3. Any vaginal discharge
4. Any chronic condition, diabetes, paraplegia, quadriplegia; cerebral palsy, meningomyelocele, spina bifida
5. Duration of symptoms
6. Possible pregnancy with high-risk complications or use of contraindicated drugs
7. Sexual activity, especially 24-48 post-vaginal intercourse
8. Method of contraception

IV. Physical Examination
A. Vital signs: temperature
B. Abdomen: any tenderness
C. Back: any costovertebral angle (CVA) tenderness or pain
D. Pelvic examination essential to rule out pelvic inflammatory disease, vaginitis, or sexually transmitted disease

V. Laboratory Examination
A. U/A: clean catch midstream urine; pyuria = > 5 WBC/hpf

B. Culture alone is sufficient on first time ever with urinary tract infection with no risk factor; all others should have culture and sensitivities
   1. Culture and sensitivities typically > 100,000 organisms felt to be diagnostic
   2. If between 10,000 and 100,000, probably significant if clinical symptoms support diagnosis
C. Note: Urine may be stored at room temperature for 1 hour or refrigerated up to 72 hours
D. Acute uncomplicated cystitis (nonpregnant woman)—dipstick; if + for nitrates and + leukocyte estrace or microscopic examination of urine show increased WBCs, consider treating presumptively

VI. Differential Diagnosis
A. Upper tract disease: pyelonephritis
B. Urethritis due to
   1. Chlamydia
   2. Bacteria from urethral manipulation causing irritation; thought to be early cystitis
C. Vaginitis
D. Pelvic inflammatory disease
E. Sexually transmitted disease
F. Interstitial cystitis
G. No recognized pathology, "honeymoon cystitis"
H. Pregnancy
I. Hormonal urethral changes

VII. Treatment
A. Antibiotics
   1. For first episode of urinary tract infection in women without risk factors: institute treatment with any of the following, provided the woman is not allergic to the drug
      a. Nitrofurantoin (Macrodantin®) 50 mg QID x 7 days and, depending on repeat culture results, possibly 25 mg QID x 7 more days or Macrobid® 100 mg BID x 7 days
      b. Trimethoprim (160 mg) sulfamethoxazole (800 mg)

(Septra DS®), Bactrim DS 1 BID x 10-14 days or Septra or Bactrim (80 mg trimetheprim 400 mg and sulfamethoxazole) 2 tabs BID x 10-14 days

   c. For uncomplicated first or second episodes, Trimethoprim (160 mg) and sulfamethoxazole (800 mg) 2 (Septra DS®) or Bactrim DS® STAT or BID for 3 days

   d. Amoxicillin 500 mg TID x 10 days

   e. Cipro® (ciprofloxacin HCL) 100 mg BID x 3 days

   f. Cefixime (Suprax®) 400 mg daily x 1 day or 200 mg BID x 1 day

   g. Monurol® (fosfomycin) 3 gm in a single dose mixed in 3-4 ounces of cold water (not recommended under age 18)

2. For reinfection of urinary tract infection in women without risk factors: same as for the first episode. Important to distinguish reinfection from relapse. Reinfection occurs within weeks to months of preceding episode, and is often caused by a new organism. Relapse is a recurrence of symptoms and infection after finishing a medication course, and is caused by the same organism as the original infection

3. For relapse in women
   a. Consider retreatment with same medication, with a test of cure 24-48 hours after completion of medication
   b. Consider change of medication with test of cure 24-48 hours after completion of medication
   c. For second relapse, consult with physician

4. For patients with risk factors (past history of pyelonephritis, known urinary tract abnormality, use of catheter, diabetes): consider referral to physician

B. For pregnant women
1. The causative pathogen in pregnant women is usually E. coli. Do culture before treatment; sensitivity only if no improvement from medication
   a. First choice: Ampicillin 250 1 QID x 10 days
   b. Second choice: Nitrofurantoin (Macrodantin®) or Macrobid® or a sulfa drug (do not use sulfa in third trimester)

   c. Do not use Septra® or Bactrim®
C. Pain relief: Phenazopyridine hydrochloride (Pyridium® Azo-Standard, Baridium, Di-Azo, Phenazo, Urodine) 200 mg TID x 24 hours; Uristat (phenazopyridine HCL 95 mg) 2 tabs TID x no more than 2 days (available OTC) (not recommended in pregnancy)
D. General measures
   1. Advise voiding before and after sex
   2. Advise adequate lubrication for sex
   3. Teaching re: hygiene, contamination
   4. Treat as above (B.) if bacteria present
   5. Consider treatment with Pyridium® or other such product only if client symptomatic in absence of pathogenic organism
   6. Cranberry juice; 6-8 glasses of water a day; ↓ bladder irritants such as caffeine, smoking; cranberry juice capsules Azo-cranberry 450 mg cranberry juice concentrate 1-4 capsules per day with meals

VIII. Complications
Pyelonephritis

IX. Consultation/Referral
A. Consider physician consult on
   1. Women with relapsed infections
   2. Women who are symptomatic after 3 days of treatment
   3. Women who have more than 3 episodes in a year

X. Follow-up
A. Follow-up culture if symptoms do not resolve after treatment
B. Consider test of cure up to 1 week after completion of medication

   Appendix JJ, on cystitis, may be photocopied or adapted for your clients.
   See Bibliography 30.

Preconception Care

I. Definition
Advanced planning aimed at reducing perinatal mortality and morbidity.

II. Etiology
Reasons for promoting preconception care (PCC) include
A. Maximize healthy life.
B. Identify any medical condition or medications in either perspective parent
C. Identify genetic disorders
D. Review past gestational and pregnancy outcome history
E. Identify high risk exposures. Tobacco, drug and alcohol use; environmental hazards, e.g., toxins, chemicals including pesticides, gases

III. History
A. Woman's medical history—including but not limited to:
    1. Diabetes   2. Phenylketonuria
    3. Cardiovascular   4. Lung
    5. Thyroid   6. Kidney
    7. Infectious disease (e.g., HIV, hepatitis B and C, toxoplasmosis, rubella, varicella, TB, STDs)
B. Obstetrical and gynecological history
    1. Contraception   2. Menstrual history
    3. Gynecological history 4. Pap smear history
    5. High-risk behavior (including STDs)
C. Immune status: need to have documentation
    1. Rubella   2. TB   3. Hepatitis B, C
    4. Varicella 5. Tetanus if ≥ 10 years
D. Drug history
    1. Current prescription medications

    2. Current over-the-counter medications
    3. Current vitamin and botanical use
    4. "Street" drug use history
E. Nutritional status
    1. Height and weight
    2. Eating habits
    3. Food allergies
    4. Caffeine and artificial sweetener intake
    5. History of being over- or underweight
    6. History of an eating disorder
    7. Current exercise habits and other physical activities
F. Genetic history
    1. May use a Genogram, identify couples with a personal or family history of problematic diseases such as:

a. Tay-Sachs	b. Thalassemia
c. Sickle-cell disease or trait	d. Phenylketonuria
e. Cystic fibrosis	f. Hemophilia
g. Mental retardation	h. Myotonic dystrophy
j. Adult polycystic kidney disease	j. Birth defects

    2. Family background
       a. Related outside marriage
       b. Ethnic background: African-American, Mediterranean, Ashkenazic Jew
G. Exposure to teratogenic toxins: areas of concern include:
    1. Exposure

a. Metals (lead)	b. Solvents
c. Gases	d. Radiation
e. Pollutants (e.g., second hand smoke)	f. Pesticides

    2. Consumption

a. Alcohol	b. Smoking

H. Social history
    1. Age
    2. Marital status
    3. Family structure
    4. Support systems
    5. Employment/financial status

6. Cultural beliefs
7. Child care issues
8. Safety issues (e.g., spousal/partner abuse)
9. Work history: exposure to chemicals, radiation; standing at work

I. Partner health history
   1. Thorough health/genetic/social history should be taken on perspective fathers. Little conclusive research has been done of how partners' exposures to chemicals/tox- ins/dr-ugs may affect fetal development. Recent studies have indicated that alcohol consumption in the month prior to conception contributes to low spermatogenesis
   2. Findings need to be integrated with maternal health history findings

IV. Physical Examination
A. Baseline height, weight, vital signs
B. General physical, including pelvic
C. Comprehensive exam based on medical history

V. Laboratory
A. Papanicolaou smear
B. Baseline studies may be considered, including:
   1. Blood Rh, type
   2. Hemoglobin/hematocrit
   3. Urinalysis
   4. RPR/VDRL
   5. Check status for
      a. Hepatitis B, C   b. Varicella
      c. Rubella   d. HIV
   6. Based on history, check:
      a. Toxoplasmosis
      b. CMV

VI. Education
A. Begin at least one month prior to planned conception
   1. Avoidance of environmental toxins
   2. Cessation of smoking and alcohol consumption

3. Begin exercise program (e.g., walking, swimming)—heart rate not to exceed 140 beats per second
4. Bring immunizations up to date. (If live vaccine used, postpone conception at least 3 months)
5. Eat a balanced diet
6. Start vitamin therapy
   a. 0.4 mg p.o. of folic acid q.d. (increase dosage for women who are at increased risk for NTD to 0.8 mg q.d.)
   b. Increase calcium intake to an equivalent of one quart of milk daily (or 1200 mg)
7. Avoid or at least decrease caffeine intake
8. Consult with primary care provider regarding prescription medications (e.g., psychotropics, antihypertensives, anticonvulsants); botanicals, vitamins
9. Avoid hot tubs, saunas (bringing body temperature above 102° F can damage the embryo)
10. Don't empty cat litter box.

VII. Referral/Consultation
A. For genetic consultation if indicated
B. Evaluation of prescriptive medication use
C. Substance abuse counseling if indicated
D. Nutritional counseling if indicated (e.g., obesity, gestational diabetes with prior pregnancies, vegetarian)
E. Community/federal programs for financial assistance if indicated
F. Domestic violence intervention

VIII. Follow-up
A. Refer for obstetrical care if pregnancy occurs (if setting does not provide care)
B. If conception does not occur within 1 year, return for further evaluation/possible referral. Consider sooner if over age 30

Appendix A may be photocopied or adapted for your clients. See Bibliography 31.

PART II. APPENDIXES

The materials in this section include clinical forms, screening tools, and patient education information.

The sections on the cervical cap and natural family planning were developed in other settings by R. Mimi Clarke Secor and the late Eleanor Tabeek with updates by Nancy Keaveney. Appendix EE was adapted from a form by Cheryl Stene Frenkel.

Alphabetical List of Appendixes

Appendix A

For Your Information: Preconception Self-Care

THE PURPOSE of preconception self-care is to help you be at your healthiest as you plan a pregnancy. Advanced planning can help reduce your risk of having a low birth weight or premature baby. Working with your clinician, you can identify any medical condition or medications you are taking that need to be considered when contemplating a pregnancy. You may also wish to have a genetic consultation if you or your partner have a family history of inherited disorders such a cystic fibrosis, Tay-Sachs disease, or hemophilia. Infections such as sexually transmitted diseases and tuberculosis may affect the health of a pregnancy, or even your ability to conceive.

Good health is important for a successful pregnancy and healthy baby. A complete health history and physical examination including a Pap smear, pelvic exam, and screening for sexually transmitted diseases, as well as other communicable diseases such as hepatitis B and C and HIV prior to conception will ensure that your body is in an optimal state for a pregnancy. Having your immunizations up to date will protect you and your baby. Evaluation of your nutritional state, diet and exercise patterns, and your toxin exposure at work and at home will help you prepare your body for conception.

Smoking and using alcohol and/or street drugs can have serious consequences for the health of a pregnancy and baby. At least one month before attempting to conceive, women who smoke, drink, or use street drugs should stop. If you use prescription or over-the-counter drugs, limit them to those your clinician approves of.

Protect yourself from exposure to toxins as much as possible.

These include pesticides, household cleaning products, gases, solvents, and radiation. Modify, undertake, or continue your program of exercise. Bring your immunizations up to date (although some are contraindicated in pregnancy, so it is best to do this 3 months before trying to conceive).

Eat a balanced diet, paying particular attention to fresh fruits and vegetables (6-8 or more servings a day); whole-grain breads, cereals, and pasta; protein (especially fish, poultry, legumes, and non-fat dairy products), and drink 6-8 glasses of water a day. Decrease or eliminate caffeine from your diet (including coffee and carbonated soft drinks). Begin taking 400 micrograms of folic acid a day—a prenatal vitamin that includes folic acid is fine. Increase your calcium intake to the equivalent of 1 quart of milk a day (1200 milligrams). In general, avoid food with lots of preservatives and artificial sweeteners.

Avoid hot tubs and saunas as these bring your body temperature above 102 degrees, which can limit or eliminate sperm production. Avoiding such excessive heat will also protect the baby once conception has occurred.

If you are on oral contraceptives, stop using them at least one month before you plan to conceive to allow your body to resume cycling. If you have Norplant implants or use Depo-Provera, have the implants removed and/or the Depo-Provera shots discontinued several months before you desire to become pregnant, as it often takes that long to resume ovulatory (fertile) cycles. You can use spermicides and condoms until you wish to try to conceive.

In order to maximize the health of their sperm, men planning to father children should stop smoking and using street drugs and avoid toxin exposure at least 3 months before attempting contraception. They should also have their infectious disease status checked through a sexually transmitted disease screen and hepatitis B and C and HIV testing. One-half of the baby's genetic material comes from the father, so he needs to be in good health.

Discuss with your partner your feelings about parenting, your expectations of him or her, and what parenting means to you. How do you expect your life to change? How will having a child change your relationship, the way your household functions, your work schedule, your expectations, and those of your partner? Who will be the primary parent? Will one or both of you have maternity/parenting leave? How will your finances be affected by having a child? How do you plan to integrate a new baby into the household with other children, extended family and other members of the household?

Planning for a pregnancy will help you be at your best when you conceive. It will also help you consider the changes pregnancy and a baby will have on your life and the lives of those close to you.

For resources on genetic counseling, nutrition, prenatal care, and prenatal classes, as well as information on conception and pregnancy, ask your clinician and check your community library, your local bookstore, and on line such as:

March of Dimes Birth Defects Foundation:

    http://www.modimes.org

Ask NOAH about: Pregnancy:

    http://www.noah.cuny.edu/pregnancy/pregnancy.html

From: Hawkins, Roberto-Nichols, & Stanley-Haney, *Protocols for Nurse Practitioners in Gynecologic Settings,* 7th edition, 2000, © The Tiresias Press, Inc.

Appendix B

Your Gynecologic Examination

SOMETIMES A WOMAN feels apprehensive about having a gynecological examination. If you understand the whole process, you'll be
better able to relax and learn how your body functions normally.
Learning about your body in a supportive atmosphere will enable you
to get and keep in touch with your own health and sexuality.

The gynecological examination includes both an external and an
internal inspection of a woman's generative organs and related structures
to determine whether they are normal or whether any growths, signs of
disease, or abnormal conditions are present. The examination may be
performed by a nurse practitioner, nurse midwife, or physician; it is
simple and painless if you are relaxed and know what to expect.

It is recommended to put nothing in your vagina during the 48 hours
before your appointment so an accurate Pap smear may be obtained (this includes having penile vaginal intercourse, vaginal medications, and birth control such as vaginal foam or film). Douching is never
recommended as a hygiene practice.

Your visit starts with filling out any necessary forms. The information requested will vary depending upon the reason for your appointment, but on your initial visit you will be asked to give information
about your present health status and any past illnesses or opera-
tions, and a family health history, as well as details about your
menstrual cycle, pregnancy history, present sexual activity, and present
or desired use of contraception.

Prior to the actual examination you will be weighed and asked to
give a urine specimen. You will then meet your clinician who will
review your history forms and discuss the reason for your visit. Next,
you will be given a paper drape and asked to get completely undressed.
Once you are on the examining table, the practitioner will take your
blood pressure and examine your heart, lungs, neck, and breasts for any
abnormal condition. At this time you can learn to do your own breast
examination. (Women should perform this simple self-examination

monthly after the menstrual period. Postmenopausal women should pick the same date each month.)

To begin the pelvic examination, you will be asked to lie on the examining table, to slide down to the end of the table, and to spread your legs and place your feet or legs in supports. To help you relax your pelvic muscles, spread your knees as wide apart as possible. The external area, the vulva, is then examined for inflammation or abnormality. A metal or plastic instrument called a speculum (which should be warm and moistened) is inserted into the vagina, gently spreading the vaginal walls apart so that the cervix (the lower portion or neck of the uterus) and vagina can be clearly seen. This shouldn't hurt because the vagina is flexible.

To detect cancer of the cervix, a Papanicolaou (Pap) smear will be taken. In this simple, painless procedure cells are gently scraped from the cervix with a flat wooden spatula and a tiny cytobrush and placed on a slide. A microscopic examination by a laboratory technician will determine the presence or absence of any cell abnormality. Cultures and smears for detection of vaginal infection or STD (sexually transmitted disease) may also be taken at this time.

After the speculum is removed, a bimanual examination is performed. Two fingers of a gloved hand (lubricated with a water soluble lubricant) are inserted into the vagina while the other hand is used to gently press on the outside lower abdominal region. By pressing up on the cervix and down on the abdomen, the practitioner can feel the size, shape, and position of the uterus. Any abnormality of the fallopian tubes, ovaries, or uterus is also checked at this time. A rectal examination is sometimes performed to check for any abnormalities and feel areas that can't be reached through the bimanual examination.

All women should have periodic gynecologic examination, but since individual needs differ, ask your practitioner about the best schedule for you. Women whose mothers used diethylstilbestrol (DES) during pregnancy should be screened for vaginal cell abnormality. You should seek consultation if you are experiencing pain, have abnormal vaginal bleeding, or suspect infection.

Whatever the reasons for your visit, remember to take the opportunity to ask any questions you might have.

From: Hawkins, Roberto-Nichols, & Stanley-Haney, *Protocols for Nurse Practitioners in Gynecologic Settings*, 2000, © The Tiresias Press, Inc.

Appendix C
Health History Form

Please fill out this confidential form so that the nurse practitioner, nurse midwife, and/or doctor can best help you meet your well woman and/or contraceptive needs.

Date __/__/__

Name _____ Date of birth __/__/__ Age___

Address _____

Where can we contact you?_____

School status and major (if applicable) _____

Occupation_____

Do you have health insurance? _____ Which? _____ _____

How did you find out about us?_____

1. Reason for appointment _____

2. Are you having any of the following now?

Frequent headaches ___   Allergies ___

Shortness of breath ___   Constipation ___

Breast lumps, discharge ___   Diarrhea ___

Seizures or fits ___   Yellow skin or eyes ___

Coughing spells ___   Crying spells ___

Dizzy spells ___   Fatigue ___

Loss of urine ___   Depression ___

Pain or swelling in legs ___   Varicose veins ___

Trouble with eyes, blurred vision, double vision ___

Weight changes—under or overweight ___

Phlebitis or clots in veins ___

Difficulty starting urination___

School or social problems ___

Concern about sexually transmitted disease, HIV/AIDS ___

Do you smoke cigarettes? ___ How many a day? ___

Do you drink alcohol? ___ How many drinks daily? ___

How many drinks weekly? ___ Do you use street drugs? ___

If yes, which and how often? _____

3. If you have ever had or still have any of the following, please describe, including date of onset, treatment, etc. Please place a check mark on the line of the *extreme left side* if your answer is yes.

	Date of Onset,
Yes	*Treatment, Other Details*

_____ rheumatic fever/frequent strep throats _____

_____ heart murmur _____

_____ nervous trouble _____

_____ German measles (Rubella) _____

_____ cancer _____

_____ high blood pressure _____

_____ stroke _____

_____ thyroid trouble _____

_____ epilepsy _____

_____ aspirin sensitivity _____

_____ asthma _____

_____ ulcer/gastrointestinal disease _____

_____ glaucoma/eye problem _____

_____ diabetes _____

_____ sickle cell anemia or trait _____

_____ hepatitis or liver problems _____

_____ infectious mononucleosis _____

_____ pelvic inflammatory disease or
        ovary/uterus problem _____

_____ hyperlipidemia (high cholesterol) _____

_____ arthritis or Lupus Erythematosus _____

_____ migraine headaches _____

_____ constipation _____

_____ urinary tract infection or
        pain and burning on urination _____

_____ vaginal infection, discharge, or sores _____

_____ abnormal Pap smear _____

_____ sexually transmitted disease including warts (HPV),
        AIDS, (HIV) _____

_____ any other illness not listed _____

4. List all the medications (prescription and non-prescription including vitamins and botanicals) you are now taking regularly_____

Are you allergic to any medication, food, other substance? _____ If yes, what? _____

If yes, what?_____

5. Have you ever been a patient in a hospital? _____ If yes, when and for what reasons? _____

6. *Family History*

Circle if any of the members of your family have:

mental depression	high blood pressure	diabetes
migraine headaches	sickle cell disease	cancer (type)
breast disease	varicose veins	phlebitis
(cancer)	hyperlipidemia	hepatitis
heart disease	(high cholesterol)	stroke
(heart attack)	lung disease/asthma	thyroid
stomach/bowel/gall	seizures (fits)	problems
bladder problems		

7. Did your mother or you ever take DES (diethylstilbestrol) or any other medicine when pregnant (with you)? _____ Please explain:_____

8. *Menstrual History*

Last period began on _____ Age when had first period

_____

Do you have cramps with your period? _____ what treatment do you use for your cramps? _____

How often do your periods occur? _____ How long does your period last? ____days. On the heaviest day of your period how many pads or tampons do you use? ____ Do you spot or bleed between your periods? _____. Have you missed a period recently? _____ Have there been any changes in your periods over the last year? _____. Do you have premenstrual symptoms? _____ including:

depression _____, fatigue _____, weight gain _____

headache_____, irritability_____, breast tenderness

_____, increased appetite ____ other _____

9. Date of last pelvic (internal) exam_____ Never had
    exam____ Date of last Pap test_____ Never had test
    _____Results_____

10. Have you in the past or are you currently using:
    douches____deodoranttampons____femininehygienesprays
    _____

11. *Sexual Activity and Birth Control*
    Are you having sexual relations now?____ How often? _____
    Have you been sexually active in the past? ____
    Age at first intercourse____ Your sexual preference: male___
    female___ both___ Do you have pain during or after sexual
    relations?____bleeding?____any other problems? _____ If
    you have a male partner, are you using any birth control
    method?____ If yes, which one(s) and for how long? ____
    Does your partner use condoms?____ If yes, how often?
    _____ Are you satisfied with your present method?____.
    Have you ever had a problem, including pregnancy, with a
    birth control method? ___ If yes, explain _____
    List in order of use
       Method   Dates of Use   Problems or Comments
      1._____
      2._____
      3._____

12. *Pregnancy History*
    Have you ever been pregnant?____ How many children born
    alive?_____ Dates of miscarriages (abortion, stillbirth)
    Number of Cesarean sections ____ When did your last
    pregnancy End? _____ Did you have any problems during
    or after your pregnancies? _____

13. Do you plan to have children in the future? _____

14. Have you ever been sexually molested/assaulted/harassed or
    been a victim of incest? _____

15. Is there violence in any of your relationships? _____

16. Are you afraid of a partner? ____

From: Hawkins, Roberto-Nichols, & Stanley-Haney, *Protocols for Nurse Practitioners in Gynecologic Settings, 7th edition,* 2000, © The Tiresias Press, Inc.

Appendix D
Gyn Annual Exam

ACCT #:_____

NAME:_____ DATE:_____ MSW FMD_____

MED PROBLEMS:_____

§: G___ P___ AGE:____ SMOKER: Y/N PkPD

LAST TETANUS BOOSTER:_____

_____

_____

_____ SIGNATURE

_____

_____

_____

_____

Q:LMP:_____ CONTRACEPTION:_____ ALLERGY:_____

LAST PAP:_____ MEDS:_____

LAST MAMMOGRAM:_____

GENERAL	NORMAL	ABNOR	HT____ WT____ BP____ URINE____
1.APPEARANCE			
2.SKIN			
3.HEAD-EENT			
4.THYROID			
5.LYMPH NODES			
6.HEART			
7.LUNGS			
8.EXTREMITIES			
9.VARICOSITIES			
10.M. SKELETAL			
11.NEUROLOGICAL			
12.ABDOMEN			

BREASTS_____

GYNECOLOGICAL EXAM

EXT. GENITALIA_____

VAGINA_____

CERVIX_____

UTERUS_____;

ADNEXA_____

RECTUM_____

Δ   DIAGNOSIS/SUMMARY:_____

P   1. EDUCATION: REVIEWED: ___ SBE ___BENEFITS OF CALCIUM
       SUPPLEMENTATION ___ RISK/BENEFIT OF:_____
       ___ SMOKING CESSATION ___ DIET AND EXERCISE
    2. TREATMENT: ___ PAP SMEAR

    _____

    _____

    3. NEXT APPT:_____

SIGNATURE:_____
        (MD/NP)

From Ellington Ob/Gyn Associates, used with permission

Appendix E

Informed Consent for Oral Contraceptives
(May also be used as informational handout)

I. Mechanism of Action
An oral, systemic method of preventing conception which acts by
A. Suppressing ovulation
B. Producing changes in the endometrium that makes it unreceptive to implantation
C. Producing a thickened cervical mucus

II. Benefits of the Method
A. Highly effective: 99.66% for combination pill (0.1 pregnancy/year); 97% for progestin only
B. Sexual spontaneity
C. Regulated menstrual flow
D. Lighter flow and less cramping
E. Decreased incidence of uterine and ovarian cancers
F. Relief of symptoms associated with peri-menopause

III. Risk of method
A. Minor side effects (these are rare and usually subside after several months of pill use; may be alleviated by changing type of pill or discontinuing pill). Listed are a few more common, although rare, side effects:
  1. Nausea (try taking pill with a meal or with milk; with severe nausea/vomiting, use back-up method of birth control such as condoms)
  2. Spotting
  3. Decreased menstrual flow and sometimes missed periods
  4. May have more problems with yeast infections or vaginal discharges
  5. Depression or mood changes
  6. Acne

    7.   Headaches (not severe)
B. Major side effects (rare in women under 40 who are non-smokers)
    1.   Blood clots in legs, lungs; stroke
    2.   Hypertension (high blood pressure)
    3.   Gallbladder disease
    4.   Heart attack (smokers age 35 and older))
    5.   Smoking doubles risk factors associated with pill use. These side effects are characterized by the following danger signals (if they occur, seek medical care *IMMEDIATELY):* pain, redness or swelling of the legs or a localized tender red spot warm to the touch may indicate a blood clot in a vein; persistent and severe headaches; chest pain and/or difficulty breathing; blurred vision, flashing vision; blindness; abdominal pain.

IV. Contraindications (reasons you may not be able to take the pill)

Woman with a history of any of the following conditions may not be able to use oral contraceptives
A.   Thromboembolic disorders (blood clot) in leg, lungs
B.   Impaired liver function at present time; liver problems
C.   Cancer of breast or reproductive system
D. Hypertension (high blood pressure); uncontrolled, or smoking and high blood pressure
E.   Hyperlipidemia (high cholesterol)
F.   Stroke
G. Coronary artery disease
H. Major surgery on legs or with prolonged immobility
I.   35 years or older and currently a heavy smoker (more than 15 cigarettes a day)
J.   Pregnancy—known or suspected
K. Undiagnosed genital bleeding
L.   Taking certain prescription drugs
M. Diabetes with vascular (blood vessel) disease
N. Headaches, migraines with neurological symptoms

V. Alternate Methods of Birth Control

A. Abstinence
B. Sterilization; natural family planning

C. Condom used with contraceptive cream, jelly or foam, contraceptive suppositories or tablets, vaginal film, contraceptive gel
D. Intrauterine device (IUD)
E. Diaphragm with contraceptive cream or jelly
F. Cervical cap
G. Norplant®
H. Female condom
I. Depo-Provera®

VI. Inquiries are encouraged. Please ask us questions; a change in decision does not create a problem

VII. Explanation of method
A. Way in which oral contraceptives are prescribed
   1. A complete physical examination is done, including blood pressure, weight, urinalysis, gynecologic examination with Papanicolaou smear (unless one was done within the past year)
   2. Review side effects and dangers of use; review packet
   3. If requested to do so by your health care provider, review and sign an informed consent for oral contraceptives
   4. You may transfer your records from another clinic or health care professional's office
B. Way in which pill is taken
   1. Start taking your first package of pills as directed by your nurse practitioner
   2. Oral contraceptive pills are *always* started initially at the same time as your period; you begin the Sunday of the week your period starts even if you are still bleeding
   3. Swallow one pill at the *same time* daily
   4. A second form of contraception is recommended for the first 7 days after starting the pill (unless specified differently)
   5. Some medications can decrease effectiveness or cause other pill-related problems (e.g., spotting). Always mention to your health care provider and pharmacist that you are on oral contraceptives prior to starting any other medication. Also tell us if you are on any medications prior to starting oral contraceptives. Use a back-up meth-

od of birth control if you have any doubts about the possibility of a drug interaction.

6. If you are taking prescribed antibiotics for an illness, you should continue your pill but use a back-up method.

7. Breakthrough bleeding (spotting) is common during the first few months a woman is on an oral contraceptive; do not be alarmed if you experience this.

   a. If you experience spotting after several months of pill use, make sure you are taking the pill correctly, as directed below. But make sure you discuss this at the time of your first pill check.

   b. If the pill is taken improperly, breakthrough bleeding may occur. You must make every effort to take your pill at the same time *every day.*

   1) If you take your pill more than 6 hours late, take the pill when you remember it; you are also advised to use a second method of birth control for the next 7 days.

   2) If you miss one pill: take the pill when you remember and then take the scheduled pill at the regular time. A second method of birth control is recommended for 7 days.

   3) If you miss 2 pills in the first 2 weeks of a pill pack: take two pills at the regular time and then take two pills at the regular time the next day, and use a second method of birth control for 7 days.

   4) If you miss 2 pills in the third week, or if you miss 3 or more pills at any time, and you start packets on Sunday, take a pill each day until Sunday, then discard the remainder of that pack and start a new pack immediately, omitting the hormone-free week. (If you don't start a new pack on Sundays, throw away rest of pill pack and start a new pack that day.) **A back-up method of birth control should be used for the first 7 days of this new pill pack.**

   5) If you miss 1 or more pills and used no back-up method and have no period, call to discuss possible pregnancy test.

   6) If you aren't sure what to do about missed pills, use a back-up method any time you have sex and keep

taking a birth control pill (hormone pill) each day
until you can talk with your health care provider.

C. Occasionally, withdrawal bleeding (your period) does not
occur during the week of non-hormone pills (placebos).
1. If this happens to you and all pills have been taken properly, continue with next pill cycle. If you miss two periods, start your third pill cycle but call your clinician
for advice.
2. If this happens to you and you have taken your pill late or
forgotten to take it, and did not use a second birth control
method, start your next pill packet but call your clinician
for advice

D. If you experience severe vomiting and/or diarrhea, use a
back-up method of birth control since the pill may not have
been absorbed properly.

I have read the above material; it has been fully explained. I have
been given the opportunity to ask questions and I understand the
information. I have chosen to use an oral contraceptive.

Signed _____ Date _____

Witness_____Date _____

Danger Signals Associated with Pill Use
Abdominal pain (severe)
Chest pain (severe) or shortness of breath
Headaches (severe)
Eye problems such as blurred vision or loss of vision
Severe leg pain (calf or thigh)
Contact us at ( )_____ if you develop any of the above
problems.
NOTE: Birth control pills can be used as emergency contra-
ception. Ask your health care provider; check directions in pill
packet; call 1888-NOT-2-LATE

From: Hawkins, Roberto-Nichols, & Stanley-Haney, Protocols for Nurse Practitioners in
Gynecologic Settings, 7th edition, 2000, ©The Tiresias Press, Inc.

Appendix F

Consent Form for Depo-Provera®
(May also be used as an informational handout)

Definition
Depo-Provera® is a hormonal substance that prevents ovulation from occurring. Injected intramuscularly every 12 weeks into the muscle of the upper arm or buttocks.

How It Works
The hormones in the injection suppress ovulation (egg production) for 12 weeks.

How Effective Is It?
Failure rate is less than one pregnancy per 100 women per year when women return for injections every 12 weeks and when injection is done in the first 5 days of menses (bleeding).

Why Choose This Method?
A. Consider use of other methods and whether their side effects make you prefer this method
B. Desire for long-term contraceptive—12-week effect
C. Desire for reversible method (ability to stop injections)
D. Desire for method disconnected from intercourse—nothing to take or put in

Why You Might Not Be a Candidate
A. Known or suspected pregnancy
B. Unexplained abnormal vaginal bleeding
C. Known breast cancer
D. Known sensitivity to Depo-Provera® or any of its ingredients (have you ever had an allergic reaction to local anesthetic at the dentist?)

Things to Consider before Choosing Depo-Provera®
A. Depression

B. Abnormal mammogram
C. Kidney disease
D. Hypertension (high blood pressure)
E. Planned pregnancy in near future
F. Gallbladder disease
G. Mild cirrhosis
H. Do you regularly use any prescription drugs—we need to check possible interactions with Depo-Provera®

Side Effects You Might Experience
A. Weight gain or loss; change in appetite
B. Menstrual irregularity—possibly no periods by second or third shot
C. Headaches
D. Abdominal bloating
E. Breast tenderness
F. Tiredness, weakness
G. Dizziness
H. Depression, nervousness
I. Nausea
J. No hair growth or loss or thinning of hair; ↑ hair growth on face or body
K. Skin rash or increased acne
L. Increased or decreased sex drive

Explanation of Method and Assessment
Depo-Provera® is injected intramuscularly in one 150 milligram dose every 12 weeks for as long as contraceptive effect is desired. It is injected in the first 5 days of the menstrual cycle (after onset of menses), within 5 days postpartum, or if breast feeding, at 6 weeks postpartum.

If time between injections is greater than 13 weeks, we would do pregnancy test before giving you the injection; we may also do a pregnancy test at 12 weeks if you have no bleeding (period).

Use of This Method and Warning Signs
1. Drug interactions are possible when using Depo-Provera® with other prescription drugs. Always check with your physician or nurse practitioner and pharmacist for such possible interactions before taking any other prescription drug; Depo-

Provera® is a medication and you need to list it in your health history.
2. Warning signs to report to your health care provider (physician or nurse practitioner):
Sharp chest pain, coughing of blood, sudden shortness of breath
Sudden severe headache, vomiting, dizziness, or fainting
Visual disturbance (double vision, blurred vision, spots before your eyes or speech disturbance (slurred, unable to speak)
Weakness or numbness in arm or leg
Severe pain or swelling in calf or leg
Unusually heavy vaginal bleeding (unlike usual periods)
Severe pain or tenderness in lower abdomen, pelvis
Persistent pain, pus, or bleeding at injection site

Follow-up Care of Yourself
A. Visit your health care provider every 12 weeks for injection
B. The visit should take place during first 5 days of your menses (period) (or at 12 weeks from last shot if no period)
C. Review any side effects or danger signs with your health care provider
D. Review your menstrual cycles with health care provider
E. Have a Pap smear every year along with a complete physical examination including pelvic and breast examinations
F. Depo-Provera® provides no protection against sexually transmitted diseases (including AIDS) or vaginal infections, so consider using condoms to protect yourself.

I have read the above and have been given a copy of this consent form and the manufacturer's information, and I agree to have Depo-Provera®.

_____
Client's signature   Date

_____
Witness's signature   Date
_____

From: Hawkins, Roberto-Nichols, & Stanley-Haney, *Protocols for Nurse Practitioners in Gynecologic Settings,* 7th edition, 2000, The Tiresias Press, Inc.

Appendix G

Informed Consent for a Diaphragm
(May also be used as an informational handout)

I. Mechanism of Action
A contraceptive diaphragm is a shallow rubber cup with a flexible rim which is placed in the vagina so as to cover the cervix. It functions as both a mechanical barrier and a receptacle for spermicidal cream or jelly which must be used to ensure effectiveness.

II. Benefits of the Method
A. Effectiveness rate ranges from 80-95%: theoretically, 95%. 80-85% use effectiveness (due to user failure)
B. No chemicals are taken internally

III. Risks of the Method
A. Allergic response to the rubber and/or spermicidal agent
B. Foul-smelling discharge from leaving diaphragm in place too long (diaphragm should not be left in place longer than 24 hours)
C. Toxic shock syndrome has been reported in association with diaphragm use during menses. To avoid this, do not leave your diaphragm in place for more than 24 hours and follow use precautions at the end of these instructions

IV. Contraindications (reasons for not using diaphragm)
A. Inability to achieve satisfactory fitting
B. You are unable to learn correct insertion technique
C. Allergy to rubber or spermicidal agent
D. Inconvenience of method (e.g., lack of sexual spontaneity, timing, messiness, etc.)
E. Repeated bladder infections (cystitis)

F. Chronic constipation ((causes discomfort for some users)

V. Alternative Birth Control Methods
A. Abstinence
B. Sterilization
C. Oral contraceptives (birth control pills, mini pills)
D. Intrauterine device
E. Norplant®
F. Condom used with contraceptive cream, foam, gel, suppositories or vaginal film
G. Cervical cap
H. Natural family planning
I. Female condom
J. Depo-Provera®

VI. Explanation of the Method
A. How a diaphragm is prescribed
   1. A complete physical examination including Papanicolaou smear is necessary unless one has been done within the past year. A pelvic examination (bimanual) will be done at the time the diaphragm is fitted
   2. If required by your health provided, review and sign an informed consent similar to this one prior to your initial prescription
B. How a diaphragm is used
   1. How it works
      a. Inserted prior to intercourse to fit snugly in vagina
      b. Holds spermicidal cream or jelly or vaginal film against cervix and kills sperm
      c. Diaphragm is to be left in place for 8 hours after last intercourse
      d. No douching for 8 hours after intercourse
      e. Prior to repeated intercourse, additional jelly or cream should be applied with applicator to outside of diaphragm or another vaginal film should be inserted
      f. Effective immediately upon insertion and up to 4 hours without adding more cream or jelly or film, or for one

intercourse (Some sources suggest 6 hours for c., d., and f.)

2. Technique for use
   a. Empty your bladder; wash your hands carefully whenever you insert or remove your diaphragm
   b. Apply approximately 1 tablespoon spermicidal cream or jelly into the dome of the diaphragm and spread around the dome; cream or jelly need not be spread on the rim or outside of diaphragm
   c. Fold in half and insert into vagina like a tampon
   d. With index finger check rim at pubic arch and make sure cervix is covered
   e. To remove (at proper time), hook finger around rim and pull diaphragm out
3. Care of diaphragm
   a. Wash with warm water and mild soap after removal
   b. Dry thoroughly
   c. Store in dry place (allowing it to dry thoroughly before putting it in a case keeps rubber in better condition longer and prevents odor; powder lightly with cornstarch)
   d. Soak in rubbing alcohol (70%) for 30 minutes after use following treatment for vaginal infection

VII. Diaphragm Check

A. We encourage you to return to the office one week after fitting for diaphragm check
B. If you lose or gain 10-15 pounds (or if diaphragm fit seems to change)
C. If you have a miscarriage, abortion, or a baby
D. If you have any kind of pelvic surgery
E. If you experience problems urinating or trouble moving your bowels with diaphragm in place

VIII. Inquiries are Encouraged

Please feel free to ask us questions at any time!
You may change your mind about a birth control method at any time.

I have read the above material; it has been explained fully. I have been given the opportunity to ask questions and I understand the information. I have chosen to use the diaphragm.

_____

Client's signature   Date

_____

Witness's signature   Date

Toxic Shock Syndrome

Toxic shock syndrome has been reported in association with diaphragm use during menses. It is recommended that if you use your diaphragm during menses, you observe handwashing recommendations carefully, use tampons only during heaviest days (not super-absorbent type—see tampon package labeling) and monitor yourself carefully for any signs of toxic shock syndrome.

Danger Signals Associated with Possible Toxic Shock Syndrome
   Fever (temperature 100° F and above)
   Diarrhea
   Vomiting
   Muscle ache
   Rash (sunburn-like)
Contact us at (__)_____if you develop any of the above problems (and don't use your diaphragm—remove at once)

If your diaphragm slips out of place or comes out, you can call 1-888-NOT-2-LATE for information on emergency contraception.

From: Hawkins, Roberto-Nichols & Stanley-Haney, *Protocols for Nurse Practitioners in Gynecological Settings, 7th edition,* 2000, The Tiresias Press, Inc.

Appendix H

Informed Consent for an Intrauterine Device (IUD)
(May also be used as informational handout)

I. Definition/Mechanism of Action
An intrauterine device consists of a sterile body placed in the uterus to prevent fertilization. This is accomplished through several mechanisms of action, depending on the type of device:
A. A local sterile inflammatory response to the foreign body (the IUD) causes a change in the cellular makeup of the uterine lining
B. A possible increase in the local production of prostaglandins may increase endometrial activity
C. Alteration in uterine and tubal transport of egg
D. Change in cervical mucus causing barrier to sperm penetration

II. Benefits of the Method
A. Encourages sexual spontaneity
B. Effectiveness rate, theoretically, 97-99%
C. Semi-permanent (depending on the type of device); replacement time varies but all devices are effective for at least one year; one device lasts 10 years

III. Risks of Method
A. Major risks
   1. Involuntary expulsion (approximately 6%)
   2. Pelvic inflammatory disease
   3. Ectopic pregnancy (outside of the uterus)
   4. Uterine perforation
   5. Pregnancy
B. Minor risks
   1. Increased menstrual flow
   2. Increased dysmenorrhea (cramps)
   3. String may cause some discomfort to partner

IV. Reasons for Not Using an Intrauterine Device (IUD)

1. Active pelvic infection (acute or subacute) including known or suspected gonorrhea or chlamydia
2. Known or suspected pregnancy
3. Recent or recurrent pelvic infection
4. Purulent cervicitis, untreated acute cervicitis, or vaginosis
5. Undiagnosed genital bleeding
6. Uterine cavity not suitable for IUD insertion
7. History of ectopic pregnancy (pregnancy outside uterus)
8. Diabetes mellitus—can use ParaGard® IUD
9. Allergy to copper (known or suspected) or diagnosed Wilson's Disease—can use Progestasert® IUD
10. Abnormal Pap; cervical or uterine cancer, precancer
11. Impaired response to infection (diabetes, steroid treatment, immunocompromised patients such as those with HIV/AIDS)
12. Presence of previously inserted IUD
13. Genital actinomycosis—chronic infection of genital area

V. Reasons IUD May not Be Best Choice or Require Careful Monitoring with Health Care Provider

1. Multiple sexual partners or partner has multiple partners
2. In very rural areas, emergency treatment difficult to obtain
3. Cervical opening resistant to inserting IUD
4. Impaired blood clotting response
5. Uterine cavity too small, too large
6. Endometriosis
7. Fibroids in uterus
8. Polyps in uterine lining (endometrium)
9. Severe dysmenorrhea (Progestasert® IUD may help)
10. Heavy or prolonged menstrual bleeding without anemia; consider oral iron or nutritional changes to prevent anemia
11. Unable to check for IUD string
12. Concerns for future fertility
13. Postpartum or infected abortion within the past 3 months
14. History of pelvic uterine infection
15. Valvular heart disease infection

VI. Alternatives

A. Abstinence

B. Sterilization

C. Birth control pills

D. Cervical Cap

E. Natural family planning

F. Depo-Provera®

G. Female condom

H. Norplant®

I. Diaphragm and spermicidal cream or jelly, film

J. Condom used with contraceptive cream, foam, suppositories, gel, or vaginal film

VII. Explanation of the Method

A. How the intrauterine device may work (no one is quite sure), but there are several theories:

1. Motility of the egg in fallopian tube is altered

2. A sterile inflammatory response to the IUD causes a change in the cells of the uterine lining

3. A change in the cervical mucus causing a barrier to sperm

B. What you should know about caring for your IUD

1. Know the type of device you have in place

2. Know when your device should be replaced

3. Learn how to check the string which extends from the center of the cervix into the vaginal canal

4. Check the string frequently the first few months and then after each period

5. Do not let your partner pull on the string

6. Never try to remove IUD yourself

7. Obtain your 6-week check-up after insertion of the device

8. Get a check-up every year including a Pap smear

9. Depending on your normal menstrual cycle, if you miss a period, consult your care provider for possible pregnancy

C. What to expect

1. Possible increase in menstrual flow, menstrual cramping
   Remember: if this condition becomes intolerable, you have the option of having your IUD removed by a clinician

D. Side effects to be reported *immediately*

1. Late period or absence of period

2. Abdominal or pelvic pain (severe)

3. Elevated temperature, chills (not due to illness)
4. Unpleasant vaginal discharge (smelly, foul, bloody, or greenish color)
5. Unusual vaginal bleeding (heavy period, clotting)

E. Insertion
1. Must be done at time of menses (your period); if inserted at end of menses, flow may become heavy again
2. Should have negative gonococcus and Chlamydia cultures prior to insertion (within 30 days)
3. Must have recent (with the year) normal Pap smear
4. May have some discomfort and dizziness with insertion
5. May have spotting for several months after insertion
6. Although the IUD is effective immediately, it is recommended that intercourse not take place for 24 hours

VII. Inquiries are encouraged! Ask us questions at any time.
I have read the above material; it has been explained fully. I have been given the opportunity to ask questions and I understand the information. I have chosen to use the IUD.

_____

    Signed   Witness

                                Date _____

Danger Signals Associated with the Use of the IUD
Late period or absence of period
Abdominal pain (severe)
Elevated temperature, chills (not due to illness, e.g., flu)
Unpleasant vaginal discharge (smelly, foul, bloody, or greenish color)
Unusual vaginal bleeding (heavy period, clotting)

Contact us or a care provider immediately if above danger signs develop!

From: Hawkins, Roberto-Nichols, & Stanley-Haney, *Protocols for Nurse Practitioners in Gynecologic Settings,* 7th edition, 2000, The Tiresias Press, Inc.

Appendix I

For Your Information:
Contraceptive Spermicides and Condoms

Spermicides

I. Definition/Mechanism of Action
Spermicides are a barrier method of birth control. All contain an inert base or vehicle and an active ingredient, most commonly a surfactant such as nonoxynol-9 which disrupts the integrity of the sperm membrane (acts as a spermicide).

II. Effectiveness and Benefits
A. Method: 96% effectiveness rate
B. User: 60% effectiveness rate
C. Inexpensive and readily available
D. Some protective effect against the transmission of sexually transmitted diseases including the AIDS virus (HIV)

III. Side Effects and Disadvantages
A. Local irritation from spermicide
B. Can necessitate interruption of love-making
C. Emotional difficulty with touching one's own body

IV. Types
A. Creams, jellies, gels   B.   Foams
C. Foaming tablets   D.   Suppositories
E. Vaginal film

V. How to Use
A. Instructions should be read prior to using any spermicide. Method of insertion, time of effectiveness, time needed prior to intercourse, etc., will vary with each type

B. Use new insertion of spermicide with each intercourse
C. After each use, wash the applicator with soap and water
D. When using a spermicide, partner should always use a condom unless you use female condom

VI. Follow-up
A. Yearly physical examination with Papanicolaou smear is recommended

Condoms

I. Definition/Mechanism of Action
Condoms are thin sheaths, most commonly made of latex (female condoms are made of polyurethane; male polyurethane condoms are now on the market) which prevent the transmission of sperm from the penis to the vagina

II. Effectiveness and Benefits
A. Method: 97-98% effectiveness rate, providing the method is used correctly
B. User: 70-94% effectiveness rate
C. Inexpensive and readily available
D. Offer protection against sexually transmitted disease. Only latex condoms provide protection against the AIDS (HIV) virus. The female condom is made of thick polyurethane so it does offer protection
E. Encourage male participation in birth control

III. Side Effects and Disadvantages
A. Allergic reaction to latex (rare). (Female condom is polyurethane as are some new male condoms)
B. Use necessitates interruption of love-making for application
C. May decrease tactile sensation
D. Psychological impotency with male condom
E. If latex allergy is a problem, double condom use is an option. If the woman is allergic, the male can wear a latex condom with a skin or polyurethane condom covering it. If the man is allergic, he can wear a polyurethane or skin condom with a

latex condom over it. Skin condoms should not be worn alone since they do not offer protection from HIV

IV. Types

Condoms vary in color, texture (smooth, studded, or ribbed), shape and price; they come lubricated and plain; some have spermicide; some are extra strength, some sheerer and thinner; some have a unique shape; some are scented

V. How to Use Male Condom

A. Always pull the male condom on an erect penis and before there is any sexual contact. Use for every act of intercourse
B. Do not pull the male condom tightly over the end of the penis; leave about an inch extra for ejaculation fluid and to avoid breakage; some condoms have a reservoir tip
C. Withdraw before the penis becomes limp and hold the open end of the condom tightly while withdrawing
D. Partner should always use a contraceptive spermicide along with condom
E. Condoms should be used only once

VI. How to Use Female Condom

The female condom comes prelubricated

A. Pinch ring at closed end of pouch and insert like a diaphragm covering the cervix; adding 1-2 drops of additional lubricant makes insertion easier and decreases or eliminates squeaking noise and dislocation during intercourse
B. Adjust other ring over labia
C. Can be inserted several minutes to 8 hours prior to intercourse
D. Remove before standing up by squeezing and twisting the Outer ring and pulling out gently

If the condom breaks or slips off, call 1-800-NOT-2-Late for emergency contraception information.

From: Hawkins, Roberto-Nichols & Stanley-Haney, *Protocols for Nurse Practitioners in Gynecologic Settings,* 7th ed., 2000, The Tiresias Press, Inc., New York: NY.

Appendix J

For Your Information: Using the Cervical Cap*

I. Definition/Mechanism of Action

The Prentif Cervical Cap is a thimble-shaped, deep-domed barrier device that fits closely over the cervix and is used with spermicidal jelly or cream. Approved by the FDA in 1988, this birth control device must be fitted by a specially trained clinician. When used consistently and carefully, the cervical cap is as effective as the diaphragm.

II. Instructions for Insertion

A. Wash your hands before handling the cap. Fill the cap 1/2 to 3/4 full of spermicidal vaginal jelly or cream. Inserting too much spermicide in the cap can interfere with the cap's suction and therefore should be avoided. Spermicide should not spill out of the cap during insertion.

B. Assume the position you plan to use when inserting the cap. Squatting shortens the vagina and lowers the cervix and may be a good position to try. Lying down may also work for you. Try different positions and remember, there is no wrong position.

C. Locate your cervix by inserting your finger into your vagina toward your tailbone. It may help to apply a small amount of lubricating jelly (like KY) to your finger before feeling for your cervix (your cervix feels like a soft nose and protrudes from the back of your vagina). Using too much lubricant may interfere with the cap's suction, so use it sparingly. The more familiar you are with your cervix, the easier inserting and removing the cap will be. Dry your fingers before handling the cap; this will make holding and inserting the cap easier. Grasp the cap and squeeze its rim together. With the other hand

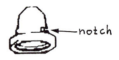

CERVICAL CAP

*This protocol was developed by R. Mimi Clarke Secor, R.N., C.S-FNP, M.Ed., M.S., Certified Family Nurse Practitioner, and is used with her permission.

separate the lips (labia) of your vagina. Direct the cap into the vagina with the rim of the cap opposite from the notch going in first; this will ensure that the notch is easy to reach so you may turn the cap later. (It is thought that doing so will improve the suction of the cap.) The opening of the cap should be held up to prevent spilling the spermicide.

E.   Once in the vagina, the cap will pop open. Quickly reposition one finger (usually the index and middle fingers work best) to either side of the thick rim and push the open part of the cap toward the cervix. (Push as far as you can until the cap stops.) Pushing the cap onto the cervix using one finger is also a good technique, but may not offer the control of the two-finger technique.

F.   Check for proper placement of the cap. This is done by tracing around the rim with your finger. If the cap is over the cervix, you will not be able to locate the cervix because it is covered by the cap. Don't worry if the soft dome of the cap feels dented or wrinkled; this is normal and not significant (either regarding the quality of the suction or the location of the cap). Don't worry if you are unable to reach the underside or the very back of the cap rim.

G.   Turning the cap may improve its suction; how far it should be turned is controversial. Turning may be accomplished by pushing the rim of the cap laterally with your fingers to either side. A one-quarter to one-half turn is probably adequate; however, some sources recommend one or two full turns

H.   If you are unable to rotate the cap at all, or very little, do not worry. The ability or inability to turn the cap is not necessarily an indication of cap suction or quality of fit.

I.   During the first few months, use a back-up method of birth control. If you are on the pill, continue taking it for a month longer until you have tried the cap in different positions of lovemaking. If you have been using a diaphragm, consider asking your partner to use a condom initially when trying different positions with the cap. Some sources recommend use of a back-up method of birth control the first six times the cap is used.

J.   If your partner is unwilling to use back-up condoms, consider the use of vaginal contraceptive film (VCF) sold over the counter at some drug stores. This is spermicidally coated gelatin paper rolled up and inserted vaginally at least five minutes before intercourse. It should not be used inside the cap as a substitute for spermicidal jelly/cream, but as a adjunct back-up method inserted after the cap is in place.

K. A diaphragm should not be used concurrently as a back-up method with the cap. However, the diaphragm may be used alternately with the cap.

L. When trying different lovemaking positions using the cap, check for proper cap placement immediately after each intercourse.

M. If you find the cap dislodged, try not to panic. Immediately insert a full applicator of spermicide high into your vagina and remain lying down for at least half an hour, preferably a full hour. Also, do not try to reposition the cap back onto the cervix, as this may cause more sperm to enter the cervical opening. Wait 8 to 12 hours to remove the cap and do not use it again until it is refitted and you have had a chance to discuss with your clinician why the dislodgement occurred.

N. Some facilities recommend use of emergency contraception if there is a possibility the cap became dislodged during intercourse, but this must be started within 72 hours of dislodgement. Contact your clinician for further information or call 1-888-NOT-2-LATE.

O. Practice using your cap. The more comfortable you are inserting and removing it, the more you will trust it as a method of contraception.

REMEMBER: Some method of birth control should be used every time you have vaginal intercourse. There is no safe time in your cycle for unprotected intercourse (unless you have been taught and are using natural family planning).

III. Additional Points on Wearing the Cap

A. You must wear the cap for at least 8 hours after penile/vaginal intercourse.

B. The FDA has approved 48 hours as the maximum time the cap may be worn (at one time). However, your clinician may suggest a maximum time limit of 24 hours (especially if you have a history of urinary or vaginal infections).

C. During your menstrual period, do not use your cap for birth control because the menstrual flow may cause the cap to dislodge.

D. Toxic shock syndrome has not been reported in women using the cap. However, the theoretical risk exists, especially in women who wear the cap in excess of 24 hours. Please discuss this information with your clinician, especially if you have further questions.*

---

*Danger signs associated with possible toxic shock syndrome: fever (temperature 100° F and above); diarrhea, vomiting, muscle ache, rash (sunburn-like).

E. The cap may be inserted many hours before intercourse, even a day before.

F. With initial use, the cap is best inserted within one hour of intercourse. If possible, insert the cap before foreplay because sexual stimulation may interfere with the insertion of the cap and the establishment of good suction. During the first few months do not wear the cap more than 24 hours at a time, and avoid repeated sexual acts and varied positions during this time. This will allow you to better monitor the cap and will minimize the variables you must examine if there is a problem.

G. With repeated intercourse (associated with ejaculation), while the cap is in place, you do not have to add extra spermicide.

IV. Other Considerations Related to Wearing the Cap

A. Partner complains. Most men do not feel the cervical cap. A few find, when they are able to feel it, that the sensation is unpleasant. Unfortunately, this problem is difficult to anticipate. Occasionally, it is the notch they feel and if you turn the cap's notch to the side, the problem may be eliminated. In some situations, trying a different cap size may help.

B. Sometimes, if a woman is not sufficiently stimulated, the man will feel both the cervix and the cap, in which case the solution is to increase the amount of foreplay before actual penile intercourse is attempted. Occasionally, only certain positions pose a problem and, by avoiding them, the cap may still be used. However, if those positions are most desired, the solution may be to use a different birth control method.

C. Reinserting the cervical cap after removal. It is recommended the cap be removed a minimum of 6-8 hours before it is reinserted.

V. Removal of the Cap

A. Assume the position you used to insert the cap. Squatting while bearing down (like having a difficult bowel movement) works well for many women. This position shortens the vagina, lowering the cervix and making the rim of the cap easier to reach.

B. Using any finger, push the rim of the cap to the side (aiming for your hip). Once the cap is loosened from the cervix, reach into the dome and remove it. You may have to struggle a bit, but don't be timid. If you continue to have difficulty removing the cap, your clinician may add a loop of nylon thread through the notch of the cap to make removal easier. This is usually a temporary solution until you develop a technique that works. Consider asking your partner to assist in removing the cap.

C. If your period starts while you are wearing the cap, wait the normal 8 hours to remove it. If the cap is unable to hold the blood, it will leak out and possibly cause the cap to come off the cervix. If this happens, simply remove the cap and wait to resume using it until your period is over. A little spotting will not usually interfere with the cap fit.

VI. Care of Your Cap

A. Wash the cap with water and mild soap. You may turn the cap inside out in order to clean the inside rim more easily; some women use a fingernail or a small brush to clean the inside rim. Dry the cap thoroughly and store it in its container. If you use an airtight container, punch some small holes in it or don't seal the lid entirely because some types of bacteria grow more readily in the absence of oxygen. Do not powder your cap.

B. If your cap develops an odor, see your clinician to check for a possible vaginal infection. Some types of infection, especially bacterial vaginosis, may cause a foul cap odor without causing you symptoms. To remove the odor, try soaking the cap for 30 minutes in soapy water or rubbing alcohol. Excessive soaking may lead to cap stretching and this may affect the fit. Rinse the cap thoroughly before reinserting it. You may need a new cap if these suggestions are not effective. Some women find the cap develops an odor if it is worn for more than 24 hours.

VII. Other Special Concerns

A. For the first few months, check the cap frequently after penile intercourse, after vaginal finger activity, bowel movements, or any other time you are nervous about the cap.

B. Weight changes do not generally affect the fit of the cap. However, if your cap behaves in an odd manner and you've had more than a 15-pound weight change, have your cap resized.

C. If you give birth vaginally, you should have your cap resized 6 to 12 weeks after delivery.

D. If you have any of the following cervical procedures (biopsy, abortion, dilation and curettage, conization, laser treatment, or cryosurgery) have your cervical cap resized. Wait at least 2 or 3 weeks to do this, or until complete healing has occurred.

E. Breast feeding may alter your cap fit, so be sure to have it refitted before and after you stop breast feeding (or any time the cap dislodges).

F. If you have been taking the birth control pill while using the cervical cap, have the cap refitted after you stop the pill. The pill may affect the cap's fit by interrupting your normal ovulatory cycle.

VIII. Follow-up

A. Within the first 3 months: follow up with your clinician to check the size and fit of the cap and your skill in using it. (You may be asked to insert the cap at home and wear it in for a visit). Do not insert your cap if you think you have a vaginal infection or if you are having problems with the cap.

B. Yearly or as recommended: a pelvic exam, Pap smear, and resizing of the cap. Bring the cap with you. According to FDA regulations, a new cap should be purchased yearly to ensure proper fit.

IX. Reasons to Temporarily Discontinue Using the Cap

A. Vaginal infection. Wait until the infection is resolved and a follow-up exam confirms this.

B. Urinary tract infection. Continuing to be sexually active while you have a urinary tract infection may slow healing and recovery.

C. Pelvic infection. Rationale is the same as for A. and B.

D. Abnormal Pap smears or conditions of the cervix such as cervicitis. The cap should not be used until your Pap smear is normal or the abnormal cervical condition is resolved.

E. Poor fit associated with such temporary situations as breast feeding or poor vaginal tone (which may improve after Kegel practice). Refitting is essential before resumption of cap use.

X. Summary

The cap is easy to use and is very effective if the instructions provided here are followed. As with any barrier method of birth control, you may become pregnant while using the cap faithfully. If you have any questions, concerns, or problems, please be sure to contact your clinician.

If your cap slips off during intercourse, call 1-888-NOT-2-LATE for emergency contraception information.

Appendix K

For Your Information:
Using the Vaginal Contraceptive Sponge

I. Definition
A. Description
    The contraceptive sponge looks like a small doughnut which measures about 1¾ of an inch in diameter. The hollow area in the center fits over the cervix. Across the bottom is a nylon tape (string) which provides for easy removal. The sponge contains a spermicide called nonoxynol-9.
B. Method of action
    1. Provides a barrier between sperm and the cervical os
    2. Traps sperm within the sponge
    3. A spermicide contained within the sponge is released over a 24-hour period to destroy the sperm

II. Effectiveness and Benefits
A. 89-90.8 method effectiveness rate, 84.5-86.7 use effectiveness
B. Readily available, over the counter, no prescription needed
C. The user may have repeated sexual intercourse within a 24-hour period without adding extra spermicide
D. It is thought that spermicides have a protective effect against the transmission of sexually transmitted diseases

III. Side Effects and Disadvantages
A. Irritation or allergic reactions to the spermicide (nonoxynol-9)
B. Inability to learn correct insertion technique
C. Difficulty removing the sponge
D. There has been some concern relating to toxic shock syndrome. Studies show that the spermicide contained in the sponge is hostile to the growth of the organism that causes toxic shock syndrome. It is recommended that it be used only with care during menses.

IV. Explanation of Method
A. How to insert (always wash hands carefully when inserting and removing sponge)

1. The sponge may be inserted any time up to 24 hours before sexual intercourse. There is no need to add additional cream or jelly once the sponge has been moistened under water and inserted into the vagina
2. Read the instructions in the package, insert carefully and follow instructions each time you use the sponge

B. How to remove
  1. Read the printed instructions carefully
  2. Remember to remove the sponge slowly to avoid tearing it
  3. Do not flush the sponge down the toilet
  4. Special removal instructions
     a. If the sponge appears to be stuck, simply relax your vaginal muscles and bear down and you should be able to remove it without difficulty
     b. The sponge may turn upside down in the vagina making the string loop more difficult to find. To find the string, run your finger around the edge on back side of the sponge until you feel the string. If you cannot find the look, grasp the sponge between your thumb and forefinger and remove it slowly
     c. The sponge can tear, so remember to remove it slowly. If it does tear and you think there may be small pieces of sponge left inside the vagina, run your finger around the upper vault of the vagina to
     remove the remaining pieces

Remember: the sponge cannot get lost in the vagina.

V. Additional information
A. Wash your hands with soap and water before inserting the sponge to avoid introducing germs into the vagina
B. It is OK to use the sponge while swimming or bathing
C. The sponge may be only used once and then should be discarded

Danger signals of Possible Toxic Shock Syndrome
Fever (temperature 101° and above)
Diarrhea
Vomiting
Muscle ache
Rash (sunburn-like)

From: Hawkins, Roberto-Nichols & Stanley-Haney, *Protocols for Nurse Practitioners in Gynecologic Settings,* 7th edition, 2000, ©The Tiresias Press, Inc.

Appendix L

For Your Information: Directions for Using Natural Family Planning to Prevent or Achieve Pregnancy

Natural family planning methods (NFP) are based on the client's knowledge about the days in the menstrual cycle when she can become pregnant. There are only a few days in the cycle when this is possible. The couple that uses one of the natural methods to prevent pregnancy makes the choice not to have intercourse during these days. Natural methods of family planning are 75% to 98% effective, depending on the method used and on how well the information about them is learned and followed. All of the modern methods of natural family planning are based upon one or more changes that occur *naturally* in a woman's body. No drugs or chemicals are used.

Commonly Used Methods of Natural Family Planning

1. Cervical mucus method—based on detectable changes in cervical mucus throughout the cycle
2. Basal body temperature method—based on changes in the temperature of the woman's body at rest
3. Symptothermal method—based on the changes in the body temperature, cervical mucus, and other bodily signs

To become knowledgeable about natural family planning methods requires instruction and can be a pleasant, healthy way to learn to avoid or achieve pregnancy and be aware of your individual fertility pattern.

---

*By the late Eleanor Tabeek, R.N., Ph.D., C.N.M., updated by Nancy Keaveney, R.N., B.S., and used with Dr. Tabeek's family's permission.

Terminology used in a Natural Family Planning Class

abstinence—not having vaginal sexual intercourse

fertile days—the days in the menstrual cycle when pregnancy (conception) is possible

genitals or genitalia—organs of the reproductive system in both male and female

genital-to-genital contact—penis *touching* or coming into close contact with the vaginal area

hormone—a substance that causes special changes in the body; may be naturally occurring or synthetically produced

infertile days—the days in the menstrual cycle when pregnancy (conception) cannot occur

menstruation—bleeding that occurs when the lining of the uterus breaks down and is released; this happens about 12-16 days after ovulation

menstrual cycle—the time from the first day of menstrual bleeding to the day *before* the next menstrual bleeding begins; may vary normally from 21 to 40 days in length

ovulation—release of the egg (ovum) from the ovary about 12 to 16 days *before* the onset of the next menstrual period (the day bleeding begins

ovum—female sex cell, egg

sperm—male sex cell (spermatozoa) found in the semen of a man

Review of the Menstrual Cycle

The menstrual cycle is controlled by hormones. The cycle begins on the *first* day of menstrual bleeding and end the day *before* menstrual bleeding begins again.

Following menstruation, eggs (ova) are usually maturing in the follicles of the ovaries as they grow, estrogen (a hormone known as the female sex hormone) is produced in increasing amounts, and certain changes take place:

1. The lining of the uterus builds up the blood supply needed for pregnancy to occur.

2. Cervical mucus changes in character to become more hospitable to sperm so sperm can live and travel in the uterus.
3. The cervix become higher in the pelvis and softer as the cervical os opens to allow sperm to enter the uterus.
4. Basal body temperature (BBT) is low.

As the time of ovulation nears, some women may experience one or more of the following changes:
1. Clearer complexion and less oily hair
2. Increase in energy level
3. Vaginal aching
4. Spotting of blood
5. Pain or aching in the pelvic area
6. Breast tenderness and/or fullness

Once ovulation has occurred, there is an increase in the production of progesterone (another hormone important to the menstrual cycle and to pregnancy), and the following changes occur during the 12-16 days before menstruation begins:
1. Basal body temperature (BBT) arises
2. Mucus becomes inhospitable to sperm so they can't live and travel into the uterus
3. Cervix becomes lower, firmer, and the opening closes to prevent sperm from going into the uterus
4. Increased progesterone maintains the lining of the uterus in place for 12-16 days

As menstruation approaches, women may also experience one or more of the following changes:
1. Cramps
2. Headaches
3. Oily hair and complexion, acne or increase in acne
4. Mood changes
5. Decrease in energy level
6. Desire to eat foods with sugar and/or salt
7. Breast tenderness
8. Pelvic aching or pain
9. Low back pain; joint pain or aches

Cervical Mucus Method

Cervical mucus is produced by tiny cells in the cervix. As the ova are maturing, the mucus will change in a special way that helps keep sperm alive and makes it easier for sperm to travel into the uterus. The mucus loses this quality within a few days after the ovum leave the ovary. The quality or condition of the cervical mucus is an excellent indicator of the days in the menstrual cycle when the woman can become pregnant.

How to check the cervical mucus

1. Begin checking the cervical mucus when the menstrual bleeding ends or becomes light enough to let you be able to see mucus.
2. Cervical mucus can be checked before or after urination.
3. Before checking, note whether the area around and in the vaginal opening feels wet or dry.
4. Fold a piece of toilet tissue and wipe over the vaginal opening. If the tissue slides across the vaginal opening, the vaginal area is wet and mucus is present. If the tissue sticks only a little to the vaginal opening, this means that the vaginal area is dry and any mucus is either crumbly, sticky, or pasty, or that no mucus is present.
5. If there is mucus on the toilet tissue, place it between two fingers and feel it by *slowly* opening the two fingers. Does it lack wetness? Is it sticky or pasty? Or does it feel slippery, wet, and stretchy?

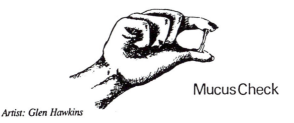

MucusCheck

Artist: Glen Hawkins

6. The woman who does not want to touch the mucus can assess the stretchiness by holding the toilet tissue in both hands, then pulling it apart.

7. Check mucus each time you use the bathroom. Remember to check in the evening, since the character of the mucus can change during the day.

How to Chart Information about the Mucus

1. A new cycle starts the first day of the menstrual bleeding, regardless of the time of the day the flow begins. Write the date that you started bleeding in the space on the Natural Family Planning Chart (see next page).
2. Record each day of bleeding with a star (*).
3. . Record any day of spotting of blood with the letter "S."
4. When the period ends, if the vaginal area is dry and *no* mucus is present *throughout* the day, this is a DRY day. Chart a dry day using the letter "D."
5. Continue to use the letter "D" each day until you see *any* kind of mucus on the toilet tissue.
6. When the vaginal area is still dry, and you see mucus that does not feel wet (but is pasty and sticky), chart this type of mucus with the letter "M."
7. Continue to use the symbol "M" each day that the mucus doesn't feel wet and the vaginal area is dry.
8. When either mucus, vaginal area, or both start to become wet, chart this by using the letter M with a circle around it (M)
9. As the time of ovulation approaches, the vaginal area will become wetter. The mucus often becomes clear and stretches like raw egg white.
10. Continue to chart M as long as the mucus and vaginal area continue to feel wet.
11. The *last* day of the wet and stretchy mucus and wet vaginal area is charted by writing an "X" through M M. The last day of wet and stretchy mucus (peak day) usually will not be noted until the following day when the mucus will not be as wet and stretchy.
12. The last day of stretchy, slippery, and wet-feeling mucus and wet vaginal sensations is called the Peak Day. On the first

Natural Family Planning Chart

day past the Peak Day, the mucus usually becomes cloudy and sticky. The mucus will lose all or most of its wet feeling and the outside of the vaginal area will feel dry again. If you are taking your basal body temperature, the Peak Day often occurs around the day the temperature rises.

Summary of Mucus Symbols

*	D	M	(M)	M̶
Menses	Dry	Mucus sticky, pasty and/or crumbly and vaginal area dry	Wet, slippery, stretchy, mucus and wet vaginal area	Last day of wet, slippery, stretchy mucus and wet vaginal area

Always chart the *most* wet-feeling mucus and wet-feeling vaginal sensations of the day.

How to Chart Other Symptoms

1. Record intercourse by a check mark (√).
2. Record any other changes in your body, e.g., pain with ovulation, breast tenderness, etc.) in the column under "Notes."
3. Until you know your mucus changes well, it is helpful to write a description of your mucus in the Notes column, e.g., sticky, white.

Basal Body Temperature (BBT) Method

Basal body temperature is the temperature of the body at rest. As the ova are maturing, the temperature is low. At some time shortly before, during, or after the ovum leaves the ovary, the temperature will usually rise about 3/10ths to 1 full degree higher than it had been. This change in temperature tells you when the ovum *has* left the ovary; that is, that ovulation has taken place.

How to Take Basal Body Temperature

1. Begin taking temperature the first day of menstrual bleeding
2. Take temperature about the same time every day, usually in the morning when you first awake.
3. Take temperature before eating, drinking, smoking, and any physical activity.
4. The thermometer can be placed in the mouth, in the vagina, or in the rectum. Always take temperature the same way every day. Record temperature on the Natural Family Planning Chart.
5. If the temperature reading on the thermometer is between two lines, record the temperature at the lower line.

Change in Daily Events

Occasionally, a woman may become ill, drink alcoholic beverages, or change the usual time she takes her temperature. Since such events or any change in lifestyle may affect the temperature, when and if they happen, take and record the temperature anyway. In the "Notes" column on the Natural Family Planning Chart, record the possible reason for any change in the usual temperature.

To record your temperature...
Circle your temperature each day on the
Natural Family Planning Chart
and connect the circles with a line.

T	**98.0**	98	98	98	98	98	98	98	98	98	98	98	98	98	98	98	98	
E		9	9	9	9	9	9	9	9	9	9	9	9	9	9	9	9	9
M		8	8	8	8	8	8	8	8	8	8	8	8	8	8	8	8	8
P		7	7	7	7	7	7	7	7	7	7	7	7	7	7	7	7	7
E		6	6	6	6	6	6	6	6	6	6	6	6	6	6	6	6	6
R		5	5	5	5	5	5	5	5	5	5	5	5	5	5	5	5	5
A		4	4	4	4	4	4	4	4	4	4	4	4	4	4	4	4	4
T		3	3	3	3	3	3	3	3	3	3	3	3	3	3	3	3	
U		2	2	2	2	2	2	2	2	2	2	2	2	2	2	2	2	
R		1	1	1	1	1	1	1	1	1	1	1	1	1	1	1	1	
E	**97.0**	97	97	97	97	97	97	97	97	97	97	97	97	97	97	97	97	
		9	9	9	9	9	9	9	9	9	9	9	9	9	9	9	9	
CYCLE DAY		1	2	3	4	5	6	7	8	9	10	11	12	13	14	15	16	1

The Cervix (Cervix Sign)

During each cycle, as the ovum is developing and maturing, the cervix is low in the vagina, the opening is closed, and the area around the opening feels firm like the tip of the nose. Around the time the ovum is getting ready to leave the ovary, the cervix will soften and the opening will become wide. These changes help sperm travel into the uterus. Within a few days after the ovum leaves the ovary (ovulation), the cervix will be lower in the vaginal canal; the area around its opening will become firm, and the opening will close up. These changes help prevent sperm from traveling into the uterus. It is not necessary to check the cervix in order to use natural family planning. However, knowing about the cervical changes can give interested women information about their fertile and infertile days.

How to Check Status of the Cervix

1. Begin checking the cervix after the menstrual bleeding ends.
2. Check the cervix while in a comfortable position such as squatting or standing with one foot on a stool or chair. Use the same position each time you check the cervix.
3. Check in the evening, and at about the *same time* each day.
4. Wash your hands before placing a finger in the vagina.
5. When feeling the cervix, check for:
    *   position in vagina: high (may be difficult to feel) or low (usually easy to feel)
    *   softness or firmness
    *   opening: open or closed
6. Chart the most fertile cervical sign of the day.

How to Chart Information about the Cervix

1. Use circles to represent the sizes of the cervical opening. Place the circles in different positions in the boxes on the Natural Family Planning Chart to represent the rising and lowering of the cervix.

⌊.⌋ low and closed |O| high and open

2. You can also use the letter "F" to represent a firm cervix and the letter "S" to represent a soft cervix:

(S) (S) (S) (S) (S) (S) (F) (F) (F)
 o   o   O O O   o
                          ●   ●
(F) (F) (F) (S) (S)
 ·   .   ●   ●   ●   ●

(Closed circles represent a closed cervical opening—as the cervix opens, the circles are larger.)

3. Another way the position of the cervix can be noted is through using arrows
   a high cervix ➤
   a lowering cervix ➤
   a cervix tilted to the side = ↓ (right side) or ↓ (left side)

Symptothermal Method
Combining use of all the information described to this point.

Natural Family Planning Rules to Prevent Pregnancy

By following the natural family planning rules, you will know on which days you are fertile or infertile during each menstrual cycle. **Note:** Please check with your instructor or health care provider before following any of the rules.

Every Other Dry Day Rule: Intercourse can take place on the evening of every other dry day until mucus is seen and/or wetness of the vaginal area experienced.

How to Determine Which Days Before Ovulation are Infertile Days

It is common for some of the man's semen to be in the woman's vagina on the day after intercourse. Therefore, if cervical mucus starts to be produced on that day, the presence of semen may prevent the woman from seeing the mucus. Since it can take up to 24 hours for semen to completely leave the vaginal area, intercourse should not take place two days in a row. Instead, the Every Other Dry Day Rule should be followed.

Remember: If cervical mucus is being produced and the couple goes ahead and has intercourse again, the woman could become pregnant. This is why abstinence from intercourse should be followed *the day after intercourse* has taken place. If the day after the abstinence day is a DRY DAY again it is safe to have intercourse on the evening of that day.

Dry Day	*Abstinence*	*Dry Day*	*Abstinence*
Intercourse	No intercourse	Intercourse	No intercourse
in the	the next day	in the evening	the next day
evening		of a dry day	

This way of timing intercourse can continue until ANY type of mucus is seen and/or the vaginal area begins to feel wet, whichever comes first. The first sign of mucus and/or a wet vaginal area IS THE BEGINNING OF THE FERTILE PHASE. When the fertile phase begins, the couple should not have vaginal intercourse until the fertile phase ends, if a pregnancy is not desired.

Rules Based on the Menses

A. It is safe to have intercourse on the first three days of the menstrual cycle if a woman is taking her basal body temperature and used the Thermal Shift Rule in the previous cycle (this is proof of ovulation), and if she is sure that the bleeding is really menstrual bleeding.

B. 21-Day Rule

1. This rule can be used to find out which days are infertile before ovulation if you know the length of your previous six consecutive menstrual cycles. These six cycles must have been your normal-usual menstrual cycles.
   Example:

   Previous six cycles:

1. June	28 days long	4. September	30 days long
2. July	29 days long	5. October	28 days long
3. August	**27 days long**	6. November	29 days long

2. Take the shortest of the six cycles and subtract 21 from this number. Example: shortest menstrual cycle: August- 27 days

3. The number of days remaining equals the number of infertile days before ovulation. Intercourse can take place at any time during these days, starting on the first day

of menstrual bleeding. Example: 27-21=6.

4. Fertile Phase begins the day after these infertile days end. Example: Abstinence begins on cycle day 7.

CAUTION: If mucus appears at any time during the infertile days, the fertile phase has started. Abstinence should begin.

C. **How to find out which days are infertile after ovulation**

1. *Peak Day Rule:* The infertile days after ovulation begin on the evening of the fourth day *after* the peak day. The peak day is the *last* day of the wet, slippery, and stretchy mucus and feelings of vaginal wetness.

   a. To use this rule, count 4 days in a row *after* the peak day. The mucus on these days must either be much less wet than it had been, be of the sticky, pasty, or crumbly type, or there may not be any mucus present. The vaginal feelings must also be dry.

   b. Mark the days after the peak day "1, "2," "3," "4."
   Example: *****DDDDMM(M)✗1234

   c. The evening of the fourth day after the peak day is the beginning of the infertile phase after ovulation according to this rule.

2. *Thermal Shift Rule:* The infertile phase after ovulation begins on the evening of the third temperature recorded above the coverline (see c. below).

   a. Watch for the first day of temperature rise. The rise is usually at least three-tenths (0.3) of a degree higher than the previous six low temperatures.

   b. Look at the 6 low temperatures recorded before the rise and find the highest of these temperatures.

   c. Draw a line (called the coverline) across the chart. This line is drawn through the temperature that is one-tenth of a degree above the *highest* of the six low temperatures.

   d. Keep taking temperature. When there are 3 recorded temperatures in a row that are above the coverline, the infertile phase after ovulation has begun.

   e. The infertile phase begins on the evening of the third temperature above the coverline.

   f. Averaging=a 0.4°F rise above the average of at least 6 normal temperatures prior to the shift.

Appendix M
Teaching Natural Family Planning to Clients: Guidelines for Instructors*

Successful use of natural family planning (NFP) is, in part, directly related to the quality of instruction provided. Because the methods are based upon clients developing an understanding of basic menstrual physiology and fertility signs, the information should be imparted clearly and simply, devoid of excessive medical terminology.

Years of experience of many NFP instructors throughout the world have shown that a person retains and understands more information about NFP when taught through an active learning process. This process involves encouraging participation of the learner through dialogue, question-and-answer sessions, and practice of the information. Consequently, the person should be instructed by an individual who is a skilled educator.

Instructors' training programs are available to health professionals both on a national and international level. The programs serve to help people develop the expertise needed to teach NFP and interpret NFP charts.

In an attempt to ensure adequate standards for preparation of instructors, objectives and guidelines have been established and are being adhered to in many of the NFP Instructor Training Programs throughout the United States. These objectives and guidelines are included here for your interest and are adapted from the guide, *Feasibility Study to Determine Quality Assurance Needs and Techniques for Natural Family Planning,* developed by Robert Kambic under HRSA Grant # FPR 000013-01-0.

Objectives, Guidelines for NFP Instructor Training Program

Fertility Awareness
1. Describe and explain male and female reproductive anatomy and physiology
2. Describe the female fertility cycle
3. Describe the role of cervical mucus, sperm, and the ovum in

---

*By the late Eleanor Tabeek, R.N., Ph.D., C.N.M., and used with her family's permission. Updated by Nancy Keaveney, RN, BS.

fertility and reproduction

Mucus Method

1. Give a general overview of the mucus method. Explain how knowing the presence and condition of the mucus can be used to plan and avoid pregnancy
2. Describe and explain techniques for becoming aware of the *sensation* of the presence of mucus at the vulva
   a. Describe how the sensation of the presence of mucus changes through the cycle
   b. Explain what it means to be dry Where are you dry? Give examples.
   c. Explain what it means to be wet. Where are you wet? Describe and explain wetness not related to cervical mucus, for example: menstrual bleeding, arousal fluids, seminal fluid
   d. Describe and explain wet and dry sensations regarding the insertion of tampons, intercourse, and wiping the vulva with tissue
   e. Describe how a woman can sense the difference between dryness and wetness and changes from dryness to wetness
   f. Describe how a woman can sense the peak of fertility and recognize it
3. Describe and explain the techniques for learning how to *observe* cervical mucus
   a. Describe how the appearance of the mucus changes through the menstrual cycle: color, texture, stretch
   b. Describe and explain what cervical mucus looks like in a changing mucus pattern
   c. Describe the appearance of discharges not related to cervical mucus
   d. Describe how to check the mucus with a tissue
   e. Describe the observations of the mucus peak
   f. Summarize the differences between internal and external mucus observation. Which method does not advocate internal observation?
4. Describe how to chart the condition of the mucus.
   a. State the number of observations to be made each day and when these observations should be charted.
   b. Explain the value of written descriptions of the mucus.
5. Explain the rules for avoiding pregnancy:
   a. during bleeding
   b. during pre-peak dry days

    c.   during changing mucus pattern
    d.   during post-peak days
    e.   during an unchanging mucus pattern
    f.   during an unchanging dry pattern
6.   Describe the rules for achieving pregnancy.

Basal Body Temperature (BBT) Method
1.   Give a general overview of the BBT method. Explain how BBT can be used to plan and avoid pregnancy.
2.   Describe and demonstrate the care and use of BBT thermometer.
3.   Illustrate charting of the BBT.
4.   Demonstrate several ways to interpret temperature rises including averaging and coverline.
5.   Describe several ways the BBT might rise including step, saw-tooth, direct.
6.   Describe and explain the BBT rules for avoiding pregnancy.

Cervix Sign
1.   Give a general overview of the cervix sign.
2.   Describe how to check the cervix.
3.   Illustrate the charting of the cervix sign
4.   Explain the cervix sign rules for avoiding pregnancy.

Calendar Method (Determining infertile days and ovulation)
1.   Give a general overview of the calendar method (determining infertile days before ovulation)
2.   Illustrate how to calculate the infertile time.
3.   Explain the rules of the calendar method for avoiding pregnancy.

The Symptothermal Method
1.   Give a general overview of the symptothermal method and its variations.
2.   Demonstrate how to combine charting of temperature and mucus for planning and avoiding pregnancy.
3.   Demonstrate how to add calculations, the cervix sign, and other minor signs to the mucus and temperature readings for planning and avoiding pregnancy.
4.   Describe and explain the use of the symptothermal method to avoid pregnancy during ovulatory and anovulatory cycles.

Styles of Teaching
1.   Describe the kinds of individuals who might come for NFP

instruction and the ways in which they might best be taught including:

   a. Postpartum women
   b. Women not breast feeding
   c. Women completely breast feeding
   d. Women partially breast feeding
   e. Women changing family planning method
   f. Premenopausal women

2. State the advantage and disadvantage of these teaching materials: slides, flip charts, teaching manuals.
3. State the advantages and disadvantages of group sessions, individual sessions, lectures, and discussions for NFP instruction.
4. Identify the advantages and disadvantages of symptothermal charting and mucus-only charting.

Follow-Up

1. Describe and explain the skills needed for interpreting the charting for symptothermal and mucus-only methods.
   a. Explain the need to interpret only the information that is on the chart and not to read something into the chart that is not recorded there.
   b. Demonstrate how to describe the charting exactly as the changes appear; the menses, number of dry days, changing mucus pattern, number of low temperatures, high temperatures; how menses confirm peak fertility and temperature changes were due to ovulation.
   c. For symptothermal charts, demonstrate how to break down the chart into its constituents and interpret each entry separately and then recombine the parts into an intelligible whole.
2. Demonstrate chart interpretation skills in mucus-only and symptothermal methods for normal ovulatory cycles and in special circumstances including:

a. complete breast feeding	h. illness
b. partial breast feeding	i. stress
c. weaning	j. poor nutrition
d. pre-menopause	k. exercise
e. post-pill status	l. chance taking with the rules
f. basic infertility patterns	
g. planning pregnancy	m. unplanned pregnancies

3. Follow up clients who are:
   a. uncertain about the methods
   b. in disagreement on their family planning intention

    c.   unhappy with available methods

    d.   discouraged in their use of NFP through the influence of friends or other professionals

    e.   not charting properly

    f.   not following the rules

Psychosocial Factors

1. Identify the characteristics of an autonomous client and explain how clients can best be helped to achieve autonomy.
2. Explain the advantages of self-monitoring and use of the method.
3. Appraise the usefulness of spouse or partner involvement in monitoring ovulatory indicators and in the practice of periodic abstinence.
4. Appraise the freedom and limitations of NFP.
5. Explain the role of the instructor with regard to encouraging the use of the infertile time for intercourse.
6. Explain effectiveness of NFP in planning and avoiding pregnancy.

Program Factors

1. Describe the kinds of follow-up records to be kept.
2. Explain the kinds of follow-up, including personal, mail, and phone, giving advantages and disadvantages of each.
3. Give examples of the client outcome definitions.
4. Describe the circumstances under which medical/social referrals are to be made.
5. Describe and summarize any outreach program.
6. Describe and summarize the financing of public and private NFP programs.

This appendix was adapted from the following materials:

McCarthy, J.J. & Martin, MC. (1977). *Fertility awareness.* Washington, D.C.: The Human Life and Natural Family Planning Foundation of America.

Basal body temperatures. (1977). Washington,D.C.: The Natural Family Planning Foundation of America, Inc.

An Introduction to Natural Family Planning for Physicians: A Manual. (1984). Los Angeles: Los Angeles Regional Family Planning Council, Inc. B. Kass'Annese, RNP, Project Director, Contract #242-84-0082, DHHS technique.

Kambic, R. *Feasibility study to determine quality assurance needs and techniques for natural family planning.* Health Resources and Services Administration Grant #FPR 000013-01-0; U.S. Public Health Service, Department of Health and Human Services.

Appendix N
Danger Assessment

Research has found several risk factors associated with the homicides (murders) of battered women. We would like you to be aware of the danger of homicide in situations of severe battering and for you to see how many of the risk factors apply to your situation. (The "he" in the questions refer to your husband, partner, ex-husband, ex-partner or whoever is currently physically hurting you).

Please check **YES** or **NO** for each question below.

YES NO

__ __ 1. Has there been more physical violence over the past year?

__ __ 2. Has the physical violence been more severe over the past year? Has a weapon or threat with a weapon been used?

__ __ 3. Does he ever try to choke you?

__ __ 4. Is there a gun in the house?

__ __ 5. Has he ever forced you into sex against your will?

__ __ 6. Does he use drugs such as "uppers" or amphetamines, speed, angel dust, cocaine, "crack," or street drugs?

__ __ 7. Does he threaten to kill you and/or do you believe he is capable of killing you?

__ __ 8. Is he drunk every day or almost every day?

__ __ 9. Does he control most of your daily activities? For instance, does he tell you who your friends can be, how much money you can have, or when you can take the car?
(If yes, but you don't let him, check here: ___

__ __ 10. Have you ever been beaten by him while you were pregnant? (If never pregnant by him, check here ___)

__ __ 11. Is he violently jealous of you? (For instance, does he say, "If I can't have you, no one can"?)

__ __ 12. Have you ever threatened or tried to commit suicide?

__ __ 13. Has he ever threatened or tried to commit suicide?

__ __ 14. Is he violent outside of the home?

__ **TOTAL YES ANSWERS**

Thank you. Please talk to your nurse, advocate or counselor about what the results of the danger assessment means in terms of your situation.

Note: Adapted from Campbell, J. (1986). Nursing Assessment for risk of homicide with battered women. *Advances in Nursing Science,* 8(4):36-51. Used with permission.

Appendix O

For Your Information: Vaginal Discharge

All women have a normal vaginal discharge called *leukorrhea;* the amount and consistency varies with each individual. This discharge is generally of a mucus-like consistency and tends to increase during the menstrual cycle up to two weeks before menstruation. A normal vaginal discharge may vary slightly in color, although it is usually clear or white, has no unpleasant odor, and it not itchy or irritating to the skin. Occasionally, a women may notice a fishy- or musty-smelling discharge if she has recently had intercourse. This may be due to dead sperm being cleansed from the vagina. If it occurs persistently, don't confuse it with a bacterial infection; have it checked. Some methods of birth control may affect the amount of normal vaginal discharge.

Hints for Prevention of Vaginal Infection

1. Even under the best conditions, vaginal infections sometimes occur. Don't panic if you discover that you have such an infection. Treat it with common sense—cleanliness, pelvic rest (no intercourse), and prescribed medications, and wear sensible clothing (cotton panties, no panty hose under slacks, no underwear to bed).

2. Cleanliness and personal hygiene are very important. Keep clean by bathing (shower or tub, but be sure you disinfect the tub before and after use) with soap and water. Vaginal deodorants can be irritating and are worthless in treating or preventing an infection. Avoid all use of feminine hygiene sprays and deodorants as well as deodorant or scented tampons, pads, panty liners, and toilet paper since these products tend to alter the natural environment of the vagina and make it more susceptible to irritation and/or infection.

3. *Douching is not recommended.* It can be harmful if done when an infection is already present. For example, the pressure of the douche solution may cause the infection to spread into the womb (uterus) and become even worse. Also, the douche solution removes the natural cleansing secretions of the vagina that normally help to maintain an environment that prevents infections. Indiscriminate douching with various commercial products may

aggravate existing conditions, set up a chemical vaginitis, or contribute to a pelvic infection.

4. To prevent both vaginal and bladder infections from occurring, wear cotton underwear and no underwear while sleeping; change tampons or sanitary napkins after each urination or bowel movement; wipe yourself in the front first and then the back after going to the bathroom; urinate after intercourse and/or genital stimulation; and drink lots of fluids—at least 6 glasses of water a day; cranberry juice may be helpful in avoiding infection.

Rules to Follow if You Have A Vaginal Infection

1. Take the entire course of medication exactly as prescribed. If you do not, the infection may "go underground" temporarily and then return and be more troublesome than before.

2. If you are treating an infection with vaginal cream or suppositories, remain lying down in bed for at least 15 minutes after insertion to allow the medication to spread deeply around the cervix, where it is needed. Standing up may cause the medicine to seep outward toward the vaginal opening.

3. Do not use tampons for protection because they will absorb the medication and reduce its effectiveness. Instead, use unscented external pads or small "mini-pads" to prevent staining underwear.

4. If you have a vaginal infection and use a diaphragm, soak diaphragm for 30 minutes with Betadyne® scrub (not solution) or 70% rubbing alcohol, after using prescribed medication for 2 days and again when medication is completed. Use alcohol for your cervical cap.

5. Sexual relations should be avoided for at least one week, and preferably throughout the entire course of treatment. Intercourse can be very irritating to the inflamed vagina and cervix during an infection and can slow down the healing process. Also, the germs that cause your infection might spread to your partner; if the partner is male, he should use a condom during the entire treatment period.

6. Insufficient lubrication prior to intercourse may contribute significantly to vaginal infections (and bladder infections). Water-soluble jelly can be used for lubrication. There are also vaginal lubricants and moisturizers especially for peri- and postmenopausal women.

From: Hawkins, Roberto-Nichols & Stanley-Haney, *Protocols for Nurse Practitioners in Gynecologic Settings*, 7th edition, 2000, © The Tiresias Press, Inc.

Appendix P
For Your Information: Candidiasis (Monilia)

I. Definition
Candidiasis, or monilia, is a yeast-like overgrowth of a fungus called Candida albicans (may also be caused by Candida tropicalis or Candida Torulopsis glabrata and rarely by other Candida species). Candida can be found in small amounts in the normal vagina but under some conditions it gets out of balance with the other vaginal flora and produces symptoms.

II. Transmission
A. Usually non-sexual
B. Some common causes of Candida overgrowth are: use of oral contraceptives; antibiotics; diabetes; pregnancy; stress; deodorant tampons and other such products

III. Signs and Symptoms
A. In the female
   1. Vaginal discharge: thick, white, and curd-like
   2. Vaginal area itch and irritation with occasional swelling and redness
   3. Burning on urination
   4. Possibly, pain with intercourse
B. In the male
   1. Itch and/or irritation of penis
   2. Cheesy material under foreskin, underside of penis
   3. Jock itch; athlete's foot

IV. Diagnosis
A. Female evaluation may include vaginal examination to check for Candida and rule out trichomoniasis, bacterial vaginosis, Chlamydia, and gonorrhea
B. Male evaluation may include:
   1. Examination of penis to check for irritation and/or cheesy materials
   2. Culture for ruling out gonorrhea and Chlamydia

3. Urinalysis

V. Treatment
Prescription medicine: _____

VI. Client Education
A. No intercourse until symptoms subside
B. Continue prescribed treatment even if menses occurs, but use pads rather than tampons
C. Ways to prevent recurrent Candida infections
  1. Bathe daily (with lots of water and minimal soap)
  2. To minimize the moist environment Candida favors, use
    a. Cotton-crotched underwear/pantyhose   (or cut out crotch of pantyhose)
    b. Loose-fitting slacks
    c. No underwear while sleeping
  3. Wipe the front first and then the back after toileting
  4. Avoid feminine hygiene sprays, deodorants, deodorant tampons/minipads, colored or perfumed toilet paper, tear-off fabric softeners in the dryer, etc., any of which may cause allergies and irritation
  5. Some women have found that vitamin C 500 mg 2-4 x each day help or taking oral acidophilous tablets 40 million to 1 billion units a day (1 tablet)
D. Over-the-counter medication. Many women choose to try an over-the-counter preparation before seeking an examination. If symptoms do not subside after 1 course of treatment (1 tube or 1 set of suppositories), having an examination for diagnosis is recommended

VII. Follow-up
Return to provider for reevaluation if symptoms persist or new symptoms occur after treatment is completed.
Special Notes: _____
Practitioner: _____

For more information call: CDC STD Hotline: 1-800-227-8922; Phone numbers of free (or almost free) STD clinics are listed in the "Community Service Numbers" in the government pages of your local phone book.
CDC http://www.cdc.gov

From: Hawkins, Roberto-Nichols & Stanley-Haney, *Protocols for Nurse Practitioners in Gynecologic Settings, 7th edition, 2000,* © The Tiresias Press, Inc.

Appendix Q
For Your Information:
Trichomoniasis ("Trich")

I. Definition
Trichomoniasis is a parasitic infection occurring in the female vagina or urethra, or male urethra and prostate. The infection is believed to be sexually transmitted although it has been identified in non-sexually active women.

II. Signs and Symptoms
A. May appear 5-30 days after contact
B. In the female, symptoms include
    1. Odorous, greenish-yellow, frothy vaginal discharge (often fishy)
    2. Painful intercourse or urination
    3. Discomfort on tampon insertion
    4. Itchiness, redness, and irritation of the vulva and upper thigh
    5. Papanicolaou smear may be abnormal
    6. Some patients may not have any symptoms
C. In the male, symptoms include:
    1. Mild itch or discomfort in penis
    2. Moisture at tip of penis disappearing spontaneously
    3. Slight early morning discharge from penis before first urination
D. Untreated symptoms in the female or male can progress to infection of neighboring urinary and reproductive organs

III. Diagnosis
A. Female evaluation may include
    1. Vaginal examination to check for trichomoniasis and to rule out yeast infections and bacterial infections such as gonorrhea or bacterial vaginosis

   2. Blood test to rule out syphilis
- B. Male evaluation may include
  1. Examination for gonorrhea or urinary tract infection
  2. Blood test for syphilis

IV. Treatment

The male should seek treatment after exposure to a partner with the infection. He may have no symptoms but could harbor the parasite in his urethra or prostate.

It is very important to report any medical conditions you have (especially seizure disorder) or medication you take regularly *before taking any treatment.*

V. Client Education

- A. Take *no alcohol* during the 48 hours after treatment (medication)
- B. For minor side effects of medication (nausea, dizziness, or metallic taste), take medication with some food or milk
- C. Advise sexual contact(s) to seek simultaneous treatment
- D. Use condoms until all partners are treated

VI. Follow-up

Return to clinic if symptoms persist or new symptoms occur.
Special notes: _____

_____

Practitioner:_____

For more information call: CDC STD Hotline: 1-800-227-8922: Phone numbers of free (or almost free) STD clinics are listed in the "Community Service Numbers" in the government pages of your local phone book.
http://www.cdc.gov

From: Hawkins, Roberto-Nichols & Stanley-Haney, *Protocols for Nurse Practitioners in Gynecologic Settings,* 7th ed, 2000, © The Tiresias Press, Inc.

Appendix R
Bacterial Vaginosis (BV)

I. Definition
Overgrowth of a variety of anaerobic bacterial, genital mycoplasmas, and gardnerella

II. Transmission
The condition can be sexually transmitted, but it may also be identified in the non-sexually active female

III. Signs and Symptoms
A. In the female
   1. Fishy, musty odor with a thin, chalk-white to gray watery vaginal discharge
   2. Discharge may cause vaginal itching and burning
   3. Burning and swelling of genitals after intercourse
   4. No symptoms in some women
B. In the male: no male version of BV has been identified

IV. Diagnosis
A. Female evaluation may include
   1. Vaginal examination to check for bacterial vaginosis
   2. Further laboratory work to rule out Candida, trichomonas, gonococcus, or Chlamydia
   3. Blood test for syphilis
B. Male evaluation: Rule out other infections such as trichomonas, gonococus, or Chlamydia

V. Treatment
A. Treatment may be by mouth or with a vaginal cream or gel
B. Treatment of partners is not recommended since studies have not shown that their treatment decreases the number of

recurrences unless partner is a woman also

C. It is very important to report any medical conditions you may have or medications you take regularly (especially for a seizure disorder) before taking any treatment.
Prescription medicine: _____

VI. Client Education

A. Sexual partners should be alerted to the diagnosis and referred for evaluation and possible treatment if the patient has other infections concurrently

B. Sexual partners should be protected by condoms until patient's treatment is over. Check with your clinician since some creams weaken the latex of condoms or vaginal diaphragms

C. Alcoholic beverages should not be consumed during or for 48 hours after oral treatment

D. Minor side effects of oral treatment may include nausea, dizziness, and a metallic taste

E. No douching with or after treatment

VI. Follow-up

Return to clinic for a re-evaluation if symptoms persist or new symptoms occur.
Special notes: _____
_____
_____

Practitioner:_____

For more information call: CDC STD Hotline: 1-800-227-8922: Phone numbers of free (or almost free) STD clinics are listed in the "Community Service Numbers" in the government pages of your local phone book.
http://www.cdc.gov

From: Hawkins, Roberto-Nichols & Stanley-Haney, *Protocols for Nurse Practitioners in Gynecologic Settings,* 7th edition, 2000, © The Tiresias Press, Inc.

Appendix S

For Your Information: Chlamydia Trachomatis

I. Definition
Chlamydia trachomatis is a sexually-transmitted disease of the reproductive tract. It is currently believed to be the most common cause of sexually transmitted disease in males and females, more common than gonorrhea.

II. Transmission
Sexual contact with 1-3 week incubation period before symptoms present

III. Signs and Symptoms
A. In the female
   1. Often no symptoms
   2. Possibly, increased vaginal discharge
   3. Cervicitis or an abnormal Papanicolaou smear
   4. Possibly, frequent uncomfortable urination
   5. Advanced symptoms include those of pelvic infection
B. In the male
   1. Possibly, thick and cloudy discharge from the penis
   2. Possibly, painful urination and/or frequent urination

IV. Diagnosis
A. Evaluation may include tests to rule out candidiasis, trichomoniasis, bacterial vaginosis, gonorrhea, syphilis, and urinary tract infection
B. Vaginal and urethral smears are examined for the Chlamydia trachomatis organism

V. Treatment

Prescription medicine: _____

_____

Take all the prescribed medicine, even though the symptoms may decrease early in treatment. Incomplete treatment gives the causative organism a chance to lie dormant and reinfect later.

VI. Client Education

A. Any sexual contacts should be advised to seek evaluation and treatment
B. Do not have intercourse until you and any sex partner(s) have completed treatment
C. In an untreated male or female the disease may progress to further reproductive infection with possible tissue scarring and infertility risks

VII. Follow-up

Return to clinic if symptoms persist or new symptoms occur.

Special notes: _____

_____

Practitioner:_____

For more information call: CDC STD Hotline: 1-800-227-8922: Phone numbers of free (or almost free) STD clinics are listed in the "Community Service Numbers" in the government pages of your local phone book.
http://www.cdc.gov

From: Hawkins, Roberto-Nichols & Stanley-Haney, *Protocols for Nurse Practitioners in Gynecologic Settings,* 7th edition, 2000, © The Tiresias Press, Inc.

Appendix T
For Your Information: Genital Herpes Simplex

I. Definition
The herpes simplex virus is one of the most common infectious agents of humans. It is transmitted only by direct contact with the virus from an active infected oral or genital lesion. The herpes simplex virus (HSV) is of two types:

HSV Type 1: *Usually* affects body sites above the waist (mouth, lips, eyes, fingers)

HSV Type 2: *Usually* involves body sites below the waist, primarily the genitals

Genital herpes may be caused by either HSV 1 or 2. If oral sex is practiced, remember that "cold sores" are herpes lesions and can be spread to the genital area. The cause, symptoms, complications, diagnosis, treatment, and client education are the same for males and females.

II. Symptoms
A. Painful, itchy sores similar to cold sores or fever blisters, surrounded by reddened skin, that appear around the mouth, nipples or genital areas 3 to 7 days after contact
B. Fever or flu-like symptoms
C. Burning sensation during urination
D. Swollen groin lymph nodes
E. Symptoms may last 2 to 3 weeks

III. Diagnosis
A. Examination based on your clinical symptoms and history
B. Laboratory analysis of discharge from the lesions to identify virus

IV. Treatment
A. Tepid bath with or without the addition of iodine solution
B. Unrestrictive clothing
C. Prevent secondary infection

D. Medication for pain
E. There are topical and oral medications that do not cure the infection but can shorten the duration and severity of symptoms and decrease recurrence. These medications may, in some cases, be taken on a long-term basis to suppress virus

V. Complications
A. Secondary infection of herpes lesions
B. Severe systemic and life-threatening infections in infants born vaginally during an episode of herpes in the mother.

VI. Recurrences
Herpes sores may never recur after the first episode or there may be occasional flare-ups, not as painful as the initial infection, lasting up to 7 days. Recurring infections may be related to stress (physical or emotional), illness, fever, over-exposure to sun, or menstruation. Recurrences are due to a reactivation of the virus already present in the nerve endings of your body.

VII. Client Education
A. After urinating, wash the genital area with cool water
B. If urinating is difficult, sit in a tub of warm water to urinate
C. Cool, wet tea bags applied to the lesions may offer some relief
D. Avoid intercourse when active lesions are present. If intercourse does occur, condoms should be used
E. Women with chronic herpes should have a Pap smear yearly.

Medication: _____

Special notes: _____

Practitioner: _____

For more information:
1. CDC STD Hotline: 1-800-227-8922: Phone numbers of free (or almost free) STD clinics are listed in the "Community Service Numbers" in the government pages of your local phone book.
2. Seek out local rap and support groups
3. Try resources on the internet. http://www.cdc.gov
   alt.support.herpes (usenet news group)

From: Hawkins, Roberto-Nichols & Stanley-Haney, *Protocols for Nurse Practitioners in Gynecologic Settings,* 7th edition, 2000, © The Tiresias Press, Inc.

Appendix U

For Your Information:
Genital Warts (Condylomata Acuminata)

I. Definition
Genital warts, or condylomata acuminata, may occur on either the male or female genital areas. The virus causing the warts is believed to be sexually transmitted, although warts have been found on individuals whose partner has no history or sign of warts.

II. Signs and Symptoms
Warts may not appear until two weeks to many months (or even years after exposure).
A. In moist areas, the warts are small, often itchy bumps, with a cauliflower-like top, appearing singly or in clusters.
B. On dry skin (such as the shaft of the penis), the warts commonly are small, hard, and yellowish-gray, resembling warts that appear on other parts of the body.
C. On the female, the warts are commonly found on or around the vaginal opening, vaginal lips, in the vagina, around the rectum, and on the cervix.
D. On the male, the warts can be found on any part of the penis and scrotum.

III. Diagnosis
A. The diagnosis is usually obvious on the basis of appearance of the warts, but sometimes a microscopic examination is necessary to identify minute lesions.
B. Laboratory tests may include checking for gonorrhea, chlamydia, and syphilis, HIV/AIDS, and a Papaniolaou smear if none within a year

IV. Treatment
A. If small, the warts may be treated by several weekly applica-

tions of medication by you or your practitioner
B. Patients with large, persistent warts or warts in the vagina or on the cervix may be referred to a physician for treatment. Some treatments include cryotherapy (freezing) and lasering the warts

V. Client Education
A. Always advise sexual partners to see a clinician for examination
B. Having warts may increase vaginal discharge; have it checked and treated
C. Treatment medication is applied weekly by the practitioner in office or clinic. *Some of the drugs used must be rinsed off in four hours. Your nurse practitioner will advise you.* Certain treatment medication should never be used in pregnant patients. If pregnancy is suspected, tell your practitioner
D. You may be given medication for self-treatment and separate instructions on how to do this.
E. Recurrence is possible without reinfection, as treatment does not always eradicate very small warts. Microscopic examination and treatment by a specialist may be necessary
F. A woman with a history of warts, especially if on the cervix, is encouraged to have an annual gynecological examination with a Pap smear as recommended by her clinician (often twice a year)

Special notes: _____

_____

Practitioner:_____

For more information and/or care for friends:
    CTD STD Hotline: 1-800-227-8922
    Phone numbers of free (or almost free) VD clinics are listed in the "Community Service Numbers" in the government pages of your local phone book.
    http://www.cdc.gov

From: Hawkins, Roberto-Nichols, & Stanley-Haney, *Protocols for Nurse Practitioners in Gynecologic Settings,* 7th edition, 2000 © The Tiresias Press, Inc.

Appendix V

For Your Information:
Self-Treatment for Genital Warts
(Condylomata Acuminata)

Condylox® is a prescription treatment for genital warts that you can use at home. Fill your Condylox prescription at any drugstore or the pharmacy in a department store. The Condylox package contains directions for use of the medication.* Please read these carefully and use the medication as directed. It is important to follow these directions and those of your health care provider to assure the maximum possible effect from the medication.

Condylox works by destroying the wart tissue. This does not happen all at once, but gradually. The wart will change in color From skin color to a dry, crusted, dead appearance and then disappear. You may feel some pain or burning when applying the Condylox as these changes occur. You may also see some redness, have some soreness or tenderness at the wart sites, and may even see small sores in that area. These symptoms usually disappear within a week after you have completed the treatment. If any of these changes are severe or concern you, stop the treatment and contact your health care provider.

Treating Your Warts

Treat your warts twice a day with Condylox. (It is okay to do so even if you get your menstrual period during the time you are treating your warts). Plan a time in the morning and again in the evening to apply the medication. Repeat the twice-a-day treat-

---

*Adapted from manufacturer's literature Oclassen Pharmaceuticals, 1990; Watson Laboratories, 1998.

ments for 3 days and then do not treat the warts again for 4 days. You can repeat this pattern of treatment—3 days of medication and then 4 days off—for up to 4 weeks. Stop the treatment, however, as soon as the warts disappear. It is important that you not treat the warts in any week for more than 3 days as such treatment will not help them to disappear faster and may cause you to have side effects from the medication.

If you have completed 4 weeks of treatment and still have warts, return to your health care provider for further evaluation and do not use Condylox until you have this check-up.

Remove any clothing over the affected area and wash your hands before treating your warts. Open the bottle of Condylox and place it on a flat surface to it will not spill while you are treating your warts. It may be helpful to use a hand mirror to locate the warts so that you can treat them. Good light is also important so that you do not get medication on skin that is free of warts.

Holding onto the bottle to steady it, dip the tip of one cotton tip applicator (Q-tip) into the medication. The tip should be wet with the medication, but not dripping. Remove any excess medication by pressing the applicator tip against the inside of the bottle. Apply the Condylox only to those areas you and your health care provider have identified as warts.

Try not to get any Condylox on any area of your skin that is not a wart. If the wart is on a skin fold, gently spread the skin with one hand to flatten out the wart and touch the medication applicator to the area with the other hand. Allow the Condylox to dry before letting skin folds relax into normal position and before putting clothing over the affected area.

After application, throw away the Q-tip. Close the bottle tightly to prevent evaporation of the medication and wash your hands carefully when you are finished with the treatment.

If you are using Condylox® gel, follow the same treatment schedule as for the liquid. Wash your hands before treating your warts. Squeeze out a small amount of gel (about half the size of a pea) onto your fingertip. Dab a small amount of the gel onto the warts or the areas your clinician has instructed you to treat. Try not to get any of the gel on normal skin areas. For warts in skin folds, spread the folds apart and apply the gel to the wart, letting the area dry before you return the skin folds to their normal position. Wash your hands carefully after completing the treatment.

The area you have treated may sting when you apply the gel. It may also become red, sore, itchy or tender after treatment.

Precautions in Self-Treatment

Condylox is intended only for treatment of venereal warts and only on the outside of the body. It is not safe to use Condylox on any other skin condition. If you have severe pain, bleeding, swelling, or itching, stop the treatment and contact your health care provider. Do not get this medication in your eyes. If you do so accidentally, flush your eyes immediately with running water and call your health care provider. The effects of Condylox on pregnancy are unknown, so it is not safe to use this medication during pregnancy.

Follow-up Care

It is important to return for a check-up as suggested by your health care provider or if you have completed 4 weeks of treatment and still have warts. If the warts reappear after you have completed treatment, contact your health care provider prior to re-starting treatment. Your partner should also be checked and treated for any warts; otherwise, you can be reinfected.

Self-treatment with Imiquimod Cream 5% (Aldara®)*

Aldara® is a prescription treatment for genital warts that you can use at home. Fill your Aldara prescription at any drugstore or pharmacy in a department store. The Aldara package contains directions for use of the medication. Please read these carefully and use the medication only as directed.

Aldara probably works by boosting your body's immune

---

*Adapted from the Aldara® manufacturer's literature, 3M Pharmaceuticals, 1998. response

response to the wart virus (there are over 80 types of wart virus, called human papilloma virus or HPV)). Aldara should be used only on warts outside the vagina, on the labia and the area around your anus.

Treating Your Warts

Careful handwashing before and after application of the cream is recommended so that you do not experience a secondary bacterial infection in the wart area and get the cream on other parts of your body. Apply Aldara three times a week just prior to your normal sleeping hours. Apply a thin layer of the cream to all external genital warts and rub it in until it is no longer visible. Leave Aldara on the skin for 6-10 hours. Don't cover the treated area. Following this treatment period, remove the cream by washing the treated area with mild soap and water. Continue treatment until the warts disappear. Do not continue treatment past 16 weeks without consulting your health care provider.

Precautions in Treatment

Aldara cream may weaken condoms and vaginal diaphragms, so do not use these while you are treating your warts. Sexual (genital contact) should be avoided while the Aldara cream is on the skin. Common reactions to Aldara include redness, burning, swelling, itching, rash, soreness, stinging and tenderness. If any of these occur, wash the cream off with mild soap and water. Do no retreat until these symptoms are gone. For any questions, call your health care provider. A very small percentage of persons have flu-like symptoms, fever, fatigue, headache, diarrhea, and/or achy joints. If you experience any of these, call your health care provider.

From: Hawkins, Roberto-Nichols, & Stanley-Haney, *Protocols for Nurse Practitioners in Gynecologic Settings,* 7th edition, 2000, © The Tiresias Press, Inc.

Appendix W
For Your Information: Gonorrhea

I. Definition
Gonorrhea is an acute infection which is spread by sexual contact and involves the genitourinary tract, throat, and rectum of both sexes. It is caused by the organism, Neisseria gonorrhoeae.

II. Important Information
A. The highest incidence of gonorrhea occurs in males between the ages of 20 and 24 and in females from 18 and 24. Gonorrhea is usually contracted from an infected person who has ignored symptoms or has no symptoms. This source can reinfect the patient, or possibly infect others, unknowingly
B. Incubation: 1-13 days. Symptoms can occur 3-30 days after sexual contact; average is 2-5 days after exposure

III. Usual Signs and Symptoms
A. Females
  1. Up to 80% have no symptoms
  2. Abnormal, thick green vaginal discharge
  3. Frequency, pain on urination
  4. Urethral discharge
  5. Rectal pain and discharge
  6. Unilateral labial pain and swelling
  7. Abnormal menstrual bleeding; increased dysmenorrhea (menstrual cramps)
  8. Lower abdominal discomfort
  9. Sore throat
B. Males
  1. 4-10% have no symptoms
  2. Frequency, pain on urination
  3. Burning sensation in the urethra
  4. Whitish discharge from the penis (early); may appear only as a drop during erection
  5. Yellow or greenish discharge from the penis (late)
  6. Sore throat

IV. Diagnosis (for Both Sexes)
A. History of sexual contact with a person known to be infected with gonorrhea
B. Smears and cultures taken from infected areas (cervix, penis, rectum, and throat)

V. Treatment for Males and Females
Antibiotics will be prescribed and are effective if taken according to directions. Be sure to tell your clinician if you are allergic to any antibiotic

VI. Complications
A. *Females:* If gonorrhea goes untreated, it may lead to pelvic inflammatory disease (PID). PID involves severe abdominal cramps, pelvic pain, and high fever that will lead to scarring and possible blockage of the fallopian tubes, the risk of tubal pregnancy, and infertility
B. *Males:* If gonorrhea goes untreated, scar tissue may form on the sperm passageway causing pain and sterility
C. *Females and males:* The infection may spread throughout the body causing arthritis, sometimes with skin lesions

VII. Patient Education (for Both Sexes)
A. All medication must be taken as directed
B. No intercourse until treatment of self and partner(s) is completed.
C. Return to the clinic for reevaluation if symptoms persist or new symptoms occur after treatment is complete.
D. **Important:**   The responsible lover informs all partners immediately upon finding out about exposure to sexually transmitted disease so that all persons involved can be evaluated adequately and treated immediately

Special notes: _____

_____

Practitioner:_____

For more information and or care of friends: CDC STD Hotline, 1-800-227-8922. For phone numbers of free (or almost free) STD clinics see the "Community Service Numbers" in the government pages of your local phone book. http://www.cdc.gov

From: Hawkins, Roberto-Nichols, & Stanley-Haney, *Protocols for Nurse Practitioners in Gynecologic Settings, 7th edition,* 2000 © The Tiresias Press, Inc.

Appendix X

Breast Self-Examination (BSE)*

Breast self-examination should be done once a month so you become familiar with the usual appearance and feel of your breasts. Familiarity makes it easier to notice any changes in the breasts from one month to another. Early discovery of a change from what is "normal" is the main idea behind BSE. The outlook is much better if you detect cancer in an early stage.

If you menstruate, the best time to do BSE is a few days after your period ends, when your breasts are least likely to be tender or swollen. If you no longer menstruate, pick a day such as the first day of the month to remind yourself it is time to do BSE.

Here is one way to do BSE:

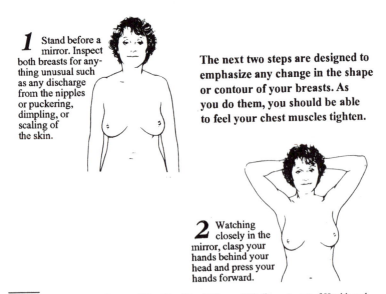

1 Stand before a mirror. Inspect both breasts for anything unusual such as any discharge from the nipples or puckering, dimpling, or scaling of the skin.

The next two steps are designed to emphasize any change in the shape or contour of your breasts. As you do them, you should be able to feel your chest muscles tighten.

2 Watching closely in the mirror, clasp your hands behind your head and press your hands forward.

---

* Adapted from *Breast Exams: What You Should Know.* U.S. Department of Health and Human Services, 1991; *How To Do Breast Self-exam,* American Cancer Society, 1999. Consult your nurse practitioner or physician about having a mammogram.

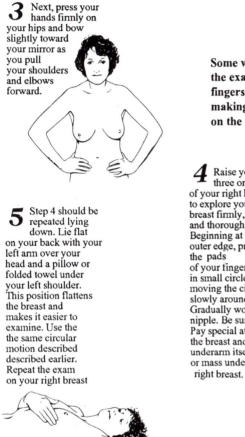

3 Next, press your hands firmly on your hips and bow slightly toward your mirror as you pull your shoulders and elbows forward.

Some women do the next part of the exam in the shower because fingers glide over soapy skin, making it easy to concentrate on the texture underneath.

5 Step 4 should be repeated lying down. Lie flat on your back with your left arm over your head and a pillow or folded towel under your left shoulder. This position flattens the breast and makes it easier to examine. Use the the same circular motion described described earlier. Repeat the exam on your right breast

4 Raise your left arm. Use three or four fingers of your right hand to explore your left breast firmly, carefully and thoroughly. Beginning at the outer edge, press the pads of your fingers in small circles, moving the circles slowly around the breast. Gradually work toward the nipple. Be sure to cover the entire breast. Pay special attention to the area between the breast and the underarm, including the underarm itself. Feel for any unusual lump or mass under the skin. Repeat on your right breast.

6 Report any lumps, thickening, discharge, or changes to your clinician. Most of these are not cancer, but you won't know f you don't ask.

7 Ages 20-39: Clinical breast examination as recommended by your clinician and your personal and family history, monthly BSE. Age 40+: Annual mammogram, annual breast examination by clinician, monthly BSE. Resources: American Cancer Society, www.cancer.org

Appendix Y

For Your Information: Colposcopy

What Is Colposcopy?

Colposcopy is a special type of diagnostic examination performed at times on women, less frequently on men. The colposcope is a microscope designed specifically for aiding the naked eye by magnifying the cervix, vagina, vulva, and anus.

Why Do You Need a Colposcopy?

You need this special examination because your practitioner suspects there may be a problem related to your cervix (the opening to your uterus), vaginal walls, vulva, or anal area based upon your initial exam. She/he may have received a report of abnormal findings from your Papanicolaou (Pap) test or may have seen some evidence of infection, inflammation, or a lesion (a sore or growth) during your exam.

If you have had an abnormal Pap smear, by using the colposcope your practitioner can examine each part of your cervix and vagina and look for abnormal appearing cells. Your cervix is made up of thousands of special cells which should have a certain pattern or structure; any changes in the expected structure require further investigation.

How Is Colposcopy Done?

It is done in much the same way as your regular gynecological exam. The only difference is that your practitioner looks at your cervix and vagina through the colposcope after inserting the vaginal speculum.

Why Else Are Colposcopies Done?

Some nurse practitioners use the colposcope for screening purposes and to identify warty lesions. She/he may need to do a more extensive exam, which may include a biopsy. She/he may also prescribe treatment if necessary.

What Is a Cervical Biopsy?

It is the removal of a small piece (or pieces) of tissue from the cervix using a specially designed instrument. This tissue is sent to the laboratory for examination.

Does the Examination Hurt?

The colposcope does not touch your body and therefore does not hurt. If your caregiver decides to perform a biopsy, you may feel a small pinch at that time only. There is no need to be tense. You will be told ahead of time if a biopsy is to be done. This procedure may be necessary to find out if there is any disease below or at the surface of your cervix.

Is There Any Vaginal Bleeding after a Biopsy?

There may be a small amount of bleeding following a biopsy. This will stop in a few minutes, with some gentle pressure. A very few patients may continue to have a small amount of bleeding afterwards, which can be easily treated. There may also be a discharge due to the medication used during the procedure.

Can a Colposcopy Be Done During Pregnancy?

Certainly. This examination is no different than the regular exam your practitioner or physician routinely performs, and it will not jeopardize your pregnancy.

How Else Can a Colposcopy Be Helpful?

With the colposcope, your care provider can identify genital warts on your cervix, in your vagina, and on your vulva. First, he/she will apply acetic acid (table vinegar) to the vulva, the walls of the vagina, and the cervix. If warts are present, they will appear white under the magnification of the colposcope, and your care provider will either locate and treat the lesions or refer you to a physician for treatment.

How Can a Colposcopy Be Helpful in Males?

Males can also have genital warts. They may be located on the shaft of the penis, at the urethral opening, on the scrotum, or around the anus. Warts are difficult to see on males with the naked eye, but with the application of acetic acid and the use of a colposcope, the most minute wart will turn white, facilitating treatment.

From: Hawkins, Roberto-Nichols, & Stanley-Haney, *Protocols for Nurse Practitioners in Gynecologic Settings,* 7th edition, 2000 © The Tiresias Press, Inc.

Appendix Z

For Your Information:
Premenstrual Syndrome (PMS)

I. Definition
The premenstrual syndrome consists of a group of behavioral and cognitive dysfunctions and physical symptoms associated with the menstrual cycle.

II. Signs and Symptoms
Usually appear one week prior to menses but may also appear up to two weeks or just several days before menses, and include:
A. Mood fluctuations
B. Depression
C. Fatigue, lethargy
D. Weight gain
E. Headache
F. Irritability
G. Breast tenderness
H. Increased appetite, craving for sweets and/or salt
I. Insomnia/sleep disturbance
J. Inability to concentrate
K. Constipation
L. Palpitations
M. Hot flashes
N. Abdominal bloating
O. Acne
P. Changes in sex drive
If you are bothered by these changes, make an appointment with your health care provider for a consultation. A complete history will be taken and a diet and exercise regimen suggested. You will be asked to document your temperature and symptoms daily using a Menstrual Cycle Daily Diary (see pages 368-369). You

will also be scheduled for a complete physical.

III. Treatment

Treatment consists of alleviating the signs and symptoms described above with a diet and exercise plan and/or medication.

A. Diet recommendation

1. Limit your consumption of refined sugar, i.e., cookies, cakes, jelly, honey
2. Limit your salt intake to 3 gm or less per day, i.e., avoid using the salt shaker
3. Limit your intake of alcohol
4. Avoid caffeine, i.e., coffee, tea, chocolate, soft drinks
5. Increase your intake of complex carbohydrates, i.e., fresh fruit, vegetables, whole grains, pasta, rice, potatoes
6. Consume moderate protein and fat. Limit your red meat consumption to 2 x weekly.

B. Exercise recommendations

Exercise 3 times per week for 30-40 minutes. Examples: brisk walking, jogging, aerobic dancing, swimming.

C. Medication

Vitamins and other medications as prescribed or recommended by your clinician.

D. Consider complementary therapies such as meditation, botanicals, aroma or muscle therapy, energy healing, acupuncture. Talk with your health care provider about these.

You may be evaluated monthly x 3 months to determine the effects of diet, exercise, vitamins, and your symptoms. If there is no improvement at that time, a more extensive work-up may be done with possible referral.

From: Hawkins, Roberto-Nichols, & Stanley-Haney, *Protocols for Nurse Practitioners in Gynecologic Settings, 7th edition,* 2000 © The Tiresias Press, Inc.

Menstrual Cycle Daily Diary

Name _____ Date of Birth _____ Last Period Began _____

Directions: Answer all questions each evening, based on the last 24 hours. For each day, indicate which symptoms occurred and indicate their severity using the following scale:

0 = No symptoms   1 = Mild   2 = Moderate   3 = Strong   4 = Very intense

Date:	1 2 3 4 5 6 7 8 9 10 11 12 13 14 15 16 17 18 19 20 21 22 23 24 25 26 27 28 29 30 31
Bleeding (0–4) or BBT Temp.	
Write in symptoms:	
1.	
2.	
3.	
4.	
5.	
6.	
7.	
8.	
9.	
10.	
11.	
12.	
13.	
14.	
15.	
16.	
17.	
18.	
19.	
20.	
21. Weight	
22. Major event of each day	

Looking back at this month, the symptoms most distressing to me were (use items from list above starting with most important):

1 2 3 4 5 6 7 8 9 10 11 12 13 14 15 16 17 18 19 20 21 22 23 24 25 26 27 28 29 30 31

Date:

8 oz. coffee (caff.)
8 oz. tea (caff.)
8 oz. hot chocolate
8 oz. decaf coffee/tea
8 oz. water/drink
cigarettes
4 oz. glasses wine
12 oz. beer
1 oz. liquor

Medication (name, mg, # pills):
1.
2.
3.
4.
5.
6.

Vitamins:
1.
2.

Over-the-counter and street drugs:
1.
2.
3.

Describe meals (time, food eaten):

Snack

Lunch

Snack

Dinner

Snack

Appendix AA

For Your Information:
After-Abortion Care

1. Someone should accompany you to the facility and wait there to take you home.
2. Normal physical activities may be resumed as soon as you feel ready.
3. You may be given some medication (methergine or ergotrate and/or an antibiotic) to take after your abortion. The first two medications will help your uterus return to its normal size and decrease bleeding. Antibiotics will help prevent infection. Follow the directions on how to take the pills. You may experience some uterine cramping (similar to menstrual cramps) with or without the methergine or ergotrate. It is okay to take acetaminophen (Tylenol, Datril, Tempra, Valadol, Valorin, Acephen) for cramps, or ibuprofen (Motrin, Advil).
4. Because of the risk of infection, it is important not to have intercourse or to insert anything into the vagina for 2-3 weeks. Other forms of sexual activity or orgasm will not be harmful to your body. Do not douche at all and do not use tampons for 2-3 weeks after the procedure, or until you stop bleeding. You may also be given 3 to 5 days of antibiotics to help prevent infection. Be sure to complete this medication.
5. Bleeding will probably cease after 3-4 days, but may last up to 3 weeks. There may be no bleeding at all. If bleeding exceeds two sanitary pads an hour or if you have a fever, call your health care provider or the facility where the procedure

was performed.

6. Menstruation (period) should resume in 4-6 weeks but may take as long as 8 weeks and as short as 2 weeks.

7. You will be given an appointment with a clinician 2-3 weeks after your abortion. The clinician will check to see that your body is back to normal and will provide you with your desired form of contraception or schedule an appointment for a diaphragm or cap fitting 6 weeks after the abortion. An IUD can be inserted immediately after or within 3 weeks of a first trimester miscarriage or abortion. Norplant can be inserted immediately (within 5 days) of an abortion. Depo-Provera may be given the day of the abortion or within 5 days of the procedure. This appointment will also give you an opportunity to discuss your feelings. A friend or partner is welcome to see the practitioner with you if you wish.

8. If you have chosen to use birth control pills, start your pills on the Sunday following the abortion procedure. If not, be sure to use another form of contraception such as spermicide and condoms when you resume sexual relations. Remember, you will probably ovulate before you resume menses; you can become pregnant any time after your abortion. If you received Depo-Provera after your abortion, it is still important to return for your after-abortion check-up 2 to 3 weeks after the procedure. You can then schedule your next Depo shot.

9. If you have a problem or concern, call the clinic or office at:
( )_____

From: Hawkins, Roberto-Nichols, & Stanley-Haney, *Protocols for Nurse Practitioners in Gynecologic Settings, 7th edition,* 2000 © The Tiresias Press, Inc.

Appendix BB

For Your Information:
Stress Incontinence (Loss of Urine)

Stress incontinence is caused by relaxation of the muscles and ligaments of the pelvic floor, that is, the muscles and ligaments that support the bladder, uterus, urethra (tube leading from the bladder to the outside), lower bowel, and vagina. Due to this relaxation, which is commonly the result of stretching due to childbirth and normal loss of muscle elasticity with aging, any stress such as laughing, coughing, or sneezing can cause involuntary loss of urine.

Urine can be irritating to the skin, so it is important to wash it off as soon as possible. The ammonia odor from urine leakage may be distressing also. Cotton underwear, the use of nondeodcrized, unscented panty liners, and use of prewetted wipes especially designed for the vaginal area will all help to prevent irritation, rashes, and cracking of skin. Skin cracking, irritation, and rashes will often increase the possibility of bacterial infection, especially in the warm, moist, genital area. Dusting with cornstarch will protect the skin from irritation. Only mild unperfumed soaps should be used, and used sparingly, as soap can be drying to skin. Perfumes (which are alcohol based) can increase the drying effect also and may cause an allergic reaction or chemical irritation to sensitive skin. Avoid bubble baths, vaginal hygiene products, and perfumed powders and talcums for the same reasons.

Diary of Incontinence

Code numbers for WHEN	*Code letters for AMOUNT*
1. coughing/sneezing	a. a drop or two
2. laughing/crying	b. a teaspoonful
3. blowing nose	c. a tablespoonful
4. climbing stairs	d. more than a tablespoonful
5. bending over	e. unable to estimate
6. sitting or resting	
7. other times	

Log of Times of Urine Loss, Circumstances of Loss, and Amount

	S	M	T	W	T	F	S
Week 1							
Week 2							
Week 3							
Week 4							

Kegal (Pelvic Floor) Exercises

Practice contracting, holding, and relaxing each time you urinate until you can stop the flow completely and start and stop at will. Then proceed to this exercise program.

Day One
Repeated contracting, holding, and relaxing of pubococcygeus muscle (muscle band of perineal area) 4 times this day, 10 contractions and 10 relaxations each time).

Day Two
Increase to 20 contractions and 20 relaxations, 4 times this day.

Day Three
Increase to 30 contractions and 30 relaxations, 4 times this day.

Day Four
Increase to 40 contractions and 40 relaxations, 4 times this day.

Day Five
Increase to 70 contractions and 70 relaxations, 4 times this day.

Continue with Day Five regime, so you are now doing the exercise 4 times each day, contracting and relaxing 70 times at each of the 4 exercise periods.

Log for Pelvic Floor Exercise
(Place a checkmark in box for each exercise period each day)

	S	M	T	W	T	F	S
Week 1							
Week 2							
Week 3							
Week 4							

You may want to ask your clinician about vaginal cones to help you practice. Graduated weighted cones are available to assist in Kegel exercises; a cone is inserted in the vagina and Kegels are performed using the cones' feedback; when weight of one cone can be maintained 15 minutes when walking or standing, move to next weight.
http://incontinent.com/home.htm

From: Hawkins, Roberto-Nichols, & Stanley-Haney, Protocols for Nurse Practitioners in Gynecologic Settings, 7th edition, 2000, ©The Tiresias Press, Inc.

Appendix CC

Informed Consent and Information Handout for Emergency Contraception (EC)

Definition
Emergency contraception (EC), often known as the "morning after pill," is the use of birth control pills to prevent pregnancy after a contraceptive method has failed or because there was no contraception.

How It Works
If used within the first 72 hours after unprotected sexual intercourse, EC probably works because of one or more of the following reasons:

• Progestational hormones in the pills interfere with the sperms' ability to travel up through the uterus and into the fallopian tube to fertilize the egg

• Estrogen hormones in the pills are thought to interfere with or disrupt ovulation (release of an egg by the ovary)

How Effective Is It?
If used within 72 hours after sex without birth control protection, EC is greater than 90% effective.

Benefits
• Pregnancy prevention
• Inexpensive
• Relatively noninvasive

Disadvantages
• Cannot be used by woman who cannot use birth control pills
• Pregnancy may occur due to:
    1. Fertilized egg already implanted in the uterus

2. Too much time between unprotected sex and taking EC
3. Failure of the emergency contraception
4. Must be used within 72 hours of unprotected sex

Risks and Side Effects
- Nausea and/or vomiting
- Breast tenderness
- Irregular bleeding
- Headache

You May Not Be Able to Take EC if You Have:
- An active liver disease
- Unexplained bleeding from the vagina
- An already established pregnancy
- History of blood clots, inflammation in the veins, or cancer of the breast, uterus or ovaries

Alternative EC
- Progestin-only oral contraceptives used as EC
- Insertion of a copper-releasing device IUD

How EC is Prescribed
- Pelvic examination as appropriate (to be determined by you and your health care provider)
- If rape or sexual assault occurred, specimens can be collected if desired by you and your health care provider
- Pregnancy test
- Testing for sexually transmitted diseases (STDs) if desired, or if recommended by health care provider
- Blood pressure

Ways in which EC is taken
1. Take _____ birth control pills within 72 hours of unprotected intercourse. Do not take the pills on a empty stomach—eat a snack such as juice or milk and crackers and take the pills 20 minutes later.
2. Take _____ birth control pills 12 hours after the first dose.
3. If you vomit within an hour after taking the birth control

pills, follow the instructions your health care provider gives you.

4. Talk with your provider about methods of contraception you might be interested in for ongoing protection. Emergency contraception is just that—for emergencies—and is not recommended for routine use. Some birth control methods can be started immediately or the day after using EC. Methods vary in how soon they become effective.

5. Report any of the warning signs listed below to your health care provider at once.

6. Six weeks after using EC, return to your health care provider for a checkup, particularly if you have not had a normal menstrual period.

I have read the above material. I have been given the opportunity to ask questions and I fully understand the information. I have chosen to use emergency contraception.

Signed_____Date_____

Witness_____Date_____

Danger Signals Associated with EC:
    Abdominal pain (severe)
    Chest pain (severe), arm pain, or shortness of breath
    Headaches (severe)
    Eye problems such as blurred or double vision, loss of vision
    Severe leg pain (calf or thigh)

Contact us at (_____)_____ if you develop any of the above danger signals.

    Emergency Contraception hot line: 800-584-9911, 888-NOT-2-LATE.

From: Hawkins, Roberto-Nichols, & Stanley-Haney: *Protocols for Nurse Practitioners in Gynecologic Settings,* 7th edition, 2000, © The Tiresias Press, Inc.

Appendix DD

Self-Assessment of AIDS (HIV) Risk*

1. Do you use injectable drugs? Does your sexual partner(s)? Do you or your partner(s) have a partner(s) who uses injectable drugs? How about in the past?
2. If you or your partner(s) use injectable drugs, do you ever share needles or syringes? How about in the past?
3. Did you or your partner(s) have a blood transfusion between 1975 and 1985 or have sexual exposure to partners who did?
4. Do you have or have you had a hemophiliac partner(s) who received blood or blood products between 1975 and 1985?
5. Do you or your partner(s) use latex condoms/female condoms whenever you have vaginal or anal sex?
6. Do you ever let your partner(s) ejaculate (cum) in your mouth?
    Do you ever have oral sex with a female partner during menses?
7. Have you ever had unprotected sex with a man who has had sex with another man?
8. Do you ever share sex toys (such as a vibrator)?
9. If you are a health-care provider, have you ever experienced a needle stick, exposure to a patient's blood, or exposure to amniotic fluid on your unprotected hands or face?
10. Are you and your partner mutually monogamous? How long have you been so?
11. Have you ever traded sex for money, shelter, food or drugs?
12. Have you ever had unwanted or forced (non-consensual) sex?

If your answer to any of the questions except 5 and 10 is yes, you may be at risk and might consider being tested.

---

*Richard S. Ferri, Ph.D., ANP, ACRN, provided invaluable input for this tool.

From: Hawkins, Roberto-Nichols, & Stanley-Haney, *Protocols for Nurse Practitioners in Gynecologic Settings,* 7th edition, 2000, © The Tiresias Press, Inc.

Appendix EE

Evaluation Tool for Protocols*

This tool is an example of an instrument that could be used both for evaluating and updating protocols, a process that should occur on an annual, or at least a regular, basis to assure that practice is based on the most recent information.

1. Does the protocol include enough background information about the contraceptive method/gyn disorder/health-care problem?

Not Nearly Enough	Not Quite Enough	Just Right	More than Enough	Much more than Enough
1	2	3	4	5

    What else should be included or left out? _____

2. Does the protocol allow the nurse practitioner freedom to individualize the protocol for each client?

Not Nearly Enough	Not Quite Enough	Just Right	More than Enough	Much more than Enough
1	2	3	4	5

    Suggestions for change: _____

3. Is the protocol appropriate for a nurse practitioner in practice as a women's health nurse practitioner?

Not at all	Probably Not	Maybe	Probably Yes	Definitely Yes
1	2	3	4	5

    Suggestions: _____

4. What are the most useful features of the protocol? _____

5. Suggestions to improve/change update it for use in practice? _____

6. Could this protocol be used/adapted for any setting? _____
7. Are there sufficient references? If not, what should be added? _____

8. Please include any comments. Thank you!

*Adapted from a form by Cheryl Stene Frenkel, R.N.C., M.S., F.N.P., and used with her permission.

From: Hawkins, Roberto-Nichols, & Stanley-Haney, *Protocols for Nurse Practitioners in Gynecologic Settings,* 7th edition, 2000 © The Tiresias Press, Inc.

Appendix FF

Vulvar Self-Examination*

How to Perform VSE...
Where To Look

POSITION. Find a comfortable, well-lighted place to sit such as a bed or a carpet. Hold a mirror in one hand. Then, expose the parts of the vulva surrounding the opening of the vagina. Once you have a good viewing position, examine the main parts of the vulva as follows:

1. Check the "mons pubis" (the area above the vagina around the pubic bone where the pubic hair is located). Look carefully for any bumps, warts, ulcers, or changes in skin color (pigmentation, especially newly developed white, red or dark areas). Then, use the finger tips to check any visible change and to sense any bump just below the surface you might feel but not see.

2. Next, check the "clitoris" and surrounding area (directly above the vagina) by looking and by touch.

3. Next, examine the "labia minora" (the smaller folds of skin just to the right and left of the vaginal opening). Look and touch by holding the skin between thumb and fingers.

4. Then look closely at the "labia majora" (the larger folds of skin just next to the labia minora). Examine both righty and left just as you did the labia minora.

5. Move down to the "perineum" (the area between the vagina and the anus). Check thoroughly.

6. Finally, examine the area surrounding the anal opening...as before by looking and by touch.

IMPORTANT NOTE: Every woman should know the parts of the vulva. (See the "Anatomy of the Vulva" drawing below.) You should also talk about VSE with your physician who can note what is "normal" for your individual anatomy. This is a good time to ask questions.

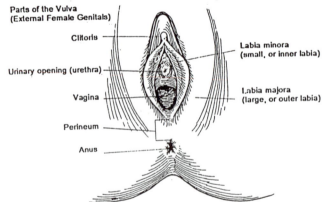

Parts of the Vulva
(External Female Genitals)

Clitoris

Urinary opening (urethra)

Vagina

Perineum

Anus

Labia minora
(small, or inner labia)

Labia majora
(large, or outer labia)

REMEMBER THE BASIC RULE: Vulvar diseases are most easily, safely, and successfully treated when discovered early. Now you know....and now you have yet another good way to help protect your own health....the monthly vulvar self examination.

*From Lawhead, R., Alan, Jr., M.D., "What Every Woman Should Know: Your Guide to the Benefits of Vulvar Self Examination," 1988, 1990, 1993, 1998. Used with permission.

Appendix GG

Constipation

Constipation is a common problem and can be related to a number of factors. First, though, it is important to clarify what is meant by the term. Irregularity is another related term—it implies that there is some standard of regularity. Although many of us have been taught that daily bowel elimination (having at least one bowel movement—BM—daily) is normal, in fact for many persons normal is every two or three days.

Constipation occurs when one's regular pattern (whatever is normal for that person) changes so that the time between bowel movements lengthens, pain and/or straining are associated with them, and/or the bowel movements are very hard. Sometimes bleeding occurs because the fecal material (the stool) is hard and the person has to strain so much that there is damage to the rectum (lowest part of the bowel) or to the opening of the intestinal track (called the anal opening). There are other causes of bleeding, too, so if you ever have bleeding with a bowel movement, you should not ignore it.

Some causes of constipation are:

- *Stress.* Stress can cause "spastic constipation" meaning tightening or spasm of the muscles in the large intestine; stress can also mean not taking time to eat properly, drink enough fluids, and/or even go to the bathroom when your body signals you.

- *Diet.* More about this later, but lack of roughage or fiber in the diet can cause constipation, as can lack of sufficient fluids, notably water.

- *Lack of Exercise.* Having no active exercise on a regular basis can cause constipation.

- *Medications.* Medications such as diuretics (water pills), iron pills, and calcium pills can cause constipation in some people, so pay attention to your body and to changes in your bowel movements when taking any medication.

■ *Symptoms.* Some diseases have constipation as a symptom, so be sure to tell your clinician if you continue to be constipated after trying the suggestions here.

What You Can Do About Constipation

1. *Eat right.* Select foods from the following groups, including lots of roughage or fiber in each day's diet:

Food Group	Foods to Emphasize	Servings per Day
breads, cereals, grains	whole wheat bread, whole grains, bran cereals, rice, wheat germ, whole wheat pasta, popcorn, oats, rice cakes, granola, wheat bran	3-4 servings a day 1 cup or more
fruits, fruit juices	dates, raisins, figs, apples, berries, melons, whole oranges, pears	3 or more fresh fruits each day
vegetables	broccoli, cauliflower, peas, green and wax beans, brussels sprouts, lettuce, spinach, cabbage, celery, asparagus, artichokes, carrots, squash, turnips	3 or more; some raw vegetables each day
miscellaneous	legumes (dried peas, kidney beans, navy beans)	varies with diet
beans, nuts	seeds, nuts	some each day

2. *Time.* Take time when your body signals you; don't put off

bowel evacuations.

3. *Fluids.* Fluid intake is very important to your general good health and especially for good bowel and bladder and kidney health. Six to 8 glasses of water a day are recommended to prepare fecal material at the proper consistency for bowel elimination. In addition to water, add fruit juices, coffee, tea, and soda; the latter three can be irritating to your bladder or stomach or both (if caffeinated), so try to keep amounts limited and don't substitute these for water.

4. *Exercise.* Regular exercise (4 to 7 times a week) is important to general good health and also helps us to keep our regular (usual for us) bowel evacuation schedule. Walking, running, bicycling, swimming, working-out, active work routine (walking a lot, lifting and moving things), dancing, skating, sports such as tennis, soccer, touch football, basketball, volleyball, handball, racquetball, all help keep our body and its functions in shape.

5. *Flavored or unflavored Metamucil* or store brand psyllium hydrophilic mucilloid fiber is useful if diet, exercise, and fluids don't work for you. Mix a tablespoon in 8 or more ounces of water. Metamucil also comes in wafers (cookies) in several flavors. You can also try over-the-counter stool softeners such as dialose, kasof, and colace. Follow directions carefully about use; it's best to discuss this with your health care provider. Stool softeners and sources of fiber are not harmful or habit forming, but you should try diet, fluids, and exercise first.

6. *Laxatives.* Laxatives, enemas, and drugs to cause you to evacuate your bowels can be harmful in the long run and should be used only after consulting a health care provider to rule out bowel disease as the cause of the constipation and after trying the measures discussed here.

From: Hawkins, Roberto-Nichols, & Stanley-Haney, *Protocols for Nurse Practitioners in Gynecologic Settings*, 7th edition, 2000, © The Tiresias Press, Inc.

Appendix HH

For Your Information: Hormone Therapy (HT)

I. Definition

Hormone therapy is the use of synthetic hormones (estrogen, progesterone, and/or testosterone) by postmenopausal women. Now known as HT, the use of hormones after menopause was once known as estrogen therapy (ET) because women were given synthetic estrogen only.

II. Reasons for Taking HT

A woman's body produces declining amounts of estrogens, progesterones and androgens during the perimenopausal period, culminating in the cessation of menstrual cycles (ovulation and bleeding). After 12 months without any bleeding (periods), you can consider that you are postmenopausal. A woman is said to have gone through surgical menopause if she has had her tubes, ovaries, and uterus removed.

Some natural estrogen production does continue after natural menopause; heavier women produce more estrogen since fat cells convert body chemicals called precursors to estrone, the most common form of natural estrogen in menopause.

Decline in natural estrogen production contributes to such menopausal symptoms as loss of elasticity of the vagina, a less lush vaginal lining causing a feeling of itching or burning or dryness, and pain around the urethra (the opening to the urinary bladder). Hot flashes or hot flushes, including night sweats, characterize menopause for some women. There may also be a relationship between menopause and loss of bone density leading to osteoporosis.

III. What You Should Know when Considering HT

HT should never be taken by women who have vaginal bleeding after menopause until the cause of the bleeding is discovered. Pregnant women or perimenopausal women who suspect pregnancy cannot take HT. If you have ever had a stroke, heart attack, or a blood clot in your legs or lungs, liver disease or any problems with the function of your liver, you may not be an HT candidate. Women with known or suspected cancer of the breast, ovaries, uterus, or cervix may not be good candidates for HT.

A number of conditions require special evaluation to determine if taking HT will be safe. These include undiagnosed vaginal bleeding, known or suspected pregnancy, a history of blood clots in your lungs or legs, known or suspected cancer of the breast or reproductive tract or malignant melanoma, history of bleeding disorder treated with blood transfusion, active gallbladder disease, family history of breast cancer, migraine headaches, elevated triglycerides and a ratio of good to bad cholesterol that is concerning, and endometriosis.

Considering HT is a decision that is yours to make if you and your clinician decide you have no contraindications to its use. To make the best decision, you and your clinician will discuss whether you are at greater risk of loss of bone density leading to osteoporosis because of your family or personal history, whether you have risk factors for developing osteoporosis, and your personal and family medical history including heart disease. Your desire for taking HT as well as your access to health care for monitoring HT will be considered. Some clinicians recommend that a sample of the lining of your uterus be analyzed before beginning HT, with a repeat of this test, called an endometrial biopsy, every year. An annual mammogram for women 40 and older as well as a Pap smear as indicated are important to your well being.

IV. Evaluating Your Physical Risks and Benefits in Taking HT

In addition to a careful personal and family history, your clinician will recommend that you have a complete physical exam including a pelvic (internal) exam and Pap smear, and testing for infections such as vaginitis, sexually transmitted diseases, and bladder infection (cystitis) if you have any signs or symptoms. Testing might also include: a mammogram if you have not had one in the past year, examination of hormone levels, an endometrial biopsy, a lipid profile to determine your cholesterol level and the ratio of low density lipids (LDL—the bad ones) to high density lipids (HDL—the good ones), a hematocrit and/or hemoglobin to see if you are anemic, a bone density scan, and an electrocardiogram (EKG) if you have never had one and/or have a family history of heart disease. Other testing will depend upon findings from the physical exam and your personal and family health history.

For some women, the benefits of taking HT outweigh the risks. For others, the risks and benefits balance, and for still others, the risks outweigh the benefits.

V. Taking HT

If your uterus has been removed (hysterectomy) you will take estrogen only without progestin. You and your clinician will decide the estrogen that you will take, both the amount and the way you take it (in pill form, the patch, or as a vaginal cream, suppository, or vaginal ring).

If you still have your uterus, you may take both estrogen and a progestin patch or pill. Some women bleed when taking progestin, so you and your clinician will need to decide what is best for you.

As androgen levels drop with menopause, some women also take a small amount of male hormone (androgen), which may help women whose menopausal symptoms are not resolved with estrogen or estrogen and progestin alone, have a decreased sense of well-being, a lower libido (sex drive), and/or generalized loss of energy (lethargy).

V. Consider Alternatives and Adjuncts to HT

All women need a diet with at least 6-8 servings of fruit and vegetables a day, several servings of complex carbohydrates such as breads and pasta, sources of protein including diary products, eggs, meat, fish and poultry, legumes such as beans and peas, and calcium. Women also need to decrease fat to 30% or less of total calories daily through using nonfat dairy products (rich in protein and calcium), limiting red meat, and eating lean meat, poultry, and fish. Whole grain pastas, cereals and breads, bran, vegetables and fruit add roughage to the diet. Most women need calcium supplements. Postmenopausal women need a total of 1500 milligrams each day of calcium as well as 400-800 international units of vitamin D. Six to eight 8-ounce glasses of water daily will help keep all tissues healthy and promote both bowel and bladder health.

Regular weight-bearing exercise and strength training is critical to maintenance of bone density; 30 to 45 minutes four to six times a week is recommended. Botanicals, Chinese remedies, vitamins, non-hormonal vaginal lubricants such as KY jelly, KY liquid, Lubrin®, Vagisil®, Replens®, and Astroglide®, naturalistic interventions, and homeopathic preparations can be helpful supplements to or alternatives to HT. Because herbs and homeopathic remedies can interact with each other and with prescription and over-the-counter medications, it is best to consult a practitioner who specializes in their use. Your local library, health food store, bookstore, and health care providers are all sources of information about caring for yourself after menopause.

Menopause: Another change of life http://www. ppfa.org.ppfa./menopub/html
National Institute on Aging: http://www. pueblo,gsa.gov/cic-text/health/other/menopause.txt
Power Surge http://www.dearest.com/refer.htm
www.allwise.com

From: Hawkins, Roberto-Nichols, & Stanley-Haney, *Protocols for Nurse Practitioners in Gynecologic Settings, 7th edition,* 2000, ©The Tiresias Press, Inc.

Appendix II
For Your Information: Osteoporosis

I. Definition

Osteoporosis is characterized by decreased bone mass (loss of bone density), deterioration of bone microarchitecture, and an increase in bone fragility and risk for bone fractures (broken bones).

II. Etiology

Humans have two types of bone—cortical and trabecular. Cortical bone is very compact; it forms the outer shell of bones and makes up 80% of the skeletons of adults. Trabecular bone, also called spongy or cancellous bone, makes up the remaining 20% and forms the interior of bones. For bones to develop properly and maintain bone mass, we need adequate calcium and phosphorus and other minerals in our diets. We also need other vitamins and adequate Vitamin D for our bodies to absorb calcium from our diets and enable the body to maintain our bones.

We reach our peak bone mass at about age 35. Estrogen seems to play a role in enabling women's bones to retain calcium and the other minerals necessary to build bone and preserve bone mass. From age 35 or so, some sources say that we lose about 2% of bone density each year. After menopause, the loss of bone mass seems to accelerate. If bone mass loss becomes too great, the woman becomes very susceptible to fractures.

III. Risk Factors

The risk of developing osteoporosis is greater for women than for men (women begin with less bone mass), and increases with age. Women who have never had children, had early menopause (before age 50), are of Northern European or Asian descent, have a thin body frame, blond or red hair, fair skin and freckles, curvature of the spine (scoliosis), are unable to digest milk or dairy products, smoke, have a high alcohol intake, low calcium diet, high salt diet, not enough Vitamin B, drink more than 2 or 3 cups of caffeinated beverages a day, do not exercise or exercise excessively, live in a northern climate, have little fluoride in their drinking water, and have a family history of osteoporosis are at greater risk than women with none of these risks.

IV. Prevention

We cannot change our heritage, family history, gender, our body build, hair or skin colors, the time at which we go through natural menopause, or our inability to drink milk or eat milk products. But we can exercise an appropriate amount, stop or never start smoking, limit alcohol intake, choose a diet with the amount of calcium we need (1200-1500 milligrams daily at ages 11-24 or when pregnant or breast feeding, 1000 milligrams between ages 25 and 49, and 1500 milligrams at age 50+), take vitamin D supplements (400-800 international units after menopause), decrease or eliminate caffeine, and decrease daily salt intake.

Calcium-rich foods include: broccoli; bok choy; collard, mustard and turnip greens; kale; and oranges. Dairy products, sardines, and salmon with bones, shrimp paste, dried anchovies, tofu, and almonds are all high in calcium. Vitamin D (400-800 international units is the recommended daily dose) can be obtained from 5 to 10 minutes in the sun each day, drinking the equivalent of a quart of vitamin D fortified milk, or taking a vitamin D supplement. Foods rich in vitamin D include fatty fish, butter, vitamin D-fortified margarine, egg yolks, and liver.

We can help prevent osteoporosis by changing what we can change in our lifestyles and by considering hormone therapy after menopause. Hormone therapy, known as HT, is not for every woman and is a decision each should make very carefully with her health care provider.

If you do not choose to use HT, in addition to all the lifestyle changes discussed above, you may also consider the use of vitamins—especially 400 units of vitamin E each day, and exploring botanicals or other homeopathic products with knowledgeable persons.

V. Treatment for Osteoporosis

If you have osteoporosis, you can prevent further loss of bone mass and, in some cases, actually restore bone mass with a regimen of exercise prescribed by a clinician specializing in osteoporosis therapy.

Calcium supplements, adequate vitamin D, hormonal and nonhormonal drug therapy, changes in lifestyle including smoking cessation, decreasing or eliminating caffeine, and lowering alcohol intake can also improve the health of your bones.

Making your home as safe as possible will help you avoid fractures. Nurses and physical therapists who specialize in working with persons with osteoporosis can help you reduce or eliminate those hazards.

From: Hawkins, Roberto-Nichols, & Stanley-Haney, *Protocols for Nurse Practitioners in Gynecologic Settings, 7th edition,* 2000, ©The Tiresias Press, Inc.

Appendix JJ
For Your Information: Cystitis (Bladder Infection)

Cystitis, a bladder infection, is usually caused by bacteria. Women are more prone to cystitis because the urethra (connection between the bladder and the outside through which we urinate or pee) is short and the vagina and rectum are close to the opening of the urethra, called the urethral meatus. However, men can also develop cystitis.

Symptoms of cystitis include:
- Frequent urination of small amounts of urine; often you will experience urgency—a feeling of needing to urinate and then just urinating a little
- Burning, pain, or difficulty in urinating
- Blood in the urine
- Pain in the lower part of the abdomen (pelvic pain) around the pubic bone
- Chills, fever

Treatment

Treatment of cystitis is with a sulfonamide or an antibiotic. It is important that you tell your clinician if you are allergic to any antibiotics or to sulfonamides so that you are given a suitable medication.

You may be asked to give what is called a clean catch urine specimen prior to the diagnosis (as opposed to just urinating in a paper cup for the specimen). For the clean catch specimen, you will be given special wipes to use on your perineal area and instructions on collecting the urine specimen in a sterile container. This specimen will be sent to the laboratory to evaluate the bacteria in the urine and to see what sulfonamides or antibiotics will be effective against the bacteria.

It is important to take the entire prescription given to you even if symptoms disappear quickly. Follow the directions for times to take the medication and try not to skip a dose as this may allow the bacteria to increase in number. You may also be given a prescription for a bladder pain medication or information about over-the-counter medication (Uristat®) to take away the bladder pain. These bladder pain medications are to be used with, and not instead of, the antibiotic or sulfonamide as they only relieve bladder pain and have no effect on the bacteria causing your cystitis.

Things You Can Do About Cystitis

There are several things you can do to avoid cystitis and to help your body heal if you have cystitis

- After going to the bathroom, wipe from front to back, or wipe the front first and then the back so as not to carry bacteria from your rectal area to the vaginal area where your urethral opening is.
- If your lovemaking includes vaginal or oral contact following anal contact, you may consider washing off your genitals and those of your partner before proceeding.
- During a tub bath, it is better not to use bath oils and bubble bath because they help bacteria travel up your urethra.
- Try to empty your bladder before sex, and after sex empty your bladder as soon as you can to wash bacteria from your urethra.
- Tight clothing, especially clothes made of synthetic fabrics such as polyester, helps bacteria grow more easily by creating a warm, dark, moist environment. Cotton underpants and loose clothing help your body breathe and discourage bacterial growth.
- Always urinate when you have the urge; don't put it off until you are desperate. Bacteria grow better in urine that is sitting in your bladder for long period of time.
- Drink 6-8 glasses of water and juice a day; cranberry juice helps to decrease cystitis. Cranberry is also available as Azo-Cranberry—cranberry juice capsules with 450 milligrams of cranberry juice concentrate; the dose is 1-4 capsules per day with meals.
- Caffeine is a bladder irritant, meaning it can cause bladder pain or spasms (cramps), so the less caffeine you take in, the less bladder irritation you will experience.
- Smoking is also very irritating to the bladder.
- A well-balanced diet including 6 or more servings of fresh fruits and vegetables a day and 3-4 servings of whole grain breads, cereals, and pasta, will increase your resistance to infection.

Cystitis is the least serious of the urinary tract infections. Untreated, it can lead to infection of the rest of the urinary tract including the ureters and kidneys. Prompt and correct treatment of cystitis will help you avoid having a more serious urinary tract infection. If your symptoms worsen or do not get better with the treatment prescribed by your clinician, call or return to the health care setting for further help.

From: Hawkins, Roberto-Nichols, & Stanley-Haney, *Protocols for Nurse Practitioners in Gynecologic Settings,* 7th ed., 2000, ©The Tiresias Press, Inc.

Appendix KK

For Your Information: Pediculosis (Lice)

I. Definition

Pediculosis means having the skin infested with lice, particularly on hairy areas such as the scalp, underarms, and the pubic area. Three types of lice prey on humans: head lice *(p. capitis),* body lice *(p. corposis),* and pubic lice or "crab lice" *(p. pubis).*

II. Transmission

Lice are transmitted by lice-infected shared clothing, bedding, brushes, towels, pillows, and upholstered furniture, or by close personal contact with an infected person. Head lice move from head to head. Adult pubic lice probably survive no more than 24 hours off their host.

III. Signs and Symptoms

A. Intense itching

B. Observing the lice or, more easily, their nits (eggs), which are greenish-white ovals attached to hair shafts—in eyebrows, eyelashes, scalp hair, pubic hair, and other body hair.

C. Known exposure to household member or intimate partner with lice

D. Crusts or scabs on body from scratching

E. Enlargement of lymph nodes (swollen glands) in the neck, an allergic response to lice

F. Body lice found on clothing, especially in the seams, as lice are rarely found on the body

G. Black dots (representing excreta) on skin and underclothing

IV. Diagnosis

See Signs and Symptoms above. Lice can best be detected by

using a magnifying glass cr microscope

V. Treatment
A. General measures
1. Wash clothing, towels, etc., with hot water, or dry clean contaminated items or run them through a dryer to destroy nits and lice; wash combs and hairbrushes in hot, soapy water. Items can also be sealed in a plastic bag for 2 weeks; lice will suffocate. Or items can be put outside in cold weather for 10 days.
2. Spray couches, chairs, car seats, and items that can't be washed or dry cleaned with over-the-counter products (A-200 Pyrinate®, Triplex®, RID, or store brand products); alternative is to vacuum carefully to pick up lice and nits.
B. Specific measures
1. Head lice
a. Thoroughly wet hair with Kwell®, Triplex Kit, Pronto, RID, or End Lice shampoo; work up lather, adding water as necessary. Shampoo thoroughly, leaving shampoo on head for 5 minutes. Pronto shampoo/conditioner can be used as an alternative to these. *OR* use Nix®, leave on 10 minutes. Kwell® cannot be used by women who are pregnant or breast feeding or for children under 2 years of age (and it requires a prescription)
b. Rinse thoroughly, towel dry
c. Remove remaining nits with fine-tooth metal comb or tweezers. Putting olive oil on the hair can help make running the comb through the hair easier
2. Body lice
a. Bathe with soap and water even if no lice are found
b. If evidence of lice is found, Kwell Lotion® may be may be applied, allowed to remain 8-10 hours, and thoroughly rinsed off
3. Pubic lice
a. Apply Kwell® shampoo, leave on 4 minutes, or apply

     A.200 Pyrinate Gel® as directed to hair and skin of pubic area

b. Rinse thoroughly
c. Repeat application in 7-10 days
d. Treat sexual partner as in a., b., c.

VI.   Client Education

A. Carefully check family and household members and close contacts for evidence of lice contamination and if found, treat as above.
B. Call your health care provider if signs of infection from scratching occur (redness, swelling of skin, discharge that looks like pus, bleeding, fever)
C. Stop using the treatment and call your health care provider if you or your family members experience sensitivity to the treatment (pain, swelling, rash)
D. Consult with your health care provider if you have lice on the eye lashes as the treatments cannot be used near eyes. Vaseline or ophthalmic (eye) ointment must be applied to the eyelashes.

VII.   Follow-up

Contact your health care provider if itching, redness or other problems listed above persist or recur.

Special notes:

Practitioner_____

From: Hawkins, Roberto-Nichols, & Stanley-Haney, *Protocols for Nurse Practitioners in Gynecologic Settings, 7th edition,* 2000, ©The Tiresias Press, Inc.

Appendix LL

For Your Information: Scabies

I. Definition
Scabies is a highly contagious skin rash whose chief symptom is itching. Scabies is caused by the scabies mite (Sarcoptes scabiei), which burrows into the skin and deposits its eggs along the tunnel it has made. The eggs hatch in 3-5 days and gather around hair follicles. Newly hatched females burrow into the skin, mature in 10-19 days, then mate and start a new cycle.

II. Transmission
A. Scabies among adults may be sexually transmitted.
B. Persons living in close proximity with others, in dormitories, and in crowded living spaces are more likely to incur scabies if one person amongst them becomes infested with the mite. Persons sharing clothing or towels are at increased risk.

III. Signs and Symptoms
A. May appear 4-6 weeks after contact with scabies from another person because it takes several weeks for sensitization to develop. In persons previously infected, symptoms may appear 1-4 days after repeat exposure to the scabies mite.
B. Itching, becoming worse at night or at times when the body temperature is raised such as after exercise. Itching begins first, before other signs and symptoms.
C. Lesions are usually on the webs between fingers, the inner aspects of the wrists and elbows, areas surrounding the surrounding the nipples, umbilicus (belly button), belt line, lower abdomen, genitalia, and cleft between the butttocks. These lesions look like little burrows about 1/2 to 3/4 inch in length ending in a raised red area (papule) or a raised area

filled with fluid (vesicle). These lesions can become scaly and become crusted over. When scratched, the areas become raw looking and become infected.

III. Diagnosis

A. Diagnosis is made through examination of lesions and of those areas of the body most frequently involved.
B. Linear burrows can be seen in the affected area.
C. Scaling, crustation lesions, furuncles (boils), and/or scratches may be visible with secondary infection.
D. When scrapings from the lesions are examined under low power with a microscope, the mites can sometimes be seen.

IV. Treatment

A. Treatments to kill mites
   1. Elimite® applied to all areas of the body from the neck down and washed off after 8-14 hours *OR*
   2. Kwell® or Scabene®, 1 ounce of lotion or 30 grams of cream applied in a thin layer to the entire body from the neck down, left on for 6-8 hours, and washed off thoroughly. These applications should not be in excess of these recommendations to avoid the possibility of damage to the nervous system from absorption through the skin. These medications should not be used for women who are pregnant or breast feeding or on children under 2 years of age. *OR*
   3. Sulfur 6% in ointment thinly applied to all areas of the body for 3 nights. Wash off previous application before applying a new one. Thoroughly wash off 24 hours after the last treatment. This treatment is less effective than the others but can be used if the others cannot be used because of pregnancy or allergy to them.
B. Treatments to relieve symptoms. Antihistamines may be taken to relieve itching. (These do not kill the mites but may make you feel better)
C. General measures to decrease risk of reinfestation

1. Clothing, towels, and bed linens should be laundered (hot cycle) or dry cleaned on day of treatment with medication.
2. If clothing items can't be washed or dry cleaned, separate them from the cleaned clothes and do not wear for at least 72 hours. Mites cannot exist for more than 2-3 days away from the body.
3. Sexual partner and close personal or household contacts within the past month should be informed and referred to a health care provider for examination and treatment.

V. Client Education
A. Follow the treatment regime carefully.
B. Itching may persist for several weeks. If you do not respond to therapy and itching persists after one week, contact your health care provider to decide if further therapy is necessary.
C. Call health care provider if the infested areas bleed, do not seem to be healing, are swollen or warm to the touch or have drainage that looks like pus. You may have a secondary infection and need additional treatment.
D. Discontinue treatment and call your health care provider if you develop a rash after using medication.

VI. Follow-up
A. Call your health care provider if
   1. Lesions do not begin to resolve with treatment or you are getting new lesions.
   2. The treatment has brought out another skin condition, one you had previously, such as eczema or psoriasis.
   3. Lesions appear to be spreading and increasing in size.
B. Return to your health care provider if symptoms persist or new symptoms occur.
C. Return to your health care provider for evaluation of the success of the treatment, the need for retreatment.

From: Hawkins, Roberto-Nichols, & Stanley-Haney, *Protocols for Nurse Practitioners in Gynecologic Settings*, 7th edition, 2000, ©The Tiresias Press, Inc.

Appendix MM

For Your Information: Syphilis

I. Definition
Syphilis is a sexually transmitted disease that can affect any organ in the body such as the bones, brain or heart. It is spread by sexual contact and can also be passed on from mother to unborn baby. It is caused by the organism Treponema pallidum (T. pallidum).

II. Important Information
A. Any sexually active person can get infected with syphilis. An untreated person can spread syphilis for one year after being infected.
B. Symptoms can occur 10-90 days after sexual contact; average is 21 days.

III. Usual Signs and Symptoms. What You May Experience
A. *Primary Syphilis.* The first sign of syphilis is a painless chancre (sore) at the site of entry of the syphilis organism. The chancre may occur on the vulva, labia, opening to vagina, clitoris, cervix, nipple, lip, roof of mouth, opening to the urethra on the head of the penis, the shaft of the penis, the anal area, or the scrotum. You may notice painful and/or swollen glands in your groin area, on your neck or under your arms. The chancre will last 1-5 weeks and will go away even if not treated. If you are not diagnosed and treated you will progress to secondary syphilis.
B. *Secondary Syphilis.* In 2-8 weeks or as long as 6 months after the chancre appears (average is 6 weeks), you will notice a rash on any part of your body. It can even appear on the palms of your hands or the soles of your feet. You may also have some hair loss so that your head has a "moth eaten" look

and you may lose part of your eyebrows. You may notice swollen glands in any part of your body, have a low-grade fever, a sore throat, headache, feel tired, have loss of appetite, and your joints may feel sore. This will last about 6 weeks and go away without treatment. If you are not diagnosed and treated you will progress to latent syphilis.

C. *Latent Syphilis.* You will have no symptoms, although 25% of persons may have a chancre again. During primary and secondary syphilis and early latency you are infectious to sexual partners. After 12 months have passed from the date of the initial infection, you are no longer infectious but the organism is in your blood. If you are not diagnosed and treated, you may remain in the latent stage for the rest of your life.

D. *Tertiary Syphilis.* One-third of persons infected with syphilis and not treated will go into the tertiary stage. In this stage your bones of skin, heart, or nervous system including your brain, can be affected. Persons with tertiary syphilis can become unable to work or care of themselves and have a shortened life.

V. Diagnosis
A. History of sexual contact with a known infected person.
B. Blood tests and examination of material from a chancre under a special microscope to see the syphilis organism.

VI. Treatment
The treatment of choice is penicillin given by injection. For those allergic to penicillin, other antibiotics can be used. The amount and treatment will depend on the stage of the syphilis.

VII. Complications
A. Progression of the disease to tertiary stage.
B. Transmission of syphilis from a woman to her unborn baby causing congenital syphilis in the baby. Congenital means "present at birth." Congenital syphilis can cause permanent damage to the baby.

VIII. Patient Education

A. Follow-up for second dose of medications as instructed by health care provider.

B. Use barrier contraception (condom) each time you have sexual intercourse.

C. Look at your partner before having sex. If you see a sore (chancre), rash, swelling or discharge, consider a check-up for both of you before having sex.

D. If you think you may have contracted syphilis or any other sexually transmitted disease (STD), avoid having sex and visit a local STD clinic

E. If you are diagnosed with syphilis, report any sexual partners to your health care provider so they can be notified and treated, or notify them to seek treatment.

F. Return for testing after treatment for primary or secondary syphilis at 3 and 6 months; for latent syphilis, at 6 and 12 months.

G. There is no immunity to syphilis, so you can be reinfected by an infected partner. Return for treatment if you believe you have been infected again.

Special Notes _____

_____

Practitioner:_____

For more information for yourself or friends:

CDC (Centers for Disease Control) STD Hotline 1-800 227-8922; on line: http://www.cdc.gov

For phone numbers of free (or almost free) STD clinics see the "Community Service Numbers" in the government pages of your local phone book.

From: Hawkins, Roberto-Nichols, & Stanley-Haney, *Protocols for Nurse Practitioners in Gynecologic Settings, 7th edition,* 2000, ©The Tiresias Press, Inc.

Appendix NN

For Your Information
Contraceptive Norplant® Implants

I. Description
The implants are 6 flexible, nonbiodegradable tubes filled with a synthetic progestin hormone designed to be released at a constant rate for 5 years. The tubes are placed under the skin on the inside of the upper arm. This method of contraception works by
A. Suppressing ovulation (release of an egg)
B. Thickening the cervical mucus making it harder for sperm to swim through
C. Making the cervical mucus more scanty
D. Suppressing the growth of the lining of the uterus (womb), making it harder for the fertilized egg to implant itself there

II. Benefits of the Method
A. 99% effective for first 5 years
B. Allows sexual spontaneity
C. Contains only a synthetic progestin, so the risk factors with estrogen do not seem to be present
D. Scanty or no menstrual flow
E. Decreased menstrual cramps
F. Decreased symptoms of endometriosis
G. No ovulation so no symptoms including pain with ovulation
H. Reversible if desired by removal of the implants
I. Smokers can use Norplant®
J. Can be used immediately after childbirth and by breast-feeding women
K. Can be used immediately after an abortion

III. Risks of the Method
A. Irregular menstrual flow either with more days of light

bleeding or no bleeding at all; heavier than usual bleeding is rare and usually lessens within a year, often in a few months
B. Possible weight gain—average over 5 years is less than 5 pounds
C. Possible breast tenderness or, rarely, breast discharge
D. Possible increase in acne
E. No protection against sexually transmitted disease unless condoms are also used
F. Depression
G. Bruising or pain associated with insertion or removal of implants; swelling or infection at site of implantation
H. Consult your health care provider about the medications you are taking since some medications may make your implants less effective
I. Initial cost is higher than other methods because of cost of insertion, but over the 5 years of the implants' life the cost is about the same as for other hormonal methods such as oral contraceptives and Depo-Provera

IV. Contraindications (Reasons You May Not Be Able to Use Norplant®)

A. *Women with any of the following should not use Norplant®:*
   1. Known or suspected pregnancy
   2. Breast cancer (or history of)
   3. Abnormal vaginal bleeding suspicious for a serious problem
B. *Women with the following need to be evaluated by their health care provider prior to having Norplant® inserted:*
   1. Abnormal mammogram
   2. Allergy or intolerance of local anesthetic
   3. High blood pressure
   4. Diabetes

V. Alternative Methods of Birth Control

A. Abstinence
B. Sterilization
C. Natural family planning
D. Condoms with contraceptive cream, foam, jelly, film or gel;

contraceptive tablets or suppositories
E. Intrauterine devices
F. Diaphragm with contraceptive cream or jelly
G. Cervical cap
H. Female condom
I. Depo-Provera®
J. Oral contraceptives ("the pill")
K. Contraceptive sponge

VI. Explanation of Method

A. Way in which Norplant® is prescribed
   1. A complete physical examination is done, including blood pressure, weight, urinalysis, gynecologic examination with Papanicolaou smear (unless done within past year)
   2. If more than 3 months since you had a complete physical, you may have a pelvic examination (bimanual)
   3. You must review and sign an informed consent prior to having Norplant® implanted.
B. Way in which Norplant® is inserted
   1. You will lie on your back on the examination table with your less dominant arm bent at the elbow and positioned so your hand is lying by your head.
   2. Your health care provider will draw an insertion map on your arm, then cleanse the area with an antiseptic solution and anesthetize the area of your arm where the Norplant® tubes will be inserted using a local anesthetic (after asking if you are allergic to local anesthetics).
   3. After making a very small incision (about ¾ of an inch), the implants will be inserted just under the skin in a fan shape, using an instrument called a trocar through which the implants will fit.
   4. After inserting all 6 implants and checking their position, your health care provider will close the small incision with a skin closure called steri-strips, cover the area with a dry dressing, and wrap your arm with gauze.
   5. You will be asked to keep the area dry for 2-3 days; you can remove the gauze after 1 day and the steri-strips after 3 days; if you have pain, call your health care provider.

6. You will experience changes in your normal menstrual cycle. If these changes seem more bothersome than described by your health care provider, call with questions.
7. You may be asked to return in 2-4 weeks and then again in 3 months to check for side effects and any problems.
8. You may return at any time but no later than 5 years after insertion for removal of the implants and replacement if you wish to continue the method.
9. Protect yourself from sexually transmitted diseases by using condoms or spermicides. You also need to use one of these back-up methods the day after Norplant® is inserted; some providers recommend using one of these methods for the first 3-7 days after insertion.
10. Be sure to call if you have any questions or problems, including depression.
11. Return for a Papanicolaou smear and pelvic and physical examinations every year, and have a mammogram per the recommendation of your health care provider.

VII. Danger Signals Associated with Norplant® Use

- Severe pain in your pelvis or lower abdomen.
- Vaginal bleeding that is unusually heavy for you.
- Change in pattern of your menstrual cycle—no menses or delayed menses after a pattern of regular menses.
- Pain in your arm at the site of the implants, or swelling, pus, bleeding or redness at the incision site.
- Shift in position of the implants, or one or more implants come out.
- Headaches that do not go away with your normal treatment, are unusually painful, are migraines, or are accompanied by visual disturbance (spots before your eyes, blurred or double vision, or loss of vision).

Contact us at (_____) _____ if you develop any of the above problems or have any questions.

From: Hawkins, Roberto-Nichols, & Stanley-Haney, *Protocols for Nurse Practitioners in Gynecologic Settings, 7th edition,* 2000, ©The Tiresias Press, Inc.

Appendix 00

Women and Heart Disease
Risk Factor Assessment*

Nonmodifiable

1. Age: postmenopausally, the risk for women increases dramatically; mortality is high for ages 35-44 and 75-84
2. Race or ethnicity: black women have a higher rate of death than white women; 5-year survival rate is lower and black women younger than 55 have >2x the death rate of white women; rates of diabetes and hypertension in black women are higher than those in white women
3. Family history of the disease
4. Gender: attenuating advantage of being a woman especially premenopausally (premenopausally, women's risk is lower than men's)
5. Socioeconomic status: inverse association with morbidity and mortality

Modifiable

1. Lifestyle
   a. Exercise: aerobic exercise can increase HDLs
   b. Nutrition: cholesterol levels, lipid profile (HDL vs. LDL); high fat vs. low fat diet; modifying effects of antioxidants
   c. Cigarette smoking
      1) Smoking and OC use increases rate of atherosclerosis
      2) Women (under 40 years old) who have MIs are mainly smokers

---

*Adapted from Rankin, S.H. (1997). Heart and soul: Evaluation of women with coronary artery disease. *Clinical Excellence for Nurse Practitioners, 1(4)*, 231-239. See also Bibliography 34.

      3) Older women who smoke have a 500% greater chance to experience sudden death than older non-smokers

      4) Acts synergistically with hyperlipidemia

  d. Hormone therapy postmenopausally

2. Internal and external environmental factors

  a. Co-morbidities: hypertension, diabetes, obesity; poor management of these chronic diseases increases risk while good management decreases risk

  b. Psychosocial concerns: stress and social support; high stress and low social support increase morbidity and mortality

  c. Access to health care: unequal access appears to be a factor in morbidity and mortality

Appendix PP
Good Idea—Stop Smoking

Smoking is the leading cause of preventable illness and early death in the United States. If you stop you can expect an increase in your life expectancy and improvement in your health.

Smokers are at greater risk for

Strokes	Cancer of the larynx
Oral cancers	Lung disease
Chronic obstructive pulmonary disease	Heart disease

Smokers also develop other smoking-related problems

Pregnancy complications

Impotence and infertility

Abnormal Papanicolaou smears (dysplasia)

Osteoporosis and bone density problems

Premature skin wrinkling

Gum disease and dental cavities

Stained teeth and bad breath

Poor circulation

Poor tolerance for exercise

High blood pressure

Family members are at greater risk for:

lung cancer and heart disease

children of smokers have higher incidences of sudden death syndrome, asthma, ear infections, colds, learning delays

The rewards of quitting are experienced quickly and long-term.

Within several weeks:

Blood pressure drops

Circulation improves

Lung function improves

Coughing, sinus infections, fatigue, and shortness of breath improve

Number of colds decreases

Energy level improves

After 1 year:
> Excess risk of heart disease improves to half that of a smoker

After 5 years:
> Lung cancer death rate decreases by almost half
> Risk of cancer of the mouth, throat and esophagus is half that of a smoker

After 5-15 years:
> Stroke risk is reduced to that of a nonsmoker

After 10 years:
> Lung cancer death rate is similar to that of a non-smoker

After 15 years:
> The risk of coronary heart disease is that of a non-smoker

Do you think you have a dependence on nicotine? Ask yourself the following questions:
- Do you smoke a cigarette first thing in the morning?
- Do you wake up to smoke a cigarette during the night?
- Do you smoke 5 or more cigarettes a day?
- Do you find it hard to not smoke in places where it is forbidden? Do you leave such places to smoke?
- Do you smoke more cigarettes in hours after you wake up than during the rest of the day?
- Do you smoke when you are ill?

If you answer yes to any of these questions you can consider yourself as having a nicotine problem

Want to quit? The following suggestions may help:
> Make the decision to stop smoking
> Think about why you want to stop smoking. Make a list of those reasons and the rewards associated with quitting. Keep this list with you and review it when you feel the urge to smoke
> Talk to your friends and family; ask for their support and encouragement
> Keep a journal. You can start it when you are making the decision to quit. Record each cigarette smoked, the time, the place, and the intensity of the craving and the reward of the cigarette. Think about the social cues associated with smoking and about how you will deal with these after you stop smoking.

Record your thoughts and feelings. Doing this can help you identify your smoking "triggers" and assist you in adapting strategies and skills to get past those triggers. Continue recording your feelings in the journal after you have quit smoking

    Avoid drinking alcohol. Alcohol will weaken your resolve

    Clean your clothes, car, drapes and furniture to rid them of the smell of smoke

    Throw out all cigarettes, ashtrays and smoking paraphernalia

    Avoid being around other smokers

    If possible, establish living space as "no smoking"

    Increase exercise level (walking, weight lifting, yoga). This assists in weight management, stress reduction, and general sense of well being

    Change your daily routine to avoid smoking triggers

    Keep oral substitutes handy. Use low calorie vegetables and fruits; sugarless gum; toothpicks

    Engage in activities that make smoking difficult, such as exercising, gardening, washing the car

    Spend time in places where smoking is prohibited

    Join a support group. Such groups are offered by Nicotine Anonymous, American Cancer Society, the America Lung Association and your local hospital.

    Make an appointment with your health care provider and talk with her/him about your desire to stop smoking. Your provider can help you choose the most appropriate method to assist in breaking your habit. Choices available include:

- Nicotine replacements: gum, transdermal patches, nasal sprays
- Zyban or Wellbutrin SR—a non-nicotine oral medication for smoking cessation treatment

Good luck in your journey to a smoke-free life. Remember, if you have a relapse and start smoking again, you can quit again. Many people need to try several times before they are successful. If this happens to you, don't be too hard on yourself. Review the above suggestions and begin again!

From: Hawkins, Roberto-Nichols, & Stanley-Haney, *Protocols for Nurse Practitioners in Gynecologic Settings, 7th edition,* 2000, ©The Tiresias Press, Inc.

BIBLIOGRAPHIES

1. Women's Health Care, Gynecologic Care, Pelvic Examination

Calle, E.E., Flanders, D., et al. (1993). Demographic predictors of mammography and Pap smear screening in US women. *American J of Public Health,* 83(1):53-60.

Collins, B.S., et al. (1997). Women, work and health: Issues and implications for worksite health promotion. *Women & Health,* 25(4):3-38.

Douglas, J.H. (1998). Female circumcision: Persistence amid conflict. *Health Care for Women International,* 19(6):477-479.

Ehrenreich, B. & English, D. (1973). Complaints and Disorders. The Sexual Politics of Sickness. Old Westbury, NY: The Feminist Press.

Ehrenreich, B. & English, D. (1973). Witches, Midwives,, and Nurses: A History of Women Healers. Old Westbury, NY: The Feminist Press.

Eliason, M., Donelan, C., & Randall, C. (1992). Lesbian stereotypes. *Health Care for Women International,* 13(2):131-144.

Farr, K.A. & Wilson-Figueroa, M. (1997). Talking about health and health care: Experiences and perspectives of Latina women in a farmworking community. *Women & Health,* 25(2):23-40.

Felton, G.M., Liu, O., et al. (1998). Health-promoting behaviors of rural adolescent women. *Women & Health,* 88(11), 67-80.

Gentry, S.E. (1992). Caring for lesbians in a homophobic society. *Health Care for Women International,* 13(2):173-180.

Hern, M.J, et al. (1998). Promoting women's health via the world wide web. *J of Obstetric, Gynecologic, and Neonatal Nursing,* 27(6):606-610.

Jacobs, D.R., Meyer, K.A., et al. (1999). Is whole grain intake associated with reduced total and cause-specific death rates in older women? The Iowa womens's health study. *American J of Public Health,* 89(3):322-329.

Keller, M.L., Duerst, B.L., & Zimmerman, J. (1996). Adolescents' views of sexual decision-making. *Image,* 28(2):125-130.

Kushnir, T., Rabinowitz, S., et al. (1995). Health responsibility and workplace health promotion among women: Early detection of cancer. *Health Care for Women International,* 16(4):329-340.

Lambden, M.P., et al., (1997). Women's sense of wellbeing before and after hyserectomy. *J of Obstetric, Gynecologic, and Neonatal Nursing,* 26(5):-540-548.

Lucas, V.A. (1992). An investigation of the health care preferences of the lesbian population. *Health Care for Women International,* 13(2):221-228.

Manderino, M .A. & Brown, M.C. (1992). A practical step-by-step approach to stress management for women. *The Nurse Practitioner,* 17(7):18, 21, 24, 27-28.

Messing, K. (1997). Women's occupational health: A critical review and discussion of current issues. *Women & Health,* 25(4):39-68.

Muscari, M.E. (1999). Adolescent health: The first gynecologic exam. *American J of Nursing,* 99(1):66, 58.

Nies, M.A., Buffington, C., et al. (1998). Comparison of lifestyles among obese and nonobese African and European American women in the community. *Nursing Research,* 47(4):251-257.

Olsson, H.M. & Gullberg, M.T. (1991). Fundamental and situational components in a strategy for attaining a positive patient experience of the pelvic examination: A conceptual approach. *Health Care for Women International,* 12(4):415-429.

Peterson-Sweeney, K.L. & Stevens, J. (1996). 13-year-old female with imperforate hymen. *Nurse Practitioner,* 21(8):90, 92-94.

Pulliam, L.W., Plowfield, L.A., & Fuess, S. (1996). Developmental care: The key to the emergence of the vital older woman. *J of Obstetric, Gynecologic, and Neonatal Nursing,* 25(7):623-628.

Reichert, G.A. (1998). Female circumcision. *AWHONN Lifelines,* 2(3):28-34.

Robertson, M.M. (1992). Lesbians as an invisible minority in the health services arena. *Health Care for Women International,* 13(2):155-163.

Rogge, S.A. (1998). Reforming managed care: Carving out women's rights in health care. *AWHONN Lifelines,* 2(6):17-18.

Ruffing-Rahal, M.A. (1998). Well-being and its shadow: Health promotion implications for older women. *Health Care for Women International,* 19(5):

Taylor, D. & Dower, C. (1997). Toward a woman-centered health care system: Women's experiences, women's voices, women's needs. *Health Care for Women International,* 18(4):407-422.

Wilbur, J., Miller, A.M., Montgomery, A. & Chandler, P. (1998). Women's physical activity patterns: Nursing implications. *J of Obstetric, Gynecologic and Neonatal Nursing,* 27(4):383-392.

Williams, J.G., Park, L.I., & Kline, J. (1995). Physicians' attitudes toward a new gynecological examination gown. *Women & Health,* 22(2):1-9.

Woods, N.F., Lentz, M. & Mitchell, E. (1993). The new woman. Health-promoting and health-damaging behaviors. *Health Care for Women International,* 14(5):389-405.

2. Methods of Family Planning

Choosing contraception for the mid-life woman. *Contraceptive Technology 1996,* 17(12):152-153.

Darney, P.D. Contraception for the dyslipidemic woman. *Dialogues in Contraception,* Spring 1995; 4(6):5-8.

Davis, A. Contraceptive choices: The adolescent years. *Dialogues in Contraception,* Spring 1995, 4(6):1-4.

Failure rates of various contraceptives. *Contraceptive Technology Update 1996,* 17(2):13-16.

Fonte, D.R. (1997). The basics of natural family planning. *Advance for Nurse Practitioners,* 5(3):37-38, 41-42

Hatcher, R.A., Trussell, J., Stewart, F., Cates, W., Stewart, G.K., Guest, F. & Kowal, D. (1998). Contraceptive Technology. New York: Ardent Media.

Guillebaud, J. (1994). Contraception. Your Questions Answered. 2nd ed. London: Churchill Livingstone.

Lethbridge, D. (1995). Fertility management in Taiwanese and African-American women. *J of Obstetric, Gynecologic, and Neonatal Nursing,* 24(5):459-463.

Lethbridge, D.J. & Hanna, K.M. (1997). Promoting Effective Contraceptive Use. New York: Springer.

Matteson, P.S. (1995). Advocating for Self: Women's Decisions Concerning Contraception. New York: Harrington Park Press.

Matteson, P.S. & Hawkins, J.W. (1993). What family planning methods women use and why they change them. *Health Care for Women International,* 14(6):539-548.

Matteson, P.S. & Hawkins, J.W. (1997). Women's patterns of contraceptive use. *Health Care for Women International,* 18(5):455-466.

Piccinino, L.J. & Mosher, W.D. (1998). Trends in contraceptive use in the United States: 1982-1995. *Family Planning Perpectives,* 30(1):4-10, 46.

Reifsnider, E. (1997). On the horizon: New options for contraception. *J of Obstetric, Gynecologic, and Neonatal Nursing,* 26(1):91-100.

Schroder, R.K. (1995). Seasonal thoughts. *Advance for Nurse Practitioners,* 3(13):17-19.

Swanson, J.M., Forrest, K., et al. (1990). Readability of commercial and generic contraceptive instructions. *Image,* 22(2):96-100.

World Health Organization. (1996). Improving Access to Quality Care in Family Planning: Medical Eligibility Criteria for Contraceptive Use. Geneva, Switzerland: World Health Organization.

3. Oral Contraception

American Health Consultants (1998). Pillpower: Oral contraceptives hold top spot in the family planning arsenal. 19(10):125-140.

Darney, P. & Klaisle, C.(1998).Contraception-associated menstrual problems: Etiology and management. *Dialogues in Contraception,* 5(5):1-6.

Davies, E.S. (1997). A new second of preventing pregnancy. *Advance for Nurse Practitioners,* 5(11):43-44, 46-47.

Gallagher, R. & Fuller, S. (1997). A new generation of oral contraceptives. *Advance for Nurse Practitioners,* 5(5):39-40.

Hahn, M.S. (1995). Should oral contraceptives be available over the counter? *Advance for Nurse Practitioners,* 3(5):24-28.

Low dose oral contraceptives don't increase stroke risk. *Contraceptive Technology Update 1996*, 17(12);148-150.

Low graduated-estrogen oral contraceptive puts new start patients on right track. *Contraceptive Technology Update 1996*, 17(12):145-147.

Nakajima, S.T. (1994). The new progestins. *Connecticut Medicine*, 58(9): 530-531.

Notelovitz, M. (1995). Contraceptive efficacy and safety of a monophasic oral contraceptive containing 150 Ug desogestrel and 30 Ug ethinyl estradiol: United States clinical experience using a "Sunday start" approach. *Fertility and Sterility*, 64(2):261-266.

Oral contraceptives and venous thromboembolism. Consensus statement. *Dialogues in Contraception*, Spring 1996, (5):1-8.

Rosenberg, M. & Meyer, A. (1998). Improving oral contraceptive compliance. *The Female Patient*, 23:83-84, 86-89, 90

Speroff, L. *(1995). Oral Contraceptive Update 1995*, 1-31.

Thijs, C. & Knipschild, P. (1993). Oral contraceptives and the risk of gallbladder disease: A meta-analysis. *American J of Public Health*, 83(8):1113-1120.

Trussel, J., Steward, F., et al. (1993). Should oral contraceptives be available without prescription? *American J of Public Health*, 83(8):1094-1099.

Wysocki, S. (1998). Improving patient success with oral contraceptives: The importance of counseling. *The Nurse Practitioner*, 23(4):55-56, 59-60.

Youngkin, E.Q. (1993). Progestogens: A look at the 'other' hormone. *The Nurse Practitioner*, 18(11):28,31,35-36,38-40.

Zachariasen, R.D. (1994). Loss of oral contraceptive efficacy by concurrent antibiotic administration. *Women & Health*, 22(1):17-26.

4. Emergency Contraception

An update on emergency contraception. (1998). *Dialogues in Contraception*, 5(6).

Ansbacher, R. (1998). Generic substitutes for brand name hormonal medications. *The Female Patient*, 22:19-21

Brown, J.W. & Boulton, M.L. (1998). Dispensation of emergency contraceptive pills in Michigan title X clinics. *American J of Public Health*, 88(9): 1380-1381.

Davies, J.E. (1997). A second chance of preventing pregnancy. *Advance for Nurse Practitioners*, 5(11):43-44, 46-47.

Chez, R.A. & Chapin, J. (1997). Emergency contraception. *Lifelines*, 1(5):28-31.

Glasier, A., Ketting, E., et al. (1996). Emergency contraception in the United Kingdom and the Netherlands. *Family Planning Perspectives*, 28:49-51.

Grossman, R.A. & Grossman, B.D. (1994). How frequently is emergency contraception prescribed? *Family Planning Perspectives*, 26(6):270-271.

Lindberg, C.E. (1997). Emergency contraception: The nurse's role in providing postcoital options. *J of Obstetric, Gynecologic, and Neonatal ursing*, 26:145-152.

Morgan, K. & Demeris, A. (1997). Emergency contraception: Preventing unintended pregnancy. *Advance for Nurse Practitioners,* 22(11):34-36, 39-40.

Narrin, D. (1994). Postcoital contraception: Has its day come? *J of Nurse-Midwifery,* 39(6):363-369.

Trussell, J., Koening, J., et al. (1997). Preventing unintended pregnancy: The cost-effectiveness of three methods of emergency contraception. *American J of Public Health,* 87(6):932-937.

Trussell, J. & Stewart, F. (1998). An update on emergency contraception. *Dialogues in Contraception,* 5(6):1-5.

Trussell, J., Stewart, F., Guest, F. & Hatcher, R.A. (1992). Emergency contraceptive pills: A simple proposal to reduce unintended pregnancies. *Family Planning Perspectives,* 26(6):269-273.

Update on Emergency Contraception. (1998). *Dialogues in Contraception,* 5(6).

Wysocki, S. (1998). Emergency contraception. *Clinician Reviews,* 8(11):53-65.

5. Diaphragm

Connell, E.B. (1990). Barrier methods of contraception. In: N.G. Kase, A.B., Weingold, & D.M. Gershenson (Eds.), Principles and Practice of Clinical Gynecology, 2nd ed., pp. 981-991. New York: Churchill Livingstone.

Connell, D.G., Grimes, D.A., & Manisoff, M.E. (1989). The Contraceptive Diaphragm. New York: Healthcare Communications Network.

Hagen, I.M. & Beach, R.K. (1980). The diaphragm: Its effective use among college women. *J of the American College Health Association,* 28:263.

Kugel, C. & Verson, H. (1986). Relationship between weight change and diaphragm size change. *J of Obstetric, Gynecologic, and Neonatal Nursing,* 15(2):123-129.

Loucks, A. (1989). A comparison of satisfaction with types of diaphragms among women in college populations. *J of Obstetric, Gynecologic, and Neonatal Nursing,* 18(3):194-200.

Pyle, C.J. (1984). Nursing protocol for diaphragm contraception. *The Nurse Practitioner,* 9(3):35-38, 40.

6. Intrauterine Devices

Grimes, D.A.(1992). Highlights from an international symposium on IUDs. *The Contraception Report,* 3(3):3-15.

Jones, H.W., Jaffe, R.B., et al. (Eds.) (1996). IUDs: A state-of-the-art conference. *Obstetrical & Gynecological Survey,* 51(12 [supp.]):S1-S72.

Kaunitz, A.M. (1997). Reappearance of the intrauterine device: A "user friendly" contraceptive. *International J of Fertility,* 42(2):120-127.

Kaunitz, A.M. (1999). Intrauterine devices: Safe, effective, and underutilized. *Women's Health in Primary Care,* 2(1):39-47.

Kimble-Hass, S.L.(1998). The intrauterine device: Dispelling the myths. *Nurse Practitioner,* 23(11):58, 63-64, 66-69, 73.

Knutson, C. (1997). A new generation of IUD use. *Advance for Nurse Practitioners,* 5(1):22-24, 27, 31.

National Institute of Child Health and Human Development. (1996). IUDs: State-of-the-art. *Clinician,* 14(5):1-24.

Nelson, A. & Schnare, S. (1996). Which patient is right for an IUD. *Office Nurse,* 1-7.

Nelson, A.L. & Sulak, P. (1998). IUD patient selection and practice guidelines. Dialogues in Contraception, 5(5):7-11.

University of Minnesota Office of Continuing Medical Education. (1996). Intrauterine contraception in the U.S.: A current perspective. Little Falls, NJ: Health Learning Systems.

7. Contraceptive Spermicides and Condoms

(1993). The female condom. *The Medical Letter on Drugs and Therapeutics,* 35(912):123.

Condom coaching, use staging for best results.(1997). *Contraceptive Technology,* 18(1):6-8.

The switch is on from contraceptive foam to film. (1993 November). *Contraceptive Technology Update,* 1-2.

Detzer, M.J., Wendt, S.J., et al. (1995). Barriers to condom use among women attending planned parenthood clinics. *Women & Health,* 23(1):91-102.

Eldridge, G.D., St. Lawrence, J.S., et al. (1995). Barriers or condom use and barrier method preferences among low-income African-American women. *Women & Health,* 23(1):73-89.

Farr, G., Gabelnick, H., et al. (1994). Contraceptive efficacy and acceptability of the female condom. *American Journal of Public Health,* 84(12):1960-1964.

Frank, M.L., Poindexter, A.N., Cox, C.A. & Bateman, L. (1995). A cross-sectional survey of condom use in conjunction with other contraceptive methods. *Women & Health,* 23(2):31-46.

Frezieres, R.G., Walsh, T.L., Nelson, A.L., Clark, V.A. & Coulson, A.H. (1998). Breakage and acceptability of a polyurethane condom: A randomized, controlled study. *Family Planning Perspectives,* 30(2):73-78.

Grimes, D.A. (1992). Contraception for women over 35: The polyurethane vaginal pouch. *The Contraception Report,* 3(2):12-14.

Hatcher, R.A. (1992). VCF: Convenient contraceptive but it may be hard to find. *Contraceptive Technology Update, 13(11):167-168.*

Miller, K.S., Levin, M.I., et al. (1998). Patterns of condom use among adolescents: The impact of mother-adolescent communication. *American J of Public Health,* 88(10):1542-1544.

Oakley, D. & Bogue, E-L. (1995). Quality of condom use as reported by female clients of a family planning clinic. *American J of Public Health,* 85(11):1526-1530.

OTC Report (1998). Spermicide Gains Popularity. *Advance for Nurse Practitioners,* 6(1):59.

Review of company data shows Avanti breaks less often than latex. (1996). *Contraceptive Technology,* 17(4):37-41.

Roye, C.F. (1998). Condom use by Hispanic and African-American adolescent girls who use hormonal contraception. *J of Adolescent Health,* 23(4): 205-211.

Soet, J.E., Delorio, C. & Dudley, W.N. (1998). Women's self-reported condom use: Intra and interpersonal factors. *Women & Health,* 27(4):19-32.

Soper, D.E., Shoupe, S., et al. (1993). Prevention of vaginal trichomoniasis by compliant use of the female condom. *Sexually Transmitted Diseases,* 20(3):137-139.

Steiner, M., Trussell, J., et al. (1994). Standardized protocols for condom breakage and slippage trials: A proposal. *American J of Public Health,* 84(12):1897-1900.

Tagg, P.I. (1995). The diaphragm: Barrier contraception has a new social role. *Nurse Practitioner,* 20(12):36, 39-42.

Trussell, J., Sturgen, K., et al. (1994). Comparative contraceptive efficacy of the female condom and other barrier methods. *Family Planning Perspectives,* 26(2):66-72.

Weir, S.S., et al. (1994). The use of nonoxynol-9 for protection against cervical gonorrhea. *American J of Public Health,* 84(6):910-914.

8. Cervical Cap

Brokaw, A.K., Baker, N.N. et al. (1988). Fitting the cervical cap. *The Nurse Practitioner* 13(7)):49-50, 52,55.

Brown, L. (1988). The cervical cap—here at last! *The Publication of the National Women's Health Network,* 13(3):1,3.

Canavan, P.A. & Lewis, C.A. (1981). The cervical cap: An alternative contraceptive. *J of Obstetric, Gynecologic, and Neonatal Nursing,* 10(4):271-273.

Cap Instruction Sheets. Cambridge, MA: Nurse Practitioner Associates of Cambridge.

Chalker, R. (1987). The Complete Cervical Cap Guide. New York: Harper and Row.

Data challenge three-month Pap smear requirement for cap users. (1989). *Contraceptive Technology Update,* 10:156-158.

Gallagher, D.M. & Richwald, G.A. (1989). Feminism and regulation collide: The Food and Drug Administration's approval of the cervical cap. *Women & Health,* 15(2):87--97.

Johnson, M.A. (1985). The cervical cap as a contraceptive alternative. *The Nurse Practitioner,* 10(1):37, 41-42,, 45.

Koch, J.P. (1982). Instructions for the Prentif Cervical Cap. (Available from 1037 Beacon Street, Brookline, MA 02146.)

Trussell, J., Strickler, J. & Vaughan, B. (1993). Contraceptive efficacy of the diaphragm, the sponge and the cervical cap. *Family Planning Perspectives* 25(3):100-105, 135.

9. Vaginal Contraceptive Sponge

Axcan Ltee. Department of Research and Development. (1996). Something new in barrier contraception: The Protectaid® contraceptive sponge. Mont-St-

Hilaire, Quebec, Canada: Axcan Ltee.

Edelman, D.A., Smith, S.C. & McIntyre, S. (1983). Comparative trial of the contraceptive sponge and diaphragm: A preliminary report. *J of Reproductive Medicine,* 28:781.

Lemberg, E. (1984). The vaginal contraceptive sponge: A new non-prescription barrier contraceptive. *The Nurse Practitioner,* 9(10):24-37.

McClure, D.A. & Edelman, D.A. (1985). Worldwide method effectiveness of the Today® Vaginal Contraceptive Sponge. *Advances in Contraception,* 1:305-311.

Murray, T. (1996). New contraceptive sponge also protects against STDs. The *Medical Post,* 32(9):1.

Sherris, J. (1984). New developments in vaginal contraception. *Population Reports,* Series H, Number 7:157-190.

Psychoyos, A. et al. (1993). Spermicidal and antiviral properties of a new vaginal contraceptive sponge (Protectaid®), containing sodium cholate (cholic acid). *Human Reproduction,* 8(6):866-869.

10. Natural Family Planning

Bitto, A., Gray, R.H., Simpson, J.L., et al. (1997). Adverse outcomes of planned and unplanned pregnancies among users of natural family planning: A prospective study. *American J of Public Health,* 87:338-343.

Diaz, S. (1989). Determinants of lactational amenorrhea. *International J of of Gynecology and Obstetrics,* Supp. 1:83-89.

Fehring, R.J. (1991). New technology in natural family planning. *J of Obstetric, Gynecologic, and Neonatal Nursing,* 20(3):199-205.

Fehring, R.J. , Lawrence, D. & Philpot, C. (1994). Use effectiveness of the Creighton model ovulation method of natural family planning. *J of Obstetric,Gynecologic, and Neonatal Nursing,* 23(4):303-309.

Fonte, D.R. (1997). The basics of natural family planning. *Advance for Nurse Practitioners,* 5(3):36-42.

Geerling, J.H. (1995). Natural family planning. *American Family Physician,* 52(6):1749-1756.

Labbok, M., Cooney, K. & Coly, S. (1994). Guidelines: Breastfeeding, family planning, and the lactational amenorrhea methods—LAM. Washington, DC: Institute for Reproductive Health, Georgetown University.

Martin, M.C. (1981). Natural family planning and instructor training. *Nursing and Health Care,* 2(10):554-556,563.

Perez, A., Labbok, M.H., et al. (1992). Clinical study of the lactational amenorrhoea method for family planning. *The Lancet,* 339:968-970.

Roth, B. (1993). Fertility awareness as a component of sexuality education. *The Nurse Practitioner,* 18(33):40,43,47-48,51-52,54.

Ryder, R.E.J. (1993). "Natural family planning": Effective birth control supported by the Catholic Church. *British Medical Journal,* 307:723-726.

Shivanandan, M. (Ed.) (1986). Breastfeeding and natural family planning: Selected papers from the Fourth National and International Symposium on Natural Family Planning. Bethesda, MD: KM Associates.

Trent, A.J. & Clark, K. (1997). What nurses should know about natural family planning. *J of Obstetric, Gynecologic, and Neonatal Nursing,* 26(6): 643-648.

Wilcox, A.J., Weinberg, C.R. & Baird, D.D. (1995). Timing of sexual intercourse in relation to ovulation. *New England J of Medicine,* 333(23):1517-1521.

11. Implants, Injectables

Counseling can boost Norplant acceptance. (1996). *Contraceptive Technology Update,* 17(6):67-68.

Cullins, V., Blumenthal, P., Remsburg, R. & Huggins, G. (1993). Preliminary experience with Norplant in an inner city population. *Contraception,* 47:193-203.

Darney, P., Atkinson, E., Tanner, S., et al. (May/June 1990). Acceptance and perceptions of Norplant among users in San Francisco, USA. *Studies in Family Planning,* 21(3):152-160.

Davidson, A.R., Kalmuss, D., Cushman, L.F., et al. (1997). Injectable contraceptive discontinuation and subsequent unintended pregnancy among low-income women. *American J of Public Health,* 87(9):1532-1534.

Frank, M.L., Bateman, L., & Poindexter, A.N. (1994). The attitudes of clinic staff as factors in women's selection of Norplant implants for their contraception. *Women & Health,* 21(4):75-88.

Haws, J.M., Butta, P.G. & Girvin, S. (1997). A comprehensive and efficient process for counseling patient desiring sterilization. *Nurse Practitioner,* 22(6):52, 55-56, 59-61, 65-66, 71.

Hinkle, L.T. (1994). Education and counseling for Norplant users. *Journal of Obstetric, Gynecologic, and Neonatal Nursing,* 23(5):387-391.

Kalmuss, D., Davidson, A., et al. (1998). Potential barriers to removal of Norplant among family planning clinic patients. *American J of Public Health,* 88(12):1846-1849.

Kaunitz, A.M. & Jordan, C.W. (1997). Two long-acting hormonal contraceptive options. *Contemporary Ob/Gyn,* (2):27-53.

Kaunitz, A.M. (1993). DMPA: A new contraception option. *Contemporary Ob/Gyn-NP,* 1(1):5-12.

Payan, J.B. (1994). Patient counseling important in Norplant use. *Advance for Nurse Practitioners,* 1(10):15-16.

Tanfer, K. (1994). Knowledge, attitudes and intentions of American women regarding the hormonal implant. *Family Planning Perspectives,* 26(2): 60-65.

Wehrle, K.E. (1994). The Norplant system: Easy to insert, easy to remove. *Nurse Practitioner,* 19(4):47-48,50-54.

Westfall, J.M. & Main, D.S. (1995). The contraceptive implant and the injectable: A comparison of costs. *Family Planning Perspectives,* 27(1):34-36.

12. Sterilization

Bhiwandiwala, P.P., Mumford, S.D., et al. (1983). Menstrual pattern changes following laparoscopic sterilization with different occlusion techniques: A review of 10,004 cases. *American J of Obstetrics and Gynecology,* 145:684.

DeStefano, F., Herzo, C., et al. (1983). Menstrual changes after sterilization. *Obstetrics and Gynecology,* 62(6): 673-681.

DeStefano, F., Perlman, J., et al. (1985). Long-term risk of menstrual disturbances after tubal sterilization. *American J of Obstetrics and Gynecology,* 152(7):835-841.

Fortney, J., Cole, L., & Kennedy, K. (1983). A new approach to measuring menstrual pattern change after sterilization. *American J of Obstetrics and Gynecology,* 147(7):830-836.

Geier, W.S. (1995). An overview of consumer-driven ambulatory surgery: Operative laparoscopy. *Nurse Practitioner,* 20(11):36, 46-51.

Lethbridge, D.J. (1992). Post-tubal sterilization syndrome. *Image,* 24(1):15-18.

Rulin, M., Davidson, A., Philliber, S., et al. (1989). Changes in menstrual symptoms among sterilized and comparison women: A prospective study. *Obstetrics and Gynecology,* 74(2):149-154.

Stergachis, A., Shy, K.K., et al. (1990). Tubal sterilization and the long-term risk of hysterectomy. *J of American Medical Association,* 264:2893-2898.

Strickler, R. (1984). Tubal ligation syndrome: Does it exist? *Postgraduate Medicine,* 75(1):233,237.

13. Infertility

Baird, D.D., Weinberg, C.R., et al. (1996). Vaginal douching and reduced fertility. *American J of Public Health,* 86(6): 844-850.

Blenner, J.L. (1992). Stress and mediators: Patients' perceptions of infertility treatment. *Nursing Research,* 41(2):92-97.

Blenner, J.L. (1991). Clomiphene-induced mood swings. *J of Obstetric, Gynecologic, and Neonatal Nursing,* 20(4):321-327.

Christian, A. (1993). The relationship between women's symptoms of endometriosis and self-esteem. *J of Obstetric, Gynecologic and Neonatal Nursing,* 22(4):370-376.

Davis, D.C. & Dearman, C.N. (1991). Coping strategies of infertile women. *J of Obstetric, Gynecologic, and Neonatal Nursing,* 20(3):221-228.

Fehring, R.J. (1990). Methods used to self-predict ovulation. *J of Obstetric, Gynecologic, and Neonatal Nursing,* 19(3):233-237.

Frank, D.I. (1990). Factors related to decisions about infertility treatment. *J of Obstetric, Gynecologic, and Neonatal Nursing,* 19(2):162-167.

Grodstein, F., Goldman, M.B. & Cramer, D.W. (1994). Infertility in women and moderate alcohol use. *American J of Public Health,* 84(9):1429-1432.

Harris, B.G., Sandelowski, M., & Holditch-Davis, D., (1991). Infertility and new interpretations of pregnancy loss. *The American J of Maternal/Child Nursing,* 16(4):217-220.

Hirsch, A.M. (1995). The long-term psychosocial effects of infertility. *J of Obstetric, Gynecologic, and Neonatal Nursing,* 24(6):517-522.

Holditch-Davis, D., Black, B.P., et al. (1994). Beyond couvade: Pregnancy symptoms in couples with a history of infertility. *Health Care for Women International,* 15(6):537-548.

Johnson, C.L. (1996). Regaining self-esteem: Strategies and interventions for the infertile woman. *J of Obstetric, Gynecologic, and Neonatal Nursing,* 25(4):291-295.

Jones, S.L. (1994). Assisted reproductive technologies: Genetic and nursing implications. *J of Obstetric, Gynecologic and Neonatal Nursing,* 23(6):492-497.

Samuels, J.I. (1995). Facing infertility. *Advance for Nurse Practitioners,* 3(5): 12-14, 16.

Sandelowski, M. (1994). On infertility. *J of Obstetric, Gynecologic, and Neonatal Nursing,* 23(9):749-752.

Sandelowski, M., Harris, B.G. & Holditch-Davis, D. (1989). Mazing: Infertile couples and the quest for a child. *Image,* 21(4):220-226.

Sandelowski, M. & Pollock, C. (1986). Women's experiences of infertility. *Image,* 18(4):140-147.

Shattuck, J.C. & Schwarz, K.K. (1991). Walking the line between feminism and infertility: Implications for nursing, medicine, and patient care. *Health Care for Women International,* 12(3):331-339.

Stanton, A.L., Tenner, H., Affleck, G., & Mendola, R. (1991). Cognitive appraisal and adjustment to infertility. *Women & Health,* 17(3):1-15.

Woods, N.F., Olshansky, E., & Drayer, M.A. (1991). Infertility: Women's experiences. *Health Care for Women International,* 12(2):179-190.

14. Vaginal Discharge, Vaginitis, Vaginosis, Herpes, Cervicitis, Hepatitis, Bartholin's Cyst, Sexually Transmitted Diseases, Lice

Allen, T. (1994). Viral hepatitis: An overview. *Advance for Nurse Practitioners,* 2(2):12-16.

Alexander, I.M. (1998). Viral hepatitis: Primary care diagnosis and management. *Nurse Practitioner,* 23(10):13-14, 17-18, 20, 25-26, 28, 31-32, 37-38, 40, 43.

American Academy of Pediatric. (1994). 1994 report of the committee on infectious disease. American Academy of Pediatrics.

Andrist, L.C. (1997). Genital herpes: Overcoming barriers to diagnosis and treatment, *American Journal of Nursing,* 97(10):16AA-16DD.

Association of Women's Health, Obstetric, and Neonatal Nurses. (1993, October). Vulvovaginitis, *Practice Resource.*

Bassa, A.G.H., Hoosen, A.A., Moodley, J. & Bramdev, A. (1993). Granuloma Inguinale (donovanosis) in women. *Sexually Transmitted Diseases,* 20(3):164-167.

Benson, L.M. (1998). Viral hepatitis. *Advance for Nurse Practitioners,* 6(6):45-47.

Bisceglie, A., et al. (1998). Hepatitis C: Uncovering an invisible epidemic. *Patient Care Nurse Practitioner,* 18-27.

Blanchard, J.F., Moses, S., Greenaway, C., Orr, P., Hammond, G.W. & Brunham, R.C. (1998). The evolving epidemiology of Chlamydial and gonococcal infections in response to control programs in Winnipeg, Canada. *American Journal of Public Health,* 88(10):1496-1502.

Bonny, A.E. & Biro, F.M. (1998). Recognizing and treating STDs in the adolescent. *Contemporary Nurse Practitioner, (Spring),* 15-24.

Burtin, P., Tzddio, A., Aribumu, O., Einarson, T.R., & Koren, G. (1995). Safety of metronidazole in pregnancy: A meta-analysis. *Obstetrics and Gynecology,* 172:525-529.

Cates, W. & Wasserheit, J. (1990). Gonorrhea, chlamydia and pelvic inflammatory disease. *Current Opinion in Infection,* 3:10-19.

Centers for Disease Control and Prevention. (1998). 1998 sexually transmitted diseases treatment guidelines. *Morbidity and Mortality Weekly Report,* 47: 1-115.

Contraception, STDs, and risk-taking behavior: Highlights from a recent ARHP conference. (1994). *The Contraception Report,* 5(3):4-7.

Davies, J.E. (1998). Close-up on the common vaginal conditions. *Advance for Nurse Practitioners,* 6(11):35-93.

Devine, P. (1998). Extrapelvic manifestations of gonorrhea. *Primary Care Update for Ob/Gyn,* 233-237.

Ebrahim, S.H., Peterman, R.A., et al. (1997). Mortality related to sexually transmitted diseases in US women, 1973-1992. *American J of Public Health,* 87(6):938-944.

Eckert, L.O. (1998). Vulvovaginal Candidiasis the manifestations, risk factors, management. An algorithm. *Obstetrics & Gynecology,* 175:757-765.

Elliott, K.A. (1998). Managing patients with vulvovaginal candidiasis. *The Nurse Practitioner,* 23(3):44-45.

Erick, L.M. (1996). Diabetes and vaginal yeast infections. *Advance for Nurse Practitioners,* 4:13.

Geiger, A.M., Foxman, B. & Gillespie, B.W. (1995). The epidemiology of vulvovaginal Candidiasis among university students. *American J of Public Health,* 85(8):1146-1148.

Holdcroft, C. (1995). New indication for oral fluconazole. *Nurse Practitioner,* 20(1):79.

King, R.R. (1997). Hepatitis C. *Advance for Nurse Practitioners,* 5(3):51-56.

King, R.R. (1999). Hepatitis C: Past, present and future issues. *Advance for Nurse Practitioners,* 5:1-52, 55-56.

Lash, D. & Garcia, T.A. (1998). Diagnosis and treatment of vaginitis: A case report. *The Famale Patient* 23:73-76, 79, 85-86, 88-89.

Lawhead, R.A. & Majmudar, B. (1990). Early diagnosis of vulvar neoplasia as a result of vulvar self-examination. *J of Reproductive Medicine,* 35(12):134-137.

Leonardo, C. & Chrisler, J.C. (1992). Women and sexually transmitted diseases. *Women & Health,* 18(4):1-15.

McGourty, M.K. (1995). Vaginal infections: Keys to treatment. *Contemporary Nurse Practitioner,* 1(3):18-23.

McQuillan, G.M., Coleman, P.J., et al., (1998). Prevalence of hepatitis B virus infection in the United States: The National Health and Nutrition Examination Survey, 1976-1994. *American J of Public Health,* 89(1):14-18.

Mertz, K.J., Levine, W.C., et al. (1997). Screening women for gonorrhea: Demographic screening criteria for general clinical use. *American J of Public Health,* 87(9):1535-1538.

Michlewitz, H., Kennison, R.D., et al. (1989). Vulvar vestibulitis - subgroup with bartholin gland duct inflammation. *Obstetrics and Gynecology,* 73(3):410.

Moraes, P.S.A. (1998). Recurrent vaginal candidiasis and allergic rhinitis: A common association. *Annals of Allergy, Asthma, and Immunology,* 81(2):165-169.

Munro, C.L. (1995). The impact of recent advances in microbiology and immunology on perinatal and women's health care. *J of Obstetric, Gynecologic, and Neonatal Nursing,* 24(6):525-531.

Murphy, P.A. & Jones, E. (1994). Use of oral metronidazole in pregnancy: Risks, benefits, and practice guidelines. *J of Nurse-Midwifery,* 39(4):214-220.

O'Connell, M.L. (1996). The effect of birth control methods on sexually transmitted disease/HIV risk. *J of Obstetric, Gynecologic, and Neonatal Nursing,* 25:476-480.

Recommendations for prevention and control of hepatitis C (HCV) infection and HCV related chronic disease. (1998). *Morbidity and Mortality Weekly Report,* 47(RR-19):1-39.

Redfern, N. & Hutchinson, S. (1994). Women's experiences of repetitively contracting sexually transmitted diseases. *Health Care for Women International,* 15(5):423-433.

Ricchini, W. (1997). Break the silence. *Advance for Nurse Practitioners,* 5(6): 55-56, 83.

Richman, S. (1998). Genital herpes presenting with leuhorrkea. *The Female Patient,* 23:63-68.

Roe, V.A. & Gudi, A. (1997). Pharmacologic management of sexually transmitted diseases. *J of Nurse-Midwifery,* 43:275-289.

Rome, E. (1998). Sexually transmitted diseases in the adolescent. *The Nurse Practitioner,* 23:15-16, 19-20, 23-24.

Rosenberg, M.J., Davidson, A.J., Chen, J., Hudson, F.N., & Douglas, J.M. (1992). Barrier contraceptives and sexually transmitted diseases in women: A comparison of female-dependent methods and condoms. *American J of Public Health,* 82(5):669-674.

Rule, C. (1994). Exposure control. *Advance for Nurse Practitioners,* 2(8):15-6, 30.

Sacks, S.L., Aoki, F.Y., et al. (1996).Patient-initiated,twice-daily oral Famciclovir for early recurrent genital herpes: A randomized, double-blind multicenter trial. *J of American Medical Association,* 276(1):44-49.

Scott, R.L. (1993). Hepatitis B. *Clinical Reviews,* 3(9):41-42, 47-50, 53-54, 57-60.

Secor, R.M. (1994). Bacterial vaginosis. *Advance for Nurse Practitioners,* 2(4):11-12, 15-16.

Selleck, C.S. (1997). Identifying and treating bacterial vaginosis. *American J of Nursing*, 97(9):16AAA-16DDD.

Semaan, S., Lauby, J. & Walls, C. (1997). Condom use with main partners by sterilized and non-sterilized women. *Women & Health*, 25(2):65-85.

Sokoloff, F. (1994). Identification and management of pediculosis. *Nurse Practitioner*, 19(8):62-64.

Soloman, A. & Smith, S. (1997). Understanding herpes simplex virus. *The Female Patient*, 23:53-56, 59-61.

Spear, P. (1994). Vaginal yeast infections. *Advance for Nurse Practitioners*, 2(7):28-29.

Spiegel, C.A. (1990). Bacterial vaginosis. *Clinical Microbiology Reviews*, 4(4):485-502.

Stover, L.C. (1997). Recurring vaginal symptoms in a 35 year-old woman: A case report. *Advance for Nurse Practitioners*, 5.

Swanson, J.M., Dibble, S.L. & Chenitz, W.C. (1995). Clinical features and psychosocial factors in young adults with genital herpes. *Image*, 27(1):16-22.

Tobin, M.J. (1995). Vulvovaginal candidiasis: Topical vs. oral therapy. *American Family Physician*, 51(7), 1715-1720.

Vander Stichele, R.H., Deqeure, E.M. & Bogaert, M. (1995). Systemic review of clinical efficacy of topical treatments for head lice. *British Medical J*, 311:604-608.

Weisman, C.S., Plichta, S., Nathanson, C.A., Ensminger, M. & Robinson, J.C. (1991). Consistency of condom use for disease prevention among adolescent users of oral contraceptives. *Family Planning Perspectives*, 23(2):71-74.

Winefield, A.D. & Murphy, S.A. (1998). Bacterial vaginosis: A review. *Clinical Excellence for Nurse Practitioners: The International J of NPACE*, 2(4):212-217.

Zhang, J., Thomas, G., et al. (1997). Vaginal douching and adverse health effects: A meta-analysis. *American J of Public Health*, 87(7): 1207-1211.

Zimmerman, H.L., Potterat, J.J., et al. (1990). Epidemiologic differences between chlamydia and gonorrhea. *American J of Public Health*, 80(11): 338-342.

15. HIV/AIDS

Binson, D., Pollack, L. & Catania, J.A. (1997). AIDS-relateld risk behaviors and safer sex practices of women in midlife and older in the U.S.: 1990-1992. *Health Care for Women International*, 18(4):343-354.

Centers for Disease Control and Prevention. (1990). Risk for cervical disease in HIV-infected women: New York City. *Morbidity and Mortality Weekly Report*, 39:846-849.

Choi, K. & Catania, J.A. (1996). Changes in multiple sexual partnerships, HIV testing, and condom use among US heterosexuals 18 to 49 years of age, 1990 and 1992. *American Journal of Public Health*, 86(4):554-560.

Colletta, L. (1997). Human papillomavirus in the woman with HIV. *Advance for Nurse Practitioners*, 5(10):16-21.

DeMarco, R.F., Miller, K.H., et al. (1998). From silencing the self to action:

Experiences of women living with HIV/AIDS. *Health Care for Women International,* 19(5):539-552.

Dykeman, M., et al. (1997). Human immunodeficiency virus. Early steps in management: Case report. *The Nurse Practitioner,* 22(3):94-96, 99-100.

Ebomoyi, E.W., Bisonette, B.S. & Ukaga, O.M. (1998). Campus courtship behavior and fear of human immunodeficiency virus infection by university students. *J of the National Medical Association,* 90(7):395-400.

Eyler, A.E. (1996). Current issues in the primary care of women with HIV. *The Female Patient,* 21:14, 16, 21, 25, 28.

Ferri, R. (1995). HIV and adolescents: A primary care perspective. *Advance for Nurse Practitioners,* 3(7):36-52.

Ferri, R., et al. (1997). Drug cocktail may restore partial immune function. *Clinician Reviews,* 7(3):189, 190, 195-196

Ferri, R., et al. (1998). HPV/HIV infections are strongly linked. *Clinician Reviews,* 8(2):111-112, 114-115.

Gavey, N. & McPhillips, K. (1997). Women and the heterosexual transmission of HIV: Risks and prevention strategies. *Women & Health,* 25(1):41-64.

Gielen, A.C., O'Campo, P., Faden, R.R. & Eke, A. (1997). Women's disclosure of HIV status: Experiences of mistreatment and violence in an urban setting. Women & Health, 25(3):19-21.

Gerchufsky, M. (1996). Issues and answers in latex sensitivity. *Advance for Nurse Practitioners,* 4(6):15-19.

Gritter, M. (1998). The latex threat. *American J of Nursing,* 98(9):26-32.

Harris, R.M. (1997). To be or not to be treated for the AIDS virus. *Nursing Research,* 46(5):293-294.

HIV/AIDS in women. (1998). *Women & Health,* 27(1/2): entire issue.

Ickovics, J.R., Morrill, A.C., et al. (1994). Limited effects of HIV counseling and testing for women: A prospective study of behavioral and psychological consequences. *J of the American Medical Association,* 272(6):413-494.

Kelly, J.A., Murphy, D.A., Washington, C.D., Wilson, T.S., Koob, J.J., Davis, D.R., Ledezema, G. & Davantes, B. (1994). The effects of HIV/AIDS intervention groups for high-risk women in urban clinics. *American J of Public Health,* 84(12):1918-1922.

Kelly, P., Holman, S., et al. (1995). Primary Care of Women and Children with HIV Infection. Boston: Jones & Bartlett.

Kitten, J.H. (1997). Health promotion in HIV: Perspectives for practitioners. *Nurse Practitioner,* 22(2):114, 116, 125.

Koniak-Griffin, D. & Brecht, M-L. (1995). Linkages between sexual risk taking, substance use, and AIDS knowledge among pregnant adolescents and young mothers. *Nursing Research,* 44(6):340-346.

Lea, A. (1994). Women with HIV and their burden of caring. *Health Care for Women International,* 15(6):489-501.

Lee, K.A., Portillo, C.J. & Miramontes, H. (1999). The fatigue experience for women with human immunodeficiency virus. *J of Obstetric, Gynecologic, and Neonatal Nursing,* 28(2):193-200.

Locher, A.W. (1996). Ethics, women with HIV, and procreation: Implications for nursing practice. *J of Obstetric, Gynecologic, and Neonatal Nursing,* 25(6):465-469.

Melroe, N.H. (1990). "Duty to Warn" vs. "Patient Confidentiality": The ethical dilemmas in caring for HIV-infected clients. *The Nurse Practitioner,* 15(2):58, 60, 65, 69.

Moneyham, L., Seals, B., Demi, A., Sowell, R., Cohen, L. & Guillory, J. (1996). Experiences of disclosure in women infected with HIV. *Health Care for Women International,* 17(3):209-221.

Nannis, E.D., Patterson, T.L. & Semple, S.J. (1997). Coping with HIV disease among seropositive women: Psychosocial correlates. *Women & Health,* 25(1):1-22.

O'Connell, M.L. (1996). The effect of birth control methods on sexually transmitted disease/HIV risk. *J of Obstetric, Gynecologic, and Neonatal Nursing,* 25(6):476-480.

Rothenberg, K.H. & Paskey, S.J. (1995). The risk of domestic violence and women with HIV infection: Implications for partner notification, public policy, and the law. *American Journal of Public Health,* 85(11):1569-1576.

Schable, B., Chu, S.Y. & Diaz, T. (1996). Characteristics of women 50 years of age or older with heterosexually acquired AIDS. *American Journal of Public Health,* 86(11):1616-1618.

Semple, S.J., Patterson, T.L., et al. & HIV Neurobehavioral Research Center Group. (1996). Social and psychological characteristics of HIV-infected women and gay men. *Women & Health,* 24(2):17-41.

Shotsky, W.J. (1996). Women who have sex with other women: HIV seroprevalence in New York State counseling and testing programs. *Women & Health,* 24(2):1-15.

Simoni, J.M., Mason, H.R.C., et al. (1996). Women living with HIV: Sexual behaviors and counseling experiences. *Women & Health,* 23(4):17-26.

Stevens, P.E. (1995). Impact of HIV/AIDS on women in the United States: Challenges of primary and secondary prevention. *Health Care for Women International,* 16(6):577-595.

Unguarski, P.J. (1997). Update on HIV infection. *American J of Nursing,* 97(1):44-52.

Warszawski, J., Meye, L. & Bajos, N. (1996). Is genital mycosis associated with HIV risk behaviors among heterosexuals? *American J of Public Health,* 86(8):1108-1111.

Wittkowski, K.M., Susser, E. & Dietz, K. (1998). The protective effect of condoms and nonoxynol-9 against HIV infection. *American J of Public Health,* 88:590-596.

Zelewsky, M.G. & Birchfield, M. (1995). Women living with the human immunodeficiency virus: Home-care needs. *J of Obstetric, Gynecologic, and Neonatal Nursing,* 24(2):257-263.

Zimmer, J.C. & Thurston, W.E. (1998). Attitudes, beliefs, and practices of nursing students concerning HIV/AIDS: Implications for prevention in women. *Health Care for Women International,* 19(4):327-342.

16. HPV, Chlamydia, Syphilis

Beutner, K.R. & Tyring, S. (1997). Human papillomavirus and human disease. *The American J of Medicine,* 102(5A):9-15.

Beutner, K.R. & Ferenczy, a. (1997). Therapeutic approaches to genital warts. *The American J of Medicine,* 102(5A):28-37.

Bosch, F.X., Munoz, N. & de Sanjose, S. (1997). Human papillomavirus and other risk factors for cervical cancer. *Biomedicine and Pharmacotherapy,* 51:268-275.

Briston, R. & Monty, F.J. (1998). Human papillomavirus molecular biology and screening applications in cervical neoplasia. *A Primer for Primary Care Physicians,* 238-246.

Carson, S. (1997). Human papillomatous virus infection update: Impact on women's health. *The Nurse Practitioner,* 22(4):24-37.

(1994). Chlamydial infection. *Clinical Reviews,* 4(7):94-96,98,101.

Downey, G.P., Bavin, P.J., et al. (1994). Relation between human papillomavirus type 16 and potential for progression of minor-grade cervical disease. *Lancet,* 344:432-435.

Ferris, D. (1998). Diagnosis and management of genital warts. *The Female Patient,* 23:68, 70, 73, 76.

Gerchufsky, M.(1996). The sexual risk more patients should know about— human papilloma virus. *Advance for Nurse Practitioners,* 4(5):20-25.

Handfield, H.H. (1997). Clinical presentation and natural course of anogenital warts. *The American J of Medicine,* 102(5A):16-20.

Hillis, S., Black, C., Newhall, J., Walsh, C. & Groseclose, S.L. (1995). New opportunities for Chlamydia prevention: Applications of science to public health practice. *Sexually Transmitted Diseases,* 22(3):197-202.

Ho, G.Y.F., Bierman, R., et al. (1998). Natural history of cervicovaginal papillomavirus infection in young women. *The New England J of Medicine,* 338(7):423-428.

Keller, M.L., Egan, J.J. & Mims, L.F. (1995). Genital human papillomavirus infection: Common but not trivial. *Health Care for Women International,* 16(4):351-364.

Koutsky, L. (1997). Epidemiology of genital human papillomavirus infection. *The American J of Medicine,* 102(5A):3-8.

Kenney, J.W. & Reuss, H. (1994). Human papillomavirus as expressed in cervical neoplasia: Evolving diagnostic and treatment modalities. *Health Care for Women International,* 15(4):287-296.

Niruthisard, S., Roddy, R.E. & Chutivongse, S. (1992). Use of nonoxynol-9 and reduction in rate of gonococcal and chlamydial cervical infections. *Lancet,* 339:1371-1374.

Oh, M.K., Smith, K.R., et al. (1998). Urine-based screening of adolescents in detention to guide treatment for gonococcal and Chlamydial infections: Translating research into intervention. *Archives of Pediatrics and Adolescent Medicine,* 152:52-56.

Palmer, J.B. & Basilere, E.J. et al. (1997). Genital wart management. *The Nurse Practitioner,* 22:52, 54, 62-63.

Reitano, M. (1997). Counseling patients with genital warts. *The American J of Medicine,* 102(5A):38-43.

Rodriquez, A.C., Meyer, W.J. & Watrobka, T. (1996). The Jarisch-Herxheimer reaction in pregnancy: A nursing perspective. *J of Obstetric, Gynecologic, and Neonatal Nursing,* 25.

Rosenberg, M.J., Long, S.O., et a. (1995). Patient-applied treatment for genital warts: Experience from a large post-marketing study. *J of Dematological Treatment,* 222-226.

Trofatter, K.F. (1997). Diagnosis of human papillomavirus genital tract infection. *The American J of Medicine,* 102(5A):21-27.

Sheahan, S.L., Coons, S.J., et al. (1994). Sexual behavior, communications, and chlamydial infections among college women. *Health Care for Women International,* 15(4):275-286.

Youngkin, E.Q. (1995). Sexually transmitted diseases: Current and emerging concerns. *J of Obstetric, Gynecologic, and Neonatal Nurses,* 24(8): 743-758.

Youngkin, E.Q., Henry, J.K. & Gracely-Kilgore, K. (1998). Women with HSV and HPV: A strategy to increase self-esteem. *Clinical Excellence for Nurse Practitioners,* 2(6):370-375.

17. Abdominal Pain and Pelvic Pain

Bernstein, J. (1995). Ectopic pregnancy: A nursing approach to excess risk among minority women. *J of Obstetric, Gynecologic, and Neonatal Nursing,* 24(9):803, 810.

Corwin, E.J. (1997). Endometriosis: Pathophysiology, diagnosis, and treatment. *The Nurse Practitioner,* 22(10):35-36, 38, 40-42, 45-46, 48-51, 55.

Dick, M.J. (1995). Assessment and measurement of acute pain. *J of Obstetric, Gynecologic, and Neonatal Nursing,* 24(9):843-848.

Grabo, T.N. & Nataupsky, L.G. (1999). Uterine myomas: Treatment options. *J of Obstetric, Gynecologic, and Neonatal Nursing,* 28(1):23-31.

Grace, V.M. (1995). Problems of communication, diagnosis, and treatment experienced by women using the New Zealand health services for chronic pelvic pain: A quantitative analysis. *Health Care for Women International,* 16(6):521-535.

Grace. V.M. (1995). Problems women patients experience in the medical encounter for chronic pelvic pain. A New Zealand study. *Health Care for Women International,* 16(6):509-519.

Igoe, B.A. (1997). Symptoms attributed to ovarian cancer by women with the disease. *The Nurse Practitioner,* 22(7):122, 127-128, 130, 133-134, 141-143.

King, M.M., Myers, C., Ling, F.W. & Rosenthal, R.H. (1991). Sociocultural and musculoskeletal factors in chronic pelvic pain. *J of Psychosomatic Obstetrics and Gynecology,* 12:87-98.

Maaiolatesi, C.R. & Peddicord, K. (1996). Methotrexate for nonsurgical treatment of ectopic pregnancy: Nursing implications. *J of Obstetric, Gynecologic, and Neonatal Nursing,* 25(3):205-208.

Marantides, D. (1997). Management of polycystic ovary syndrome. *The Nurse Practitioner,* 22(12):34, 36-38, 40-41.

Peters, A.A.W. et al. (1991). A randomized clinical trial to compare two different approaches in women with chronic pelvic pain. *Obstetrics and Gynecology,* 77:740.

Norbryhn, G.A. (1995). Treating chronic pelvic pain nonsurgically. *Contemtemporary Nurse Practitioner,* 1(3):38-40, 43-47.

Stabile, I. & Grudzinskas, J.G. (1990). Ectopic pregnancy: A review of incidence, etiology, and diagnostic aspects. *Obstetrics and Gynecological Survey,* 5(6):335-347.

Star, W.L. & Stiles-Donnelly, R. (1993). Managing chronic pelvic pain. *Contemporary Ob/Gyn-NP,* 2(2):10-13, 17.

Stone, R. (1996). Primary care diagnosis of acute abdominal pain. *Nurse Practitioner,* 21(12):19-20, 23-26, 28-30, 35-39.

Summitt R.L. & Ling, F.W. (1991). Urethral syndrome presenting as chronic pelvic pain. *J of Psychosomatic Obstetrics and Gynecology,* 12 (supplement):77-86.

Zadinsky, J.K. & Boyle, J.S. (1996). Experiences of women with chronic pelvic pain. *Health Care for Women International,* 17(3):223-232.

18. Pelvic Inflammatory Disease (PID)

Griffith, C.J. (1995). Pelvic inflammatory disease. *Advance for Nurse Practitioners,* 3(8):33-36.

Hillis, S.D., Joesoef, R., et al. (1993). Delayed care of pelvic inflammatory disease as a risk factor for impaired fertility. *American J of Obstetrics and Gynecology,* 168(5):1503-1509.

Ivey, J.B. (1997). The adolescent with pelvic inflammatory disease: Assessment and management. *The Nurse Practitioner,* 22(2):78, 81-82, 84, 87-88, 90-91.

Kottmann, L.M. (1995). Pelvic inflammatory disease: Clinical overview. *J of Obstetric, Gynecologic, and Neonatal Nursing,* 24(8):759-767.

19. Breast Conditions, Mammography

Andersen, M.R. & Urban, N. (1998). The use of mammography by survivors of breast cancer. *American J of Public Health,* 88(11):1713-1715.

Arnold, G. & Neiheisel, M.B. (1997). A comprehensive approach to evaluating nipple discharge. *The Nurse Practitioner,* 22(7):96, 98-102, 105-111.

Baron, R.H. & Walsh, A. (1995). 9 facts everyone should know about breast cancer. *American J of Nursing,* 95(7):29-33.

Brown, L.W. & Williams, R.D. (1994). Culturally sensitive breast cancer screening programs for older Black women. *Nurse Practitioner,* 19(3):21, 25-26,31,35.

Bullough, B., et al., (1990). Methylxanthines and fibrocystic breast disease: A study of correlations. *The Nurse Practitioner,* 15(3):36, 38, 43-44.

Cady, B., Steele, G., et al., (1994). Evaluation of Common Breast Problems: A Primer for Primary Care Providers. The Society of Surgical Oncology and the Commission on Cancer of the American College of Surgeons for the Centers for Disease Control and Prevention. 3:125-139.

Chaliki, H., Loader, S., et al. (1995). Women's receptivity to testing for a genetic susceptibility to breast cancer. *American J of Public Health,* 85(8):1133-1135.

Champion, V. & Miller, A.M. (1996). Recent mammography in women aged 35 and older: Predisposing variables. Health Care for Women International,

17(3):233-245.

Champion, V.L. & Scott, C.R. (1997). Reliability and validity of breast cancer screening belief scales in African-American women. *Nursing Research*, 1(7): 331-337.

Cockey, C.D. (1997). News from the front: This nurse soldier is waging war on breast cancer. *Lifelines*, 1(5):39-45.

Crane, L.A., Kaplan, C.P., et al. (1996). Determinants of adherence among health department patients referred for a mammogram. *Women & Health*, 24(2):43-64.

Dumble, L.J. (1996). Dismissing the evidence: The medical response to women with silicone implant-related disorders. *Health Care for Women International*, 17(6):515-525.

Ernster, V.L. (1997). Mammography screening for women aged 40 through 49—A guidelines saga and a clarion call for informed decision making. *American J of Public Health*, 87(7):1103-1106.

Goldman, S. (1994). Evaluating breast masses. *Contemporary Ob/Gyn-NP*, 2(1):8-13,17.

Haas, B.K. (1997). The effect of managed care on breast cancer detection, treatment, and research. *Nursing Outlook*, 45(4):167-172.

Houn, F., Bober, M.A., et al. (1995). The association between alcohol and breast cancer: Popular press coverage of research. *American J of Public Health*, 85(8):1082-1086.

Jacobson, J.A., Danforth, D.N., et al. (1995). Ten-year results of a comparison of conservation with mastectomy in the treatment of stage I and II breast cancer. *New England J of Medicine*, 332(14):907-911.

Jacobson, N. (1998). The socially constructed breast: Breast implants and the medical construction of need. *American J of Public Health*, 88(8):1254-1261.

Janz, N.K., Schottenfeld, D., et al. (1997). A two-step intervention to increase mammography among women aged 65 and older. *American J of Public Health*, 87(10):1683-1686.

King, E.S., Rimer, B.K., et al. (1994). Promoting mammography use through progressive interventions: Is it effective? *American J of Public Health*, 84(1):104-106.

Kuhrik, N.S., Bohner, D.G., et al. (1994). Evaluating women with fibrocystic breast condition. *American J of Nursing*, 94(7):16A-16D.

Lauver, D. (1994). Care-seeking behavior with breast cancer symptoms in Caucasian and African-American women. *Research in Nursing and Health*, 17:421-431.

Lauver, D. & Angerame, M. (1990). Overadherence with breast-examination recommendations, *Image*, 22(3):148-152.

Lauver, D. & Keena, C. (1991). Identifying women's descriptions of breast tissue for the promotion of breast self-examination. *Health Care for Women International*, 12(1):73-83.

Lauver, D. & Tak, Y. (1995). Optimism and coping with a breast cancer symptom. *Nursing Research*, 44(4):202-207.

Lierman, L.M., Young, H.M., et al. (1994). Effects of education and support on breast self-examination in older women. *Nursing Research*, 43(3):158-163.

Logothetis, M.L. (1995). Women's reports of breast implant problems and silicone-related illness. *J of Obstetric, Gynecologic, and Neonatal Nursing,* 24(7):609-616.

MacFarlane, M.E. & Sony, S.D. (1992). Women, breast lump discovery and associated stress. *Health Care for Women International,* 13(1): 23-32.

McCance, K.L. & Jorde, L.B. (1998). Evaluating the genetic risk of breast cancer. *The Nurse Practitioner,* 23(8):14, 16, 19-20, 23-27.

McCool, W.F. (1995). Barriers to breast cancer screening in older women. *J of Nurse-Midwifery,* 39(5):283-299.

McKeon, V.A. (1998). The breast cancer prevention trial. *AWHONN Lifelines,* 2(5):20-25.

Mast, M.E. (1998). Survivors of breast cancer: Illness uncertainty, positive reappraisal, and emotional distress. *Oncology Nursing Forum,* 25(3):555-562.

Maxwell, A.E., Bastani, R., et al. (1998). Mammography utilization and related attitudes among Korean-American women. *Women & Health,* 27(1):89-107.

Miller, A.M. & Champion, V.L. (1996). Mammography in older women: One-time and three-year adherence to guidelines. *Nursing Research,* 45(4):239-245.

Nicholson, A. (1996). Diet and the prevention and treatment of breast cancer. *Alternative Therapies,* 2(6):32-38.

Northouse, L.L., Jeffs, M., et al. (1995). Emotional distress reported by women and husbands prior to a breast biopsy. *Nursing Research,* 44(4):196-201.

Olson, K.L. & Morse, J.M. (1996). Explaining breast self-examination practice. *Health Care for Women International,* 17(6):575-591.

Partin, M.R., Korn, J.E. & Slater, J.S. (1997). Questionable data and preconceptions: Reconsidering the value of mammography for American Indian women. *American J of Public Health,* 87(7):1100-1102.

Pasacreta, J.V. (1997). Depressive phenomena, physical symptom distress, and functional status among women with breast cancer. *Nursing Research,* 46(4): 214-221.

The perils of breast examination. (1995). *Insurance Quarterly,* 2(1):3-7.

Planned Parenthood Women's Health Letter: Making Decisions about Mammography: March, 1995.

Price, J. & Purtell, J.R. (1997). Prevention and treatment of lymphedema after breast cancer. *American J of Nursing,* 97(9):34-37.

Schumann, D. (1994). Health risks for women with breast implants. *Nurse Practitioner,* 19(7):19-20,23-25,29-30.

Seckel, M.M. & Birney, M.H. (1996). Social support, stress, and age in women undergoing breast biopsies, CNS: *The J for Advanced Nursing Practice,* 10(3):137-143.

Shapiro, T.J. & Clark, P.M. (1995). Breast cancer: What the primary care provider needs to know. *Nurse Practitioner,* 20(3):36, 39-40, 42, 45-46, 48-50, 52-53

Skaer, T., Robison L.M., Sclar, D.A. & Harding, G.H. (1996). Financial incentive and the use of mammography among Hispanic migrants to the United States.(1994). *Health Care for Women International,* 17(4):281-291.

Skinner, C.S., et al. (1994). Physicians' recommendations for mammography:

Do tailored messages make a difference? *American J of Public Health,* 84(1):43-49.

Speigel, K.K. (1997). On your markers: Research advances in breast cancer in women. *Lifetines,* 1(5):33-38.

Taplin, S.H., Anderman, C., et al. (1994).Using physician correspondence and postcard reminders to promote mammography use. *American J of Public Health,* 84(4):571-574.

Thomas, L.R., Fox, S.A., et al. (1996). The effects of health beliefs on screening mammography utilization among a diverse sample of older women. *Women & Health,* 24(3):77-94.

Thune, L., Brenn, T., et al. (1997). Physical activity and the risk of breast cancer. *The New England J of Medicine,* 336(18):1269-1274.

Tulman, L. & Fawcett, J. (1996). Lessons learned from a pilot study of biobehavioral correlates of functional status in women with breast cancer, *Nursing Research,* 45(6):356-358.

Urban, N. et al. (1994). Mammography screening: How important is cost as a barrier to use? *American J of Public Health,* 84(1):50-55.

Weber, E.S. (1997). Questions & answers about breast cancer diagnosis. *American J of Nursing,* 97(10):34-38.

Zapka, J.G., Bigelow, C., Hurley, T., Ford, et al., (1996). Mammography use among sociodemographically diverse women: The accuracy of self-report. *American J of Public Health,* 86(7):1016-1021.

20. DES Exposure

Bekker, M.H.J., Van Heck, G.L. & Vingerhoets, A.J.M. (1996). Gender-identity, body experience, sexuality, and the wish for having children in DES-daughters. *Women's Health,* 24(2):65-82.

Kaufman, R.H., Adam, E., et al. (1981). Upper genital tract changes and pregnancy outcome in offspring exposed in utero to diethylstilbestrol. *Obstetrical and Gynecological Survey,* 36(3):137-140.

Havens, C.S., Sullivan, N.D. & Titton, P. (Eds.) (1991). Manual of Outpatient Gynecology. 2nd ed. Boston: Little Brown.

Niculescu, A.M. (1985). Effects of in utero exposure to DES on male progeny. *J of Obstetric, Gynecologic, and Neonatal Nursing,* 14(6): 468-470.

Reagan, J.W. & Olaizola, M.Y. (1980). Using cytology to study DES daughters. *Contemporary Ob/Gyn,* 15:95-110.

Rivlin, M.E., Morrison, J.C. & Bales, G.W. (1990). Manual of Clinical Problems in Obstetrics and Gynecology. 3rd ed. Boston: Little Brown.

Wetherill, P.S. (1980). DES exposure: A continuing disaster. *Women & Health,* 5(2):91-93.

Vieriralves-Wiltgen, C. & Engle, W.F. (1988). Identification/management of DES-exposed women. *The Nurse Practitioner,* 13(11):15-16,19-20,22,27.

21. Cervical and Vulvar Aberrations, Papanicolaou Smears, and Colposcopy

Agency for Health Care Policy and Research. (1999). Evaluation of Cervical Pathology. Bethesda, MD: US Department of Health and Human Services.

American Society for Colposcopy and Cervical Pathology. (1996). Management guidelines for follow-up of atypical squamous cells of undetermined significance (ASCUS). *The Colposcopist,* 27(1):1-9).

(1993). The Bethesda system for reporting cervical/vaginal cytologic diagnoses. *ACTA Cytologica,* 37(2):115-124.

Beach, R.K. (1996). Why teenage girls need yearly Pap smears. *Contemporary Adolescent Gynecology,* 2(1):4-21.

Becker, T.M., et al. (1994). Sexually transmitted diseases and other risk factors for cervical dysplasia among southwestern Hispanic and non-Hispanic white women. *J of the American Medical Association,* 271:1181-1188.

Burnhill, M. & Beardsley, L. (1996). Pap laboratory update. *Insurance Quarterly,* 12(3).

Byrnes, E.C. (1998). A new age in Pap testing. *Advance for Nurse Practitioners,* 6(11):65-66, 92.

Crowther, M.E. (1995). Is the nature of cervical carcinoma changing in young women? *Obstetric and Gynecologic Survey,* 50:71-82.

de Sanjose, S., Bosch,.X., Munoz, N., et al. (1996). Socioeconomic differences in cervical cancer: Two case-controlled studies in Colombia and Spain. *American J of Public Health,* 86(11):1532-1538.

Epperson, W.J. & Pfenninger, J. (1998). Electrosurgery for cervical intraepithelial neoplasia. *The Female Patient,* 23:28, 30, 35-36, 38, 41-44, 46.

Ferreira, S.E. (1998). Cervical intrepithelial neoplasia diagnosis: Emotional impact and nursing implications. *Clinical Excellence for Nurse Practitioners: The International J of NPACE,* 2(4):218-224.

Foulks, M.J. (1998). The Papanicolaou smear: Its impact on the promotion of women's health. *J of Obstetric, Gynecologic, and Neonatal Nursing,* 27(4):367-373.

Frye, C.A. & Weisberg, R.B. (1994). Increasing the incidence of routine pelvic examinations: Behavioral medicine's contribution. *Women & Health,* (1):33-55.

Gitsch, G., Kainz, C., et al. (1992). Oral contraceptives and human papilloma virus infection in cervical intraepithelial neoplasia. *Archives of Gynecology and Obstetrics,* 252:25-30.

Hall, D. (1996). Lichen sclerosus: Early diagnosis is the key to treatment. *Nurse Practitioner,* 21(12):57-58, 61-62.

Harmon, M.P., Castro, F.G. & Coe, K. (1996). Acculturation and cervical cancer: Knowledge, beliefs, and behaviors of Hispanic women. *Women and Health,* 24(3):37-57.

Heller, D. (1997). The Pap smear in identification of inflammatory conditions *The Female Patient,* 22:61-64, 67-68.

Ho, G.Y.E., Bierman, R., et al. (1998). Natural history of cervicovaginal papillomavirus infection in young women. *New England J of Medicine,* 338:423-428.

Klemm, P.R. & Guarnieri, C. (1996). Cervical cancer: A developmental perspective. *J of Obstetric, Gynecologic, and Neonatal Nursing,* 25(7):629-634.

Kurman, R.J., Henson, D.E., et al. (1994). Interim guidelines for management of abnormal cervical cytology. *J of the American Medical Association,* 271(23):1866-1869.

Larsen, N.S. (1994). Invasive cervical cancer rising in young white females. *J of the National Cancer Institute, 86:6-7.*

Lauver, D. & Rubin, M. (1991). Women's concerns about abnormal Papanicolaou test results. *J of Obstetric, Gynecologic, and Neonatal Nursing,* 20(2):154-159.

Lavin, C., Goodman, E., et al. (1997). Follow-up of abnormal Papanicolaou smears in a hospital-based adolescent clinic. *J of Pediatric Adolescent Gynecology,* 10:141-145.

Lungu, O., Sun, X.W., Felix, J., et al.(1992). Relationship of human papillomavirus type to grade of cervical intraepithelial neoplasia. *J of the American Medical Association,* 267:2493-2496.

Mandelblatt, J., Freeman, et al. (1997). The costs and effects of cervical and breast cancer screening in a public hospital emergency room. *American J of Public Health,* 87(7): 1182-1189.

Mashburn, J., Scharbo-DeHann, M. (1997). A clinician's guide to Pap smear interpretation. *The Nurse Practitioner,* 22(4):115-118, 124, 126-127.

Mitchell, M.F., et al. (1998). A ramdomized clinical trial of cryotherapy, laser vaporizer, and loop electrosurgical excision for treatment of squamous intraepithelial lesions of the cervix. *Obstetrics and Gynecology,* 92(5):737-744.

Modesitt, S., et al. (1998). Vulver intraepithelial neoplasia III: Occult cancer and the impact of margin status recurrence. *Obstetrics and Gynecology,* 92(6):262-265.

Morris, D.L., McLean, C.H., et al. (1998). A comparison of the evaluation and treatment of cervical dysplasias by gynecologists and nurse practitioners. *The Nurse Practitioner,* 23(4):101-102, 108-110, 113-114.

Munoz, N. & Bosch, F.X. (1996). The causal link between HIV and cervical cancer and its implications for prevention of cervical cancer. *Bulletin of the Pan American Organization, 30:362-377.*

Nugent, L.S. & Clark, R. (1996). Colposcopy: Sensory information for client education. *J of Obstetric, Gynecologic, and Neonatal Nursing,* 25(3):225-231.

Palank, C. (1998). An introduction to colposcopy concepts, controversies and guidelines for practice. *Advance for Nurse Practitioners,* 6:44-48, 50, 91.

Rajaram, S.S., et al. (1997). A biographical disruption: The care of an abnormal Pap smear. *Health Care for Women International,* 18(6):521-531.

Rubin, M. (1999, February 17-19). New technologies for cervical screening. Can we afford to use them? Can we afford not to use them? Presentation at the 23rd Annual Post-Graduate Seminar for Nurse Practitioners in Women's Health Care. Philadelphia

Rubin, M.M. & Lauver, D. (1990). Assessment and management of cervical intraepithelial neoplasia. *Nurse Practitioner,* 15(10):23-24, 26-28, 30-31.

Schaffer, S.D. & Philput, C.B. (1992). Predictors of abnormal cervical cytology: Statistical analysis of human papillomavirus and cofactors. *The Nurse Practitioner,* 17(3):46-48, 50.

Secor, R.M.C., guest editor. (1992). Entire issue devoted to vulvar and vaginal conditions. *Nurse Practitioner Forum,* 3(3).

Secor, R.M.C. & Fertitta, L. (1992). Vulvar vestibulitis syndrome. *Nurse Practitioner Forum,* 3(3):161-168.

Slade, C. (1998). HPV and cervical cancer. *Advance for Nurse Practitioners,* 6(3):39-40, 42, 54-54.

Spadt, S.K. (1995). Suffering in silence, managing vulvar pain patients. *Contemporary Nurse Practitioner,* 1(6):32-38.

Stevens, S.A., Cockburn, J., Hirst, S. & Jolley, D. (1997). An evaluation of educational outreach to general practitioners as part of a statewide cervical screening program. *American J of Public Health,* 87(7):1177-1181.

Stone, K.M., Zaidi, A., et al. (1995). Sexual behavior, sexually transmitted diseases, and risk of cervical cancer. *Epidemiology,* 6: 409-411.

Tomaino-Brunner, C., Freda, M.C., Damus, K. & Runowicz, C.D. (1998). Can precolposcopy education increase knowledge and decrease anxiety? *Journal of Obstetric, Gynecologic, and Neonatal Nursing,* 27(6):636-645.

Wahman, A. & Begneud, W.P. (1998). Keratosis on Papanicolaou smear: An indication for colposcopy? *Primary Care Update Ob-Gyn,* 5(6):296-299.

Washburn, J. & Scharbo-DeHann, M. (1997). A clinician's guide to Pap interpretation. *The Nurse Practitioner,* 22(4):115-118, 124, 126-127.

Winegardner, M.F. (1998). The atypical pap smear: New concerns. *The Clinical Advisor,* 26-29.

Wright, V.C. (1995). Guidelines for colposcopic investigations of lower genital intraepithelial neoplasia. *Advance for Nurse Practitioners,* 3(3):28-31.

Wright, T.C., Ellerbrock, T.V., et al., & the New York Cervical Disease Study. (1994). Cervical intraepithelial neoplasia in women infected with human immunodeficiency virus: Prevalence, risk factors, and validity of Papanicolaou smears. *Obstetrics & Gynecology,* 84:591-597/

Wright, T.C., Gagnon, S.E., Richart, R.M., et al. (1992). Treatment of cervical intraepithelial neoplasia using the loop electrosurgical excision procedure. *Obstetrics & Gynecology,* 79:173-178.

Yaeger, K. (1994). Colposcopy. *Advance for Nurse Practitioners,* 2(7):21-24.

Yoder, L. & Rubin, M.C. (1992). The epidemiology of cervical cancer and its precursors. *Oncology Nursing Forum,* 19(3):485-493.

22. Menses and Menstrual Disorders, Endometrial Biopsy

Boyle, J.S., Gramling, L.F. & Voda, A.M. (1996). Eskimo women and a menstrual cycle study: Some ethnographic notes. *Health Care for Women International,* 17(4):331-342.

Cahill, C.A. (1998). Differences in cortisol, a stress hormone in women with turmoil-type premenstrual syndrome. *Nursing Research,* 47(5):278-284.

Chandraiah, S. (1998). Premenstrual syndrome—an update. *Resident & Staff Physician,* 67-70.

Chang, A.M., Holroyd, E. & Chau, J.P. (1995). Premenstrual syndrome in employed Chinese women in Hong Kong. *Health Care for Women International,* 16(6):551-561.

Choung, C.J, Pearsall-Otey, L.R. & Rosenfeld, B.L (1995). A practical guide to relieving PMS. *Contemporary Nurse Practitioner,* 1(3):31-34, 36-37.

Chrisler, J.C. & Levy, K.B. (1990). The media construct a menstrual monster: A content analysis of PMS articles in the popular press. *Women & Health,* 16(2):89-104.

Chrisler, J.C. & Zittel, C.B. (1998). Menarche stories: Reminiscences of college students from Lithuania, Malaysia, Sudan, and the United States. *Health Care for Women International,* 19(4):303-312.

Cumming, C.E., Urion, C., Cumming, D.C. & Fox, E.E. (1994). "So mean and cranky, I could bite my mother": An ethnosemantic analysis of women's descriptions of premenstrual change. *Women & Health,* 21(4):21-41.

Dealy, M. (1988). Dysfunctional uterine bleeding in adolescents. *The Nurse Practitioner,* 23(5):12-13, 16, 18-20, 22-23.

Estok, P.J. & Rudy, E.B. (1994). Nutrient intake of women runners and nonrunners. *Health Care for Women International,* 15(5):435-451.

Estok, P.J., Rudy, E.B., Kerr, M.E. & Menzel, L. (1993). Menstrual response to running: Nursing implications. *Nursing Research,* 42(3):158-165.

Garner, K. (1994). Use of GnRH agonists. *Journal of Obstetric, Gynecologic, and Neonatal Nursing,* 23(7):563-570.

Gurevich, M. (1995). Rethinking the label: Who benefits from the PMS construct? *Women & Health,* 23(2):67-98.

Jarrett, M., Heitkemper, M.M. & Shaver, J.F. (1995). Symptoms and self-care strategies in women with and without dysmenorrhea. *Health Care for Women International,* 16(2):167-178.

Johnson, J. & Whitaker, A.H. (1992). Adolescent smoking, weight changes, and binge-purge behavior: Associations with secondary amenorrhea. *American Journal of Public Health,* 82(1):47-54.

Koff, E. & Rierden, J. (1995). Early adolescent girls' understanding of menstruation. *Women & Health,* 22(4):1-19.

Lewis, L.L. (1995). One year in the life of a woman with premenstrual syndrome: A case study. *Nursing Research,* 44(2):111-115.

McMaster, J., Cormie, K. & Pitts, M. (1997). Menstrual and premenstrual experiences of women in a developing country. *Health Care for Women International,* 18(6):533-541.

Marean, M., Fox, E.E., et al. (1998). Irritability and sociability in women with symptomatic premenstrual change. *Women & Health,* 27(1):65-71.

Mashburn, J. (1993). Endometrial biopsy in the office setting. *J of Nurse-Mid wifery*, 28(2 supplement), 31S-35S.

Mastrangelo, R. (1994). Taming the beast known as PMS. *Advance for Nurse Practitioners*, 2(10):10-14.

Mauri, M. (1990). Sleep and the reproductive cycle: A review. *Health Care for Women International*, 11(4):409-421.

Mehring, P., (1997). Uterine bleeding: Evaluating this common complaint. *Advance for Nurse Practitioners*, 5:27-28, 31-32.

MishelD.R. & Kaunitz, A.M. (1998). Devices for endometrial sampling. *J of Reproductive Medicine*, 43(3):180-184.

Morse, G. (1999). Positively reframing perceptions of the menstrual cycle among women with premenstrual syndrome. *J of Obstetric, Gynecologic, and Neonatal Nursing*28(2):165-174.

Samadi, A.R., Lee, N.C., et al. (1996). Risk factors for self-reported uterine fibroids: A case-control study.*American J of Public Health*, 86(6):858-862.

Schnare, S. (1994). Endometrial biopsy. *Contemporary Ob/Gyn-NP*, 1(1):5-7.

Seideman, R.Y. (1990). Effects of a premenstrual syndrome education program on premenstrual symptomatology. *Health Care for Women International*, 11(4):491-501.

Severy, L.J., Thapa, S., Askew, I. & Glor, J. (1993). Menstrual experiences and beliefs: A multicountry study of relationships with fertility and fertility regulating methods. *Women & Health*, 20(2):1-20.

Smith, C.B. (1998). Pinpointing the cause of abnormal uterine bleeding. *Women's Health in Primary Care*, 1(10):835-844.

Ugarriza, D.N., Klingner, S. & O'Brien, S. (1998). Premenstrual syndrome: Diagnosis and prevention. *Nurse Practitioner*, 23(9):40, 45, 49-50, 55

van den Akker, O., Sharifian, N., Packer, A. & Eves, F. (1995). Contribution of generalized negative affect to elevated menstrual cycle symptom reporting. *Health Care for Women International*, 16(3):263-272.

Woods, N., Taylor, D., et al. (1998). Perimenstrual symptoms and health-seeking behavior. *Western J of Nursing Research*, 14:418-439.

23. Toxic Shock Syndrome

Colbry, S.L. (1992). A review of toxic shock syndrome: The need for education still exists. *The Nurse Practitioner*, 17(9):39-40,43.

Creehan, P.A. (1995). Toxic shock syndrome: An opportunity for nursing intervention. *J of Obstetric, Gynecology, and Neonatal Nursing*, 24(6): 557-561.

Hanrahan,, S.N. (1994). Historical review of menstrual toxic shock syndrome. *Women & Health*, 21 (2/3):141-165.

Helgerson, S.D. (1981). Toxic shock syndrome. Tampons, toxins, and time: The evolution of understanding an illness. *Women & Health*, 6(3/4):93-104.

Oram, D. & Beck, J. (1981). The tampon: Investigated and challenged. *Women & Health* 6(5/4):105-122.

Petitti, D.B. & Reingold, A.L (1991). Recent trends in the incidence of toxic shock syndrome in northern California. *American J of Public Health*, 81(9):1209-1211.

24. Abortion

Cates, W., Grimes, D.A. & Hogue, L.L. (1995). Topics for our times: Justice Blackman and legal abortion—a besieged legacy to women's reproductive health. *American J of Public Health,* 85(9):1204-1206.

Dipierri, D. (1994). RU486, Mifepriston: A review of a controversial drug. *The Nurse Practitioner,* 19(6):59-61.

Donaldson, K., Briggs, J. et al. (1994). RU486: An alternative to surgical abortion. *J of Obstetric, Gynecologic, and Neonatal Nursing,* 23(7):555-559.

Ellertson, C. (1997). Mandatory parental involvement in minors' abortions: Effects of the laws in Minnesota, Missouri, and Indiana. *American J of Public Health,* 87(8):1367-1374.

Levine, P.B., Staiger, D., Kane, T.J. & Zimmerman, D.J. (1999). Roe v Wade and American fertility. *American J of Public Health,* 89(2):199-203.

McFarlane, D.R. & Meier, K.J. (1994). State abortion funding policies in 1990. *Women & Health,* 22(1):99-115.

Mertus, J.A. (1990). Fake abortion clinics: The threat to reproductive self-determination. *Women & Health,* 16(1):95-113.

Mueller, L. (1991). Second-trimester termination of pregnancy: Nursing care. *J of Obstetric, Gynecologic, and Neonatal Nursing,* 20(4):284-289.

Rogers, J.L., Stoms, G.G. & Phifer, J.L. (1989). Psychological impact of abortion: Methodological and outcomes summary of empirical research between 1966-1988. *Health Care for Women International,* 10(4):347-376.

Russo, N.F., Horn, J.D. et al. (1993). Childspacing intervals and abortion among Blacks and Whites: A brief report. *Women & Health,* 20(3): 43-51.

RU486 Fact Sheet. (1993). New York: Planned Parenthood Federation of America.

Slonim-Nevo, V. (1991). The experiences of women who face abortions. *Health Care for Women International,* 12(3):283-292.

Slonim-Nevo, V., Anson, J. & Sova, J. (1995). Delayed abortion among teenagers: Can a population at risk be identified? *Health Care for Women International,* 16(2):101-112.

Wells, N. (1991). Pain and distress during abortion. *Health Care for Women International,* 12(3):292-302.

Wyatt, L., Wyatt, G.E., Morgan, J., et al., (1995). Office abortion services for women: Private physician providers. *Women & Health,* 23(2):47-65.

25. Abuse, Sexual Assault, and Battering

Brasseur, J.W. (1994). The battered woman: Identification and intervention. *Clinician Reviews,* 4(9):45-47,49,53-56,58-60,64-65,,69-70,73-74.

Burgess, A.W. & Fawcett, J. (1996). The comprehensive sexual assault assessment tool, *Nurse Practitioner,* 21(4):66, 71-72, 74-76, 78, 83, 86

Chez, N. (1994). Helping victims of domestic violence. *American J of Nursing,* 94(7):33-37.

Eby, K.K., Campbell, J.C., Sullivan, C.M. & Davidson, W.S. (1995). Health effects of experiences of sexual violence for women with abusive partners. *Health Care for Women International,* 16(6):563-576.

Esparza, D.V. & Esperat, M.C.R. (1996). The effects of childhood sexual abuse on minority adolescent mothers. *J of Obstetric, Gynecologic, and Neonatal Nursing,* 25(4):321-328.

Fairchild, D.G., Fairchild, M.W. & Stoner, S. (1998). Prevalence of adult domestic violence among women seeking routine care in a native American health care facility. *American J of Public Health,* 88(10):1515-1517.

Farley, M. & Keaney, J.C. (1997). Physical symptoms, somatization, and dissociation in women survivors of childhood sexual assault. *Women & Health,* 25(3):33-45.

Fishwick, N.J. (1998). Assessment of women for partner abuse. *J of Obstetric, Gynecologic, and Neonatal Nursing,* 27(6):661-670.

Forjuoh, S.N., Cohen, J.H. & Gondoff, E.W. (1998). Correlates of injury in women with partners enrolled in batterer treatment programs. *American J of Public Health,* 88(11):1705-1708.

Furniss, K.K. (1993). Screening for abuse in the clinical setting. *AWHONN's Clinical Issues in Perinatal and Women's Health Nursing,* 4(3):402-406.

Gerbert, B., Johnston, et al. (1996). Experiences of battered women in health care settings: A qualitative study. *Women & Health,* 24(3):1-17.

Gerlock, A.A. (1997). New directions in the treatment of men who batter women. *Health Care for Women International,* 18(5):481-493.

Glass, N. & Campbell, J.C. (1998). Mandatory reporting of intimate partner violence by health care professionals: A policy review. *Nursing Outlook,* 46:279-283.

Heritage, C. (1998). Working with childhood sexual abuse survivors during pregnancy, labor, and birth. *J of Obstetric, Gynecologic, and Neonatal Nursing,* 27(6):671-677.

Keenan, C.K., El-Hadad, A. & Balian, S.A. (1998). Factors associated with domestic violence in low-income Lebanese families. *Image,* 30(4):357-362.

Landenburger, K.M. (1998). The dynamics of leaving and recovering from an abusive relationship. *J of Obstetric, Gynecologic, and Neonatal Nursing,* 27(6):700-706.

Limandri, B.J. & Tilden, V.P. (1996). Nurses' reasoning in the assessment of family violence. *Image,* 28(3):247-252.

McFarlane, J. & Parker, B. (1994). Preventing abuse during pregnancy: An assessment and intervention protocol. *The American J of Maternal/Child Nursing,* 19(6):321-324.

McGrath, M.E., Hogan, J.W. & Peipert, J.F. (1998). A prevalence survey of abuse and screening for abuse in urgent care patients. *Obstetrics & Gynecology,* 91(4):511-514.

McMurray, A. (1997). Violence against ex-wives: Anger and advocacy. *Health Care for Women International,* 18(6):543-556.

Mahony, D.L. & Campbell, J.M. (1998). Children witnessing domestic violence: A developmental approach. *Clinical Excellence for Nurse Practitioners,* 2(6):362-369.

Merritt-Gray, M. & Wuest, J. (1995). Counteracting abuse and breaking free: The process of leaving revealed through women's voices. *Health Care for Women International,* 16(5):399-412.

Mitchell, C.A. & Smyth, C. (1994). A case study of an abused older woman. *Health Care for Women International,* 15(6):521-535.

Nelson, J.A (1997). Gay, lesbian, and bisexual adolescents: Providing esteem-enhancing care to a battered population. *Nurse Practitioner,* 22(2):94, 99, 103, 106, 109.

Parker, B. & McFarlane, J. (1991). Identifying and helping battered pregnant women. *The American J of Maternal/Child Health,* 16(3):161-164.

Parker, B. & Ulrich, Y. Nursing Research Consortium on Violence and Abuse (1990). A protocol of safety: Research on abuse of women. *Nursing Research,* 39(4):248-250.

Phillips, D.S.H. (1998). Culture and systems of oppression in abused women's lives. *J of Obstetric, Gynecologic, and Neonatal Nursing,* 27(6):678-683.

Read, J.P., Stern, A.L., et al. (1997). Use of a screening instrument in women's health care: Detecting relationships among victimization history, psychological distress, and medical complaints. *Women & Health,* 25(3):1-17.

Roberts, G.L., Williams, G.M., et al. (1998). How does domestic violence affect women's mental health? *Women & Health,* 28(1):117-129.

Roberts, S.J. (1996). The sequelae of childhood sexual abuse: A primary care focus for adult female survivors. *Nurse Practitioner,* 21(12):42, 49-50, 52.

Roussillon, J.A. (1998). Adult survivors of childhood sexual abuse: Suggestions for perinatal caregivers. *Clinical Excellence for Nurse Practitioners,* 2(6):329-337.

Ruckman, L.M. (1992). Rape: How to begin the healing. *The American J of of Nursing,* 92(9):48-51.

Ryan, J. & King, M.C. (1998). Scanning for violence. *AWHONN Lifelines,* 2(3):36-41.

Schafer, J., Caetano, R. &Clark,C.L. (1998). Rates of intimate partner violence in the United States. *American J of Public Health,* 88(11):1702-1704.

Schaffer, S.D. & Zimmerman, M.L. (1990). The sexual addict: A challenge for the primary care provider. *The Nurse Practitioner,* 15(6):25-26,28,33.

Schnitzer, P.G. & Runyan, C.W. (1995). Injuries to women in the United States: An overview. *Women & Health,* 23(1):9-27.

Widom, C.S. & Kuhns, J.B. (1996). Childhood victimization and subsequent risk for promiscuity, prostitution, and teenage pregnancy: A prospective study. *American J of Public Health,* 86(11):1607-1612.

Wingood, G.M. & DiClemente, R.J. (1997). The effects of an abusive primary partner on condom use and sexual negotiation practices of African-American women. *American J of Public Health,* 87(6):1016-1018.

26. Sexuality and Sexual Dysfunction

Alteneder, R.R. & Hartzell, D. (1997). Addressing couples' sexuality concerns during the childbearing period: Use of the PLISSIT model. *J of Obstetric, Gynecologic, and Neonatal Nursing,* 26(6):651-658.

Boston Women's Health Book Collective, (1998). Our Bodies, Ourselves for the New Century. A Book By and For Women. New York: Simon & Schuster.

Buenting, J.A. (1992). Health life-styles of lesbian and heterosexual women. *Health Care for Women International,* 13(2):165-171.

Finan, S.L. (1997). Promoting healthy sexuality. Guidelines for early through older adulthood. *Nurse Practitioner,* 22(12):54, 56, 59-60, 63-64.

Hitchcock, J.M. & Wilson, H.S. (1992). Personal risking: Lesbian self-disclosure of sexual orientation to professional health care providers. *Nursing Research,* 41(3):178-183.

Hutchinson, M.K. (1999). Individual, family, and relationship predictors of young women's sexual risk perceptions. *J of Obstetric, Gynecologic, and Neonatal Nursing,* 28(1):60-67.

Johnson, B.K. (1998). A correlational framework for understanding sexuality in women age 50 and older. *Health Care for Women International,* 19(6):553-364.

Jones, K.D., Lehr, S.T. & Hewell, S.W. (1997). Dyspareunia: Three case reports. *J of Obstetric, Gynecologic, and Neonatal Nursing,* 26(1): 19-23.

Kennison, R.D. & Fertita, L.L. (1990). Taking a woman's sexual history. *Medical Aspects of Human Sexuality,* 24(11):58-60.

Kurtz, M.E., Wyatt, G. & Kurtz, J.C. (1995). Psychological and sexual well-being, philosophical/spiritual views, and health habits of long-term cancer survivors. *Health Care for Women International,* 16(3):253-262.

Marin, B.V., Tschann, J.M., Gomez, C.A. & Kegeles, S.M. (1993). Acculturation and gender differences in sexual attitudes and behavior. Hispanic vs non-Hispanic white unmarried adults. *American J of Public Health,* 83(12):1759-1761.

Misener, T.R., Sowell, R.L., Phillips, K.D. & Harris, C. (1997). Sexual orientation: A cultural diversity issue for nursing. *Nursing Outlook,* 45(4):178-181.

Mueller, I.W. (1997). Common questions about sex and sexuality in elders. *American Journal of Nursing,* 97(7):61-64.

Robohm, J.S. & Buttenheim, M. (1996). The gynecological care experience of childhood virgins: Genital sexual activities of high school students who have never had vaginal intercourse. *American J of Public Health,* 86(11): 1570-1576.

Sarazin, S.K. & Seymour, S.F. (1991). Causes and treatment options for women with dyspareunia. *The Nurse Practitioner,* 16(10):30,35-36,38,41.

Schnare, S. (1993). Evaluation and treatment of diminished libido in women. *Contemporary Ob/Gyn-NP,* 1(11):3-4.

Stevens-Simon, C. (1993). Clinical application of adolescent female sexual development. *The Nurse Practitioner,* 18(12):18,21,25-27,29.

Sulpizi, L.K. (1996). Issues in sexuality and gynecologic care of women with developmental disabilities. *J of Obstetric, Gynecologic, and Neonatal Nursing,* 25(7):609-614.

Webster, D.C. (1997). Recontextualizing sexuality in chronic illness: Women and interstitial cystitis. *Health Care for Women International,* 18(6):575-

589.
Williamson, M.L. (1992). Sexual adjustment after hysterectomy. *J of Obstetric, Gynecologic, and Neonatal Nursing,* 21(1):42-47.
Wilmoth, M.C. (1996). The middle years: Women, sexuality, and the self. *J of Obstetric, Gynecologic, and Neonatal Nursing,* 25(7):615-621.
Woodson, S.A. (1997). Sexual health across the lifespan. *Lifelines,* 1(4):34-39.

27. Peri- and Postmenopausal Care, Hormone Therapy

Aber, C.S., Arathuzik, D. & Righter, A.R. (1998). Women's perceptions and concerns about menopause. *Clinical Excellence for Nurse Practitioners: The International J of NPACE,* 2(4):232-238.
Andrews, W.C. (1995). Continuous combined estrogen/progestin hormone replacement therapy. *Nurse Practitioner,* 20 (11 supplement):1-11.
Archer, D.F. (1998). The progestin dilemma: Protecting the endometrium without compromising adherence. *International New Proceedings J,* 11(1):19-26.
Archer, D.F., Pickar, J.H. & Bottiglioni, F. (1994). Bleeding patterns in post-menopausal women taking continuous combined or sequential regimens of conjugated estrogens with medroxyprogesterone acetate. *Obstetrics & Gynecology,* 83(5):686-692.
Bell, M.L. (1995). Attitudes toward menopause among Mexican American women. *Health Care for Women International,* 16(5):425-435.
Bernhard, L.A. & Sheppard, L. (1993). Health, symptoms, self-care, and dyadic adjustment in menopausal women. *J of Obstetric, Gynecologic, and Neonatal Nursing,* 22(5):456-461.
Benner, F. (1998). Quality of life and new delivery systems: individualizing election regimes. *International New Proceedings J,* 11(1):29-36.
Bueche, M.N. & Gelser, L.J. (1997). Women's lived experience of perimeno-pause. *Clinical Excellence for Nurse Practitioners,* 1(7):437-443.
Burger, H.G. (1998). HRT and the endocrinology of the menopause. *Menopausal Medicine,* 6(4):5-8
Carlson, E.S., Li, S. & Holm, K. (1997). An analysis of menopause in the popular press. *Health Care for Women International,* 18(6):557-564.
Carlson, E.S. & Li, S. (1998). Androgen therapy for menopausal women. *Clinical Excellence for Nurse Practitioners,* 2(6):324-328.
Carr, B.R. (1998). HRT: Lessons in serum lipids and cardiovascular risk. *International Proceedings J,* 1:1-9.
Chang, C. & Chang, C.H. (1996). Menopause and hormone using experiences of Chinese women in Taiwan. *Health Care for Women International,* 17(4):307-318.
Cornell, S. (1997). Another use for estrogen. *Advance for Nurse Practitioners,* 5:49-50, 53.
Donnelly, V., O'Connell, P.R. & Herlihy, C. (1997). The influence of oestrogen replacement on faecal incontinence in postmenopausal women. *British J of Obstetrics and Gynecology,* 104:311-315.
Ellis, J. & Kanusky, C. (1996). Addressing women's midlife concerns. *Advance*

for Nurse Practitioners, 4(5):45-50.

Folsom, A.R., Mink, P.J., Seller, T.A., et al.,(1995). Hormonal replacement therapy and morbidity and mortality in a prospective study of postmenopausal women. *American J of Public Health,* 85(8):1128-1132.

Gambell, R.D. (1998). Overcoming the side effects of hormone replacement therapy. *Women's Health in Primary Care,* 160-163, 167-168.

Gannon, L. & Stevens, J. (1998). Portraits of menopause in the mass media. *Women and Health,* 27(3):1-15.

Gelford, M.M. (1998). Altering HRT for individual needs. *ACOG Clinical Review,* 3(4):1-2.

George, T. (1996). Women in a South Indian fishing village: Role identity, continuity, and the experience of menopause. *Health Care for Women International,* 17(4):271-279.

Hautman, M.A. (1996) Changing womanhood: Perimenopause among Filipina-Americans, *J of Obstetric, Gynecologic, and Neonatal Nursing,* 25(8): 667-673.

Hollenbach, K.A., Barrett-Connor, E., Edelstein, S.L. & Holbrook, T. (1993). Cigarette smoking and bone mineral density in older men and women. *American J of Public Health,* 83(9):1265-1270.

Im, E. & Lipson, J.G. (1997). Menopausal transition of Korean immigrant women: A literature review. *Health Care for Women International,* 18(6):507-520.

Jacobson, B.H., Aldana, S.G., Adams, T.B. & Quirk, M. (1996). The relationship between smoking, cholesterol, and HDL-C levels in adult women. *Women & Health,* 23(4):27-38.

Kaplan, H., Abisia, M.L. (1997). In transition. *Advance for Nurse Practitioners,* 5:29-33

King, K.M. (1996). Estrogen replacement therapy and coronary heart disease in postmenopausal women. *Health Care for Women International,* 17(3):247-254.

Learn, C.D. (1998). Appraising the menopause web. *Lifelines,* 2(4):40-44.

Li, S., Lanuza, D., Gulanick, M., Penckofer, S. & Holm, K. (1996). Perimenopause: The transition into menopause. *Health Care for Women Internationall,* 17(4):293-306.

Mayes, S.J. (1998). Testosterone for female libido. *The Clinical Advisor for N.P.,* 34.

McDonnell, D.P. (1998). Selective estrogen receptor modulators (Serms). *Menopausal Medicine,* 6(4).

McKeon, V.A.. (1994). Hormone replacement therapy: Evaluating the risks and benefits. *J of Obstetric, Gynecologic, and Neonatal Nursing,* 23(8):647-657.

Mestel, R. (1997). A safer estrogen. *Health,* 72-75.

Nand, S.L., et al. (1998) Bleeding pattern and endometrial changes during continuous combined hormone replacement therapy. *Obstetrics & Gynecology,* 91(5):678-864.

National Institutes of Health. (1997). The Women's Health Initiative: Study Protocol and Policies, Vol. 1. Bethesda, MD : N I H

Newton, K. et al. (1998). Hormone replacement therapy and tertiary prevention of coronary heart disease. *Menopausal Medicine,* 6(1):5-9.

Norman, D.J. (1997). Variations on traditional HRT. *Advance for Nurse Practitioners,* 5(11):34-37.

Perz, J.M. (1997). Development of the menopause symptom list: A factor analytic study of menopause associated symptoms. *Women & Health,* 25(1):53-69.

Peters, S. (1998). Menopause: A new era. *Advance for Nurse Practitioners,* 6(7):61-64.

Poma, P. (1997). A simple strategy for managing perimenopausal bleeding. *Contemporary Nurse Practitioner,* 2(3):21-22, 24-26.

Sanders, S.L. (1995). A protocol for HRT. *Advance for Nurse Practitioners,* 3(9):41-42.

Scharbo-Dehaan, M. (1994). Management strategies for hormonal replacement therapy. *Nurse Practitioner,* 19(12):47-52, 55-57.

Scharbo-Dehaan, M. (1996). Hormone replacement therapy. *Nurse Practitioner,* 21(12, part 2):1-15.

Shaw, C.R. (1997). The perimenopausal hot flash: Epidemiology, physiology, and treatment. *The Nurse Practitioner,* 22(3):55-56, 61-66.

Shephard, M.A. (1998). Serum estrogen levels and cognition. *Journal Watch Women's Health,* 3(9):68.

Simon, J.A. (1998). Effects of progestins and progesterone on CNS function. *Menopausal Medicine,* 4(8):8-12.

Snabes, M. (1998). Clinical use of serms in postmenopausal women. *Menopausal Medicine,* 6(2):4-7.

Sullivan, J.M. (1998). The role of estrogen in secondary prevention of cardiovascular events. *Menopausal Medicine,* 6(3):7-10.

Taylor, M. (1998). Alternative to conventional hormone replacement. *Menopausal Medicine,* 6(3).

Thomas, S.P. & Atakan, S. (1993). Trait anger, anger expression, stress, and health status of American and Turkish midlife women. *Health Care for Women International,* 14(2):129-143.

Thorneycroft, I.H. (1998). Assessing bone resorption levels to predict skeletal response to HRT. *International New Proceedings Journal,* 11(1):10-18.

Toronto Women's Health Network. (1996, September). Hormone replacement therapy: The good, the bad, and the confusing.

Triadafilopoulos, G., Finlayson, M.A. & Grellet, C. (1998). Bowel dysfunction in postmenopausal women. *Women & Health,* 27(4):55-66.

Turner, C. (1994). Pharmacologic highlights: Hormone replacement therapy: Its use in the management of acute menopausal symptoms. *J of the American Academy of Nurse Practitioners,* 6(7):318-320.

Vassilopopulsis, R. (1998). Hormone replacement therapy after breast cancer diagnosis and treatment. *Menopausal Medicine,* 6(1):1-5.

Wagner, P.J., Kuhn, S., Petry, L.J. & Talbert, F.S. (1996). Age differences in attitudes toward menopause and estrogen replacement therapy. *Women & Health,* 23(4):1-16.

Wasaha, S. & Angelopoulos, F.M. (1996). What every woman should know about menopause. *American J of Nursing,* 96(1):24-32.

Wehrle, K.E. (1996). Perfect timing for a healthy life: What to expect during perimenopause. *Advance for Nurse Practitioners,* 4(11):18-27.

Westermann, C. (1997). Pharmacology and selection of postmenopausal estrogen replacement therapy. *The Female Patient,* 22:15-19, 22.

Wilbur, J., Holm, K. & Dan, A. (1992). The relationship of energy expenditure to physical and psychologic symptoms in women at midlife. *Nursing Outlook,* 40(6):269-276.

Wood, N.J. (1992). The use of vaginal pessaries for uterine prolapse. *The Nurse Practitioner,* 17(7):31,35,38.

Woods, N.F. & Mitchell, E.S. (1997). Women's image of midlife: Observations from the Seattle midlife women's health study. *Health Care for Women International,* 18(5):439-453.

Writing group for the PEPI trial. (1995). Effects of estrogen or estrogen/progestin regimens on heart disease risk factors in postmenopausal women. *J of the American Medical Association,* 273(3):199-208.

Youngkin, E.Q. (1990). Estrogen replacement therapy and the estradenn transdermal system. *The Nurse Practitioner,* 15(5):19-20,26,31.

28. Osteoporosis

Ailinger, R.L. & Emerson, J. (1998). Women's knowledge of osteoporosis. *Applied Nursing Research,* 11(3):111-114.

Brager, R. (1997). Alendronate treatment for osteoporosis. *Advance for Nurse Practitioners,* 5(3):28-34.

Delmas, P.D., Bjarnason, N.H., Mitlak, B.H., Ravoux, A., et al. (1997). Effects of reloxifene on bone mineral density, serum cholesterol concentrations, and uterine endometrium in a postmenopausal women. *New England J of Medicine,* 337:1641-1647.

Damond, S. (1998). Calcium and magnesium update. *Women's Health Alternatives,* 7-8.

Eiken, P., Nielson, S.P. & Kolthoff, N.C. (1997). Effects on bone mass after eight years of hormonal replacement therapy. *British J of Obstetrics and Gynecology,* 104(6):702-707.

Feskanich, D., Willett, W.C. et al. (1997). Milk, dietary calcium, and bone fractures in women: A 12-year prospective study. *American J of Public Health,* 87(6):992-997.

Galsworthy, T.D. & Wilson, P.L. (1996). Osteoporosis: It steals more than bone. *American J of Nursing,* 96(6):26-33.

Kessenich, C.R. (1998). Raloxifene: A new class of anti-estrogens for the prevention of osteoporosis. *Nurse Practitioner,* 23(9):91-93.

Kessenich, C.R. (1996). Breaking the osteoporosis cycle. *Advance for Nurse Practitioners,* 4(8):16-20

Kessenich, C.R. (1996). Update on pharmacologic therapies for osteoporosis. *Nurse Practitioner,* 21(8):19-20, 22-24.

Kim, S.H., Morton, D.J. & Barrett-Connor, E.L. (1997). Carbonated beverage consumption and bone mineral density among older women: The Rancho Bernardo Study. *American J of Public Health,* 87:276-279.

Kupecz, D. (1996). Alendronate for the treatment of osteoporosis. *Nurse*

Practitioner, 21(1):86, 88-89.

Licata, A.A. (1999). Update on osteoporosis: Strategies for prevention and treatment. *Women's Health in Primary Care,* 2(3):229-243.

Massachusetts Medical Society (publishers of the New England J of Medicine and Journal Watch). (1998). Raloxifene: A future alternative to estrogen. *Journal Watch. Women's Health,* 3(1):1-2.

McClung, B.L. (1999). Using osteoporosis management to reduce fractures in elderly women. *Nurse Practitioner,* 24(3), 26-27, 32, 35-36, 38, 41-41.

Matsumoto, D., Pun, K.K., Nakatani, M., et al., (1996). Cultural differences in attitudes, values, and beliefs about osteoporosis in first and second generation Japanese-American women. *Women & Health,* 23(4):39-56.

Overgaard, K., Hansen, M.A., Jensen, S.B. & Christiansen, S. (1992). Effect of salcatonin intranasally on bone mass and fracture rates in established osteoporosis: A dose-response study. *British Medical J,* 305:556-561.

Rosenblatt, K. (1998). Osteoporosis: Current status of screening, prevention, and therapy. *Primary Care,* 10(3):53-54.

Setter S. (1998). Improving compliance with estrogen therapy for osteoporosis. *The Female Patient,* 23:1-52, 54, 57-58, 60, 62.

Soroko, S., Holbrook, T.L., Edelstein, ScM. & Barrett-Connor, E. (1994). Lifetime milk consumption and bone mineral density in older women. *American J of Public Health,* 84(8):1319-1322.

Walsh et al. (1998). Does Raxoxifene measure up to HRT? *Clinical Review,* 8(9):44-45.

Whiting, S. (1998). Pharmacology update (1997) calcium supplementation. *J of the American Academy of Nurse Practitioners,* 9(4):187-190.

Whitmore, S. (1998). Rebuilding bone—an overview of developments in osteoporosis management. *Advance for Nurse Practitioners,* 6(9):30.

Woodhead, G.A. & Moss, M.M. (1998). Osteoporosis: Diagnosis and prevention. *Nurse Practitioner,* 23(11):18, 23-24, 26-27, 31-32, 34-35.

Zhang, J., Feldblum, P.J. & Fortney, J.A. (1992). Moderate physical activity and bone density among perimenopausal women. *American J of Public Health,* 82(5):736-741.

29. Stress Incontinence

Brink, C.A., Wells, T.J., et al. (1994). A digital test for pelvic muscle strength in women with urinary incontinence. *Nursing Research,* 43(6):352-356

Cyarapata, B. (1997). Urinary incontinence: Proactive management. *Contemporary Nurse Practitioner,* 2(4):16-18, 20-22, 24-26.

Czarapata, B.J.R. & McKillips, K.J. (1997, April). Silent suffering. Helping women find the path to continence. *Lifelines,* 1:28-34.

Davila, G.W. (1996). Introl bladder neck support prosthesis: A nonsurgical urethropexy. *J of Endourology,* 10(3):293-296.

Dougherty, M.C., Dwyer, J.W., Pendergast, J.F., Tomlinson, B.U., et al., (1998). Community-based nursing continence care for older rural women. *Nursing Outlook,* 46(5):233-244.

Foldspang, A., Mommsen, S. & Djurhuus, J.C. (1999). Prevalent urinary incontinence as a correlate of pregnancy, vaginal childbirth, and obstetric techniques. *American J of Public Health,* 89(2):209-212.

Gallo, M.L., Fallon, P.J. & Staskin, D.R. (1997). Urinary incontinence: Steps to evaluation, diagnosis, and treatment. *Nurse Practitioner,* 22(2):21-22, 24, 26, 28, 31-33

Griffin, C., Dougherty, M.C. & Yarandi, H. (1994). Pelvic muscles during rest: Responses to pelvic muscle exercise. *Nursing Research,* 43(3):164-167.

Hudacek, S. (1995). Evaluation and treatment of urinary incontinence: A primary care approach. *Nurse Practitioner,* 20(2):74-77.

Jirovec, M.M., Wyman, J.F. & Wells, T.J. (1998). Addressing urinary incontinence with educational continence-care competencies. *Image,* 30(4):375-378.

Miller, J.L. & Bavendam, T. (1996). Treatment with the Reliance® urinary control insert: One-year experience. *J of Endourology,* 10(3):287-292.

Newman, D.K. (1998). Controversies in incontinence. *The Clinical Letter for Nurse Practitioners,* 2(6):1-7.

Nygaard, I. (1994). Nonsurgical therapy for SUI. *Contemporary Ob/Gyn-NP,* 2(1):18-24.

Rabin, J.M. (1997). The "Femassist" a new device for the treatment of female urinary incontinence. *Advance for Nurse Practitioners,* 5(4), 199

Ravalli, R. & Brettschneider, N. (1996). Nursing assessment and management strategies for urinary incontinence. *J of Endourology,* 10(3):297-300.

Sampselle, C.M., Burns, P.A., Dougherty, M.C., Newman, D.K., et al. (1997). Continence for women: Evidence-based practice. *J of Obstetric, Gynecologic, and Neonatal Nursing,* 26(4):375-385.

Versi, E., et al. (1998). New external urethral occlusive device for female urinary incontinence. *Obstetrics & Gynecology,* 2(2):286-291.

Wyman, J.F., Elswick, R.K., Ory, M.G., Wilson, M.S. & Fantl, J.A. (1993). Influence of functional, urological, and environmental characteristics on urinary incontinence in community-dwelling older women. *Nursing Research,* 42(5):270-275.

30. Urinary Tract Infection

Bromberg, W. (1998). Urinary tract infections. *Clinical Advisor,* 60-64.

Czarapata, B.J.R. (1996). Interstitial cystitis and vulvodynia. *Advance for Nurse Practitioners,* 4(10):21-23.

Duffield, P. (1996). Managing urinary tract infections, part I: Diagnosing and treating adults. *American J of Nursing,* 96(9):16b-16d.

Foxman, B. (1990). Recurring urinary tract infection: Incidence and risk factors. *American J of Public Health,* 80(33):331-333.

Freeman, S.B. (1995). Common genitourinary infections. *J of Obstetric, Gynecologic, and Neonatal Nursing,* 24(8):735-742.

Hassay, K.A. (1994). Urinary discomfort. *Advance for Nurse Practitioners,* 2(5):9-11,37.

Hassay, K.A. (1995). Effective management of urinary discomfort. *Nurse Practitioner,* 20(2):36, 39-40, 42-44, 46-47.

Leiner, S. (1995). Recurrent urinary tract infections in otherwise healthy adult women. *Nurse Practitioner,* 20(2):48, 51-52, 54-56.

Polivka, B.J., Nickel, J.T. & Wilkins, J.R. (1997). Urinary tract infection during pregnancy: A risk factor for cerebral palsy. *J of Obstetric, Gynecologic, and Neonatal Nursing,* 26(4):405-413.

Pollen, J.J. (1995). Short-term course for uncomplicated cystitis. *Contemporary Nurse Practitioner,* 1(4):21-30.

Sale, P.G. (1995). Genitourinary infection in older women. *J of Obstetric, Gyne cologic, and Neonatal Nursing,* 24(8):769-775.

Webster, D.C. & Brennan, T. (1994). Use and effectiveness of physical self-care strategies for interstitial cystitis. *Nurse Practitioner,* 19(10):55-61.

Webster, D.C. & Brennan, T. (1995). Use and effectiveness of psychological self-care strategies for interstitial cystitis. *Health Care for Women International,* 16(5):463-475.

31. Pre-Conception Care

ACOG. (1995). Planning for Pregnancy, Birth and Beyond, 2nd ed.

Bassetti, M. (1996). Offering a head start to a healthy pregnancy: The role of folic acid. *Advance for Nurse Practitioners,* 4(7):22-31.

Bauer, W.S. & Ludka, D.A. (1995). Getting pregnancy off to a good start—before it starts. *Contemporary Nurse Practitioner,* 1(4):16-26.

Bonin, M.M., Bretzlaff, J.A., Therrien, S.A. & Rowe, B.H. (1998). Knowledge of periconceptional folic acid for the prevention of neural tube defects: The missing link. *Archives of Family Medicine,* 7(5):438-442.

Moos, M-K. (1994). Conception. *Advance for Nurse Practitioners,* 2(6):9-10.

Perry, L.E. (1996). Preconception care: A health promotion opportunity. *Nurse Practitioner,* 21(11):24, 26, 32, 34, 39-41.

Rogers, J. & Davis, B.A. (1995). How risky are hot tubs and saunas for pregnant women? *The American J of Maternal/Child Nursing,* 20(3):137-140.

Romanczuk, A.N. & Brown, J.P. (1995). Folic acid will reduce risk of neural tube defects. *The American J of Maternal/Child Nursing,* 19(6):331-334.

Sussman, Jr. & Levett, B.B. (1989). Before You Conceive. New York: Bantam

Tinkle, M.B. & Sterling, B.S. (1997). Neural tube defects: A primary prevention role for nurses. *J of Obstetric, Gynecologic, and Neonatal Nursing,* 26(5):503-512.

32. Complementary/Alternative Therapies

Collins, C. (1998). Yoga: Intuition, preventive medicine, and treatment. *J of Obstetric, Gynecologic, and Neonatal Nursing,* 27(5):563-568.

Complementary Medicine. www.pitt.edu/wcbw/altm.htm

Engebreston, J. & Wardell, D. (1993). A contemporary view of alternative healing modalities. *Nurse Practitioner,* 18(9):51-55.

Foster, S. & Tyler, V.E. (1999). Tyler's Honest Herbal. Binghamton, NY: Haworth Herbal Press.

George, D. (1997). Antioxidants: Can they reverse the aging process? *Clinical Excellence for Nurse Practitioners: The International J of NPACE,* 1(5):289-293.

Glisson, J., Crawford, R., & Street, S. (1998). Review, critique, and guidelines for the use of herbs and homeopathy. *Nurse Practitioner,* 34(4):44, 46, 53, 60, 65-67.

Kendig, S. & Sanford, D.G. (1998). Alternative aging. *AWHONN Lifelines,* 2(3):55-58.

Marcus, C.L. (1999). Alternative medicine: The AMA reviews scientific evidence. *Clinical Reviews,* 9(2):87-90.

Robbers, J.E. & Tyler, V.E. (1999). Tyler's Herbs of Choice. Binghamton, NY: Haworth Herbal Press.

Schirner, G. (1998). Alternative Medicine. Med 2000, Inc., pp. 1-102.

Starn, J.R. (1998). Energy healing with women and children. *J of Obstetric, Gynecologic, and Neonatal Nursing,* 27(5):576-584.

Tiedje, L.B. (1998). Alternative health care: An overview. *J of Obstetric, Gynecologic, and Neonatal Nursing,* 27(5):557-562.

Tyler, V.E. (1993). The Honest Herbal. Pharmaceutical Products Press.

Whiting, S., et al. (1997). Caclcium supplementation. *J of the Americn Academy of Nurse Practitioners,* 9(4):187-190.

Youngkin, E.Q. & Israel, D.S. (1996). A review and critique of common herbal alternative therapies. *Nurse Practitioner,* 21(10): 39, 43-44, 46, 49-52.

33. Smoking Cessation

Andrews, J. (1998). Optimizing smoking cessation strategies. *Nurse Practitioner,* 23(8):47-48, 51-52, 57-58, 61-62, 64, 67.

Hershberger, P. (1998). Smoking and pregnant teens. *Lifelines,* 2(4):26-32.

Jacobson, B.H., Aldana, S.G., Adams, T.B., & Quirk, M. (1996). The relationship between smoking, cholesterol, and HDL-C levels in adult women. *Women & Health,* 23(4):27-38.

Jensen, P.M. & Coambs, R.B. (1998). Health and behavioral predictors of success in an intensive smoking cessation program for women. *Women and Health,* 21(1):57-72.

Kilby, J.W. (1997). A smoking cessation plan for pregnant women. *J of Obstetric. Gynecologic, and Neonatal Nursing,* 26(4):397-402.

Krawiec, J.V. & Pohl, J.M. (1997). Smoking cessation and nicotine replacement therapy: A guide for primary care providers. *American J for Nurse Practitioners,* 1(10):15-33.

Leccese, C. (1998). To each his own. *Advance for Nurse Practitioners,* 6(4):67-70.

Lindell, K.O. & Reinke, L.F. (1999). Nursing strategies for smoking cessation. *The American Nurse* (Supp.) 31(2):A1-A8.

National Institutes of Health, National Heart, Lung and Blood Institute. (1993). Nurses: Help your patients stop smoking. Bethesda, MD: National Institutes of Health.

Pohl, J.M. & Caplan, D. (1998). Smoking cessation: Using group intervention methods to treat low-income women. *Nurse Practitioner,* 23(12):13, 17-18, 20, 25-27, 31-32, 37

Scheibmeir, M. & O'connell, K.A. (1997). In harm's way: Childbearing women and nicotine. *J of Obstetric, Gynecologic, and Neonatal Nursing,* 26(4):477-

484.

Secker-Walker, R.H., Solomon, L.J., Geller, B.M., Flynn, B.S., Worden, J., et al. (1997). Modeling smoking cessation: Exploring the use of a videotape to help pregnant women quit smoking. *Women & Health,* 25(1):23-35.

34. Women and Heart Disease

Arnold, E. (1997). The stress connection: Women and coronary artery disease. *Critical Care Nursing Clinics of North America,* 9(4):565-575.

Arnstein, P.M., Buselli, E.F. & Rankin, S.H. (1996). Women and heart attacks: Prevention, diagnosis, and care. *Nurse Practitioner,* 21(5):57-67.

Brezinka, V. & Kittel, F. (1996). Psychological factors of coronary artery disease in women: A review. *Social Science and Medicine,* 42(10):1351-1365.

Cole, S.R., McDermott, R.J. & Drimmer, A. (1996). Educational components of secondary prevention of heart disease in phase II cardiac rehabilitation programs. *International J of Rehabilitation and Health,* 2(3):210.

Eaker, E.D., Johnson, W.D., Loop, F.D. & Wenger, N.K. (1992). Heart disease in women: How different? *Patient Care,* 2(15):199-202.

MooreS.M. (1996). Women's views of cardiac rehabilitation programs. *J of Cardiopulmonary Rehabilitation,* 16(2):123-129.

Moore, S.M. & Kramer, F.M. (1996). Women's and men's preferences for cardiac rehabilitation program features. *J of Cardiopulmonary Rehabilitation,* 16(3):163-168.

Moore, S.M., Ruland, C.M.. Pashkow, F.J. & Blackburn, G.G. (1998). Women's patterns of exercise following cardiac rehabilitation. *Nursing Research,* 47(6):318-324.

Murdaugh, C. (1990). Coronary artery disease in women. *J of Cardiovascular Nursing, 4(4):35, 44, 46-47.*

Nikiforov, S.V. & Mamaev, V.G. (1998). The development of sex differences in cardiovascular disease mortality: A historical perspective. *American J of Public Health,* 88(9):1348-1353.

Poduri, A. & Grisso, J.A. (1998). Cardiovascular risk factors in economically disadvantaged women: A study of prevalence and awareness. *J of the National Medical Association,* 90(9):531-536.

Rankin, S.H. (1997). Heart and soul: Evaluation of women with coronary artery disease. *Clinical Excellence for Nurse Practitioners,* 1(4):231-234.

Rimm, E.B., Willett, W.C., et al. (1998). Folate and vitamin B6 from diet and supplements in relation to risk of coronary heart disease among women. *The J of the American Medical Association,* 279(5):359-364.

Thurau, R. (1997). Perceived gender bias in the treatment of cardiovascular disease. *J of Cardiovascular Nursing,* 15(4):124-126.

Turner, S.L. & Bechtel, G.A. (1999). Homocysteine and the heart. *Advance for Nurse Practitioners,* 7(3):71-73.

Wenger, N.K. (1993, December). Coronary heart disease in women: an overview (myths, misperceptions, and missed opportunities). *Cardiovascular Review and Rehabilitation,* 24-41.

Index